Exercise in Modern Medicine

EDITED BY

Barry A. Franklin, Ph.D.
Director, Cardiac Rehabilitation and Exercise Laboratories
Division of Cardiovascular Diseases
William Beaumont Hospital
Royal Oak, Michigan
Associate Professor of Physiology
Wayne State University School of Medicine
Detroit, Michigan

Seymour Gordon, M.D.
Medical Director, Cardiac Rehabilitation and Exercise Laboratories
Division of Cardiovascular Diseases
William Beaumont Hospital
Royal Oak, Michigan
Clinical Professor of Health Sciences
Oakland University
Rochester, Michigan

Gerald C. Timmis, M.D.
Clinical Professor of Health Sciences
Oakland University
Rochester, Michigan
Medical Director of Clinical Research
Division of Cardiovascular Diseases
William Beaumont Hospital
Royal Oak, Michigan

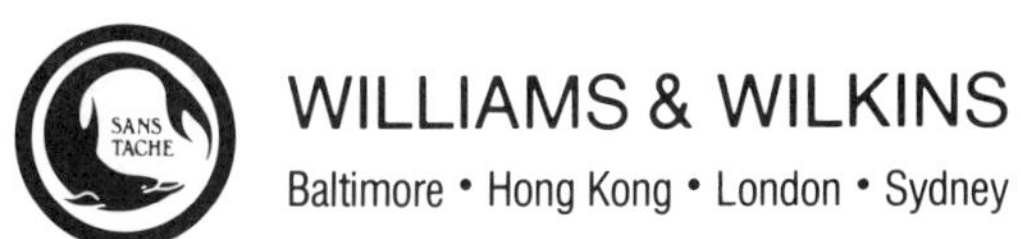

WILLIAMS & WILKINS
Baltimore • Hong Kong • London • Sydney

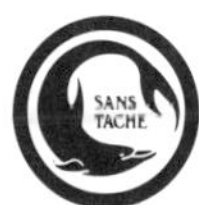

Editor: Nancy Collins
Associate Editor: Carol Eckhart
Copy Editor: Harry Finkelstein
Design: Saturn Graphics
Illustration Planning: Wayne Hubbel
Production: Anne G. Seitz

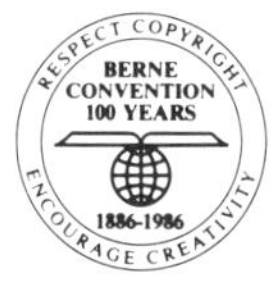

Accurate indications, adverse reactions, and dosage schedules for drugs are provided in this book, but it is possible that they may change. The reader is urged to review the package information data of the manufacturers of the medications mentioned.

Printed in the United States of America

Library of Congress Cataloging-in-Publication Data

Exercise in modern medicine / edited by Barry A. Franklin, Seymour
Gordon, Gerald C. Timmis.
p. cm.
Includes index.
ISBN 0-683-03350-6
1. Exercise therapy. 2. Exercise. I. Franklin, Barry A.
II. Gordon, Seymour. III. Timmis, Gerald C.
[DNLM: 1. Exercise Therapy. WB 541 E954]
RM725.E92 198
615.8′24—dc19
DNLM/DLC
for Library of Congress 88-184
CIP
88 89 90 91 92
1 2 3 4 5 6 7 8 9 10

9

Exercise in Modern Medicine

To my lovely wife, Linda, who has helped in so many ways, to turn my dreams into reality, and to my wonderful children, Michael and Laura, the "joy" of my life.

BAF

To my wife, Marilynn, and children, Nancy, Richard, and Carol, for their patience, understanding, love, and support.

SG

To my Dorothy, as always.

GCT

Foreword

Physicians today are in the forefront of research regarding the values and problems involved in the prescription of exercise for the well and the sick. They have become integral parts of the multidisciplinary team that investigates, prescribes, and monitors exercise as a preventive and therapeutic means.

To be noninjurious to the subject and effective for the purposes intended, exercise must be prescribed specifically according to the subject's age, physical characteristics, sex, previous exercise experience, and functional capacity. Special deficits or defects resulting from congenital deformities, injury or chronic disease, and the needs and contraindications imposed by these conditions must also be taken in account. The fundamentals of exercise prescription and training for apparently well persons are easily accessible today and are generally familiar to many physicians involved in primary care. Great attention has been devoted to the use of exercise in the therapy of the cardiac patient, and much experience has been accumulated. Its use for persons with cardiovascular conditions other than coronary heart disease, for chronic obstructive pulmonary disease and asthma, and for chronic renal disease, diabetes, and other less common forms of chronic disease is less well understood and is not familiar to many physicians and exercise specialists. Special prescriptions and precautions are necessary for the pregnant, the obese, and the elderly.

This book has the special purpose of providing a single source of information for physicians and exercise specialists and of relating principles and recommendations regarding these special conditions to the standards that have been established for healthy people. This book makes a substantial contribution to the continuing development of exercise science which has resulted in a gradual perceptual change in life-style for a large segment of our population.

Allan J. Ryan, M.D.
Director
Sports Medicine Enterprise
Minneapolis, Minnesota

Preface

"We doctors can now state from our experience with people, both sick and well, and from a growing series of scientific researches that 'keeping fit' does pay richly in dividends of health and longevity."

Paul Dudley White, M.D.

Interest in the essential medical role of exercise testing, training, and prescription has continued to escalate. Patients are enthusiastic about regular exercise as a self-improvement technique. Moreover, physicians have embraced the use of exercise in the prevention, diagnosis, and treatment of a variety of clinical conditions and chronic health problems.

Although there are numerous books on exercise testing and training for presumably healthy adults and cardiac patients, we recognized the need for, and value of, a comprehensive reference source that would address the requirements of special patient populations.

This virtual pharmacopoeia of exercise guidelines, geared especially toward the primary care physician and other members of the health care team, should prove helpful in more clearly defining the benefits and limitations of exercise testing and training in the evaluation and management of a broad spectrum of patients, including those with coronary heart disease, nonischemic heart disease, peripheral vascular disease, obesity, diabetes, chronic obstructive pulmonary disease, asthma, and cystic fibrosis, as well as those who are pregnant, elderly, or wheelchair-confined.

Each chapter contains guidelines for exercise testing and prescription, information highlighting chronic adaptations to training, and special exercise precautions, limitations, and problems unique to each type of patient. In addition, the first chapter provides a generic overview of exercise physiology as it applies to exercise testing and prescription, whereas the last chapter outlines practical and effective strategies for enhancing patient compliance.

Our acknowledgments begin with the patients, support staff, administration, and physicians of the William Beaumont Hospital. Together we have developed a productive research laboratory and a successful cardiac rehabilitation program, the essence of which this book partially seeks to capture.

Several key people at William Beaumont Hospital helped to chart the course of this long journey and most certainly reduced the potential for misadventure. We would like to express our appreciation to Pat Bagamery for the administrative coordination of the text; she served as liaison among editors, authors, and publisher, overseeing the style requirements, proofreading, and checking of references—critical and laborious tasks that are required for the production of a multiauthored text. Special thanks also go to Brenda White who, with a unique sense of pride and dedication, meticulously orchestrated the word processing and editing, and to Patricia Banks, an extraordinarily talented graphic artist, for the detailed drawings and figures that she prepared for several of the chapters. Furthermore, we express our gratitude to Nancy Collins and Carol Eckhart, our editors, and to Anne Seitz, our production sponsor at Williams & Wilkins, for their patience, encouragement, and expertise.

Finally, we would like to thank the contributors who painstakingly worked to summarize, in a clear and concise manner, the latest research findings in each area, with specific reference to patient care and application. It has been an honor for us to collaborate with this prestigious group of scientists, clinicians, researchers, and teachers who are authorities in their respective fields.

Barry A. Franklin, Ph.D.
Seymour Gordon, M.D.
Gerald C. Timmis, M.D.

Contributors

R. James Barnard, Ph.D.
(Chapter 5)
Professor, Departments of Kinesiology and Medicine
University of California
Los Angeles, California
Director of Research
Pritikin Research Foundation
Santa Monica, California

Michael J. Belman, M.D.
(Chapter 9)
Associate Director
Division of Pulmonary Diseases
Cedars-Sinai Medical Center
Los Angeles, California

Steven N. Blair, P.E.D.
(Chapter 2)
Director of Epidemiology
Institute for Aerobics Research
Dallas, Texas

James F. Clapp III, M.D.
(Chapter 14)
Professor, Department of Obstetrics and Gynecology
The University of Vermont
College of Medicine
Burlington, Vermont

Glen M. Davis, Ph.D.
(Chapter 13)
Assistant Professor
Department of Health, Physical Education and Recreation
University of North Texas
Denton, Texas

Herbert A. deVries, Ph.D.
(Chapter 12)
Professor Emeritus
University of Southern California
South Laguna, California

Barry A. Franklin, Ph.D.
(Chapters 1 and 3)
Director, Cardiac Rehabilitation and Exercise Laboratories
Division of Cardiovascular Diseases
William Beaumont Hospital
Royal Oak, Michigan
Associate Professor of Physiology
Wayne State University School of Medicine
Detroit, Michigan

Larry W. Gibbons, M.D.
(Chapter 2)
Director
The Cooper Clinic
Dallas, Texas

Roger M. Glaser, Ph.D.
(Chapter 13)
Professor of Physiology and Biophysics
Wright State University School of Medicine
Senior Research Health Scientist
Veterans Administration Medical Center
Director of Clinical Studies
Rehabilitation Institute of Ohio
Miami Valley Hospital
Dayton, Ohio

Seymour Gordon, M.D.
(Chapters 1 and 3)
Medical Director, Cardiac Rehabilitation and Exercise Laboratories
Division of Cardiovascular Diseases
William Beaumont Hospital
Royal Oak, Michigan
Clinical Professor of Health Sciences
Oakland University
Rochester, Michigan

James M. Hagberg, Ph.D.
(Chapter 7)
Associate Professor
Center on Aging
University of Maryland
College Park, Maryland

John A. Hall, M.S.
(Chapter 5)
Programs Director
Director, Peripheral Vascular Diagnostic Laboratory
Pritikin Longevity Center
Santa Monica, California

Herman K. Hellerstein, M.D.
(Chapter 3)
Professor Emeritus
Case Western Reserve University
School of Medicine
Attending Physician
University Hospitals of Cleveland
Cleveland, Ohio

Richard M. Lampman, Ph.D.
(Chapter 8)
Associate Research Scientist
Division of Cardiology, Department of Internal Medicine
Director, Work Performance Laboratory
University of Michigan
Ann Arbor, Michigan

Arthur S. Leon, M.D.
(Chapter 6)
Professor and Director, Applied Nutrition Physiology Section
Division of Epidemiology
School of Public Health
University of Minnesota
Minneapolis, Minnesota

John E. Martin, Ph.D.
(Chapter 15)
Professor
Doctoral Training Facility
Psychology Annex for Research and Training
San Diego State University
San Diego, California

T. William Moir, M.D.
(Chapter 4)
Professor of Medicine
Case Western Reserve University
School of Medicine
University Hospitals of Cleveland, Division of Cardiology
Cleveland, Ohio

Bruce G. Nickerson, M.D.
(Chapter 10)
Director, Pulmonary Function Laboratory
Children's Hospital of Oakland
Oakland, California

Patricia A. Nixon, Ph.D.
(Chapter 11)
Exercise Physiologist
Pulmonary/Cystic Fibrosis Division
Department of Pediatrics
Children's Hospital of Pittsburgh
Pittsburgh, Pennsylvania

David M. Orenstein, M.D.
(Chapter 11)
Associate Professor of Pediatrics
Director, Pulmonary Division
Director, Cystic Fibrosis Center
Children's Hospital of Pittsburgh
University of Pittsburgh
Pittsburgh, Pennsylvania

David E. Schteingart, M.D.
(Chapter 8)
Professor of Internal Medicine, Medical School
Division of Endocrinology and Metabolism, Department of Internal Medicine
University of Michigan Medical Center
Ann Arbor, Michigan

Gerald C. Timmis, M.D.
(Chapters 1 and 3)
Clinical Professor of Health Sciences
Oakland University
Rochester, Michigan
Medical Director of Clinical Research
Division of Cardiovascular Diseases
William Beaumont Hospital
Royal Oak, Michigan

Contents

CHAPTER 1

Fundamentals of Exercise Physiology: Implications for Exercise Testing and Prescription

Barry A. Franklin, Ph.D.
Seymour Gordon, M.D.
Gerald C. Timmis, M.D.

Aside from the energy required for physical activity, individuals expend considerable energy even at complete rest, including the energy required for digestion, absorption, assimilation of food nutrients, glandular function, establishment of appropriate electrochemical gradients along the cell membrane, and for the synthesis of new chemical compounds (1). Our cells do not directly use the nutrients obtained from the breakdown of food for their immediate supply of energy. Instead, the food we eat is converted through a series of chemical reactions to an energy-rich compound, adenosine triphosphate, referred to hereafter as ATP, which serves as the "fuel" for all the energy-requiring processes within the cell. Figure 1.1 illustrates a simplified structure of an ATP molecule.

The energy needs of exercising human muscle may increase up to 120-fold in the transition from rest to maximal physical exertion (2). Because the available stores of ATP are extremely limited, and capable of providing energy to maintain vigorous activity for several seconds only, ATP must be constantly resynthesized to provide a continuous supply of energy. Therefore, working muscles must possess a tremendous capacity for increasing their metabolic rate in order to produce enough ATP to allow increased activity to continue. This capacity relies heavily on the respiratory and cardiovascular systems for the delivery of oxygen and nutrients and for the removal of waste products to maintain the internal equilibrium of the cells.

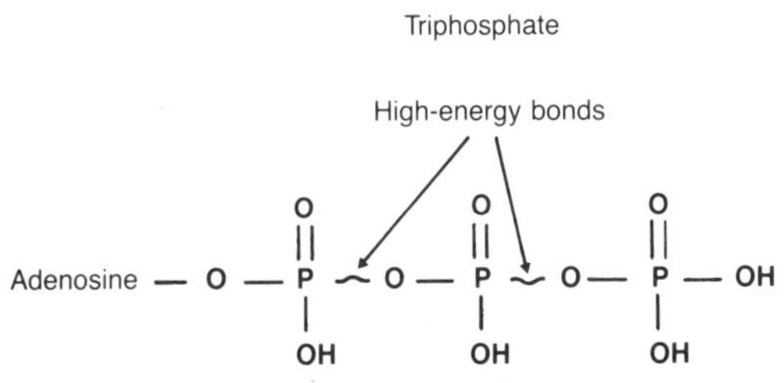

Figure 1.1. Simplified structure of an ATP molecule. The symbol ∼ represents the high-energy bonds.

A study of exercise physiology, therefore, includes the acute and chronic physiologic adaptations that the body makes in order to cope with the increased energy demands imposed by physical activity. An important aim of the immediate adaptations, involving all tissue and organ systems in the body, is to supply sufficient ATP to maintain the work rate of exercising muscles.

The purpose of this chapter is to review basic terminology and fundamentals of exercise physiology, with specific reference to energy production, aerobic versus anaerobic metabolism, the relationship between muscle fiber type and performance, the physiologic significance of the maximal oxygen consumption ($\dot{V}O_2max$), normal cardiorespiratory responses to submaximal and maximal exercise, substrate utilization, and the gas-exchange anaerobic threshold. Such background information is clinically relevant to the following chapters and is vital to the reader's understanding of the role of exercise physiology in the interpretation of clinical exercise testing and the prescription of exercise in health and disease.

ENERGY SYSTEMS FOR EXERCISE

The energy (ATP) required for muscle contraction or other forms of biologic work is produced by anaerobic and aerobic energy pathways.

Anaerobic Production of ATP

Anaerobic pathways supply ATP when the demand for energy exceeds the availability of oxygen. This form of energy production supplies a *rapid* source of ATP for brief physical exertion of near-maximal intensity, such as a 440-yard run, 100-yard swim, running up several flights of stairs, and other activities that produce exhaustion quickly.

ATP may be synthesized anaerobically (in the absence of oxygen) via (*a*) the splitting of a phosphate molecule from another energy-rich compound, creatine phosphate, or CP, and (*b*) the breakdown of carbohydrate within the cell through a series of chemical reactions known as glycolysis. It should be emphasized, however, that carbohydrates are the only food that can provide energy anaerobically for the formation of ATP.

The resynthesis of ATP is possible if sufficient energy is available to rebond one phosphate (P) molecule to an adenosine diphosphate (ADP) molecule. The breakdown of CP, stored in muscles in considerably larger quantities than ATP, can supply this energy. However, the energy released from the breakdown of stored ATP and CP will sustain vigorous exercise for only several seconds.

Glycolysis, involving the breakdown of a 6-carbon glucose molecule into two 3-carbon molecules of pyruvic acid, occurs within the cellular fluids and results in the production of two molecules of ATP. However, these two ATP molecules represent only about 5% of the potential ATP that can be produced when the glucose molecule is completely degraded to carbon dioxide and water during subsequent *aerobic* reactions. In addition to the low ATP yield, anaerobic glycolysis results in the conversion of pyruvic acid to lactic acid. As work intensity increases, the level of lactic acid rises sharply and fatigue soon occurs. Nevertheless, anaerobic metabolism provides a rapid source of ATP, which is particularly important at the beginning of exercise and during high-intensity activity that can only be sustained for brief periods. As exercise time increases, the relative contribution of anaerobic energy sources decreases (Fig. 1.2) (3).

Aerobic Production of ATP

Because the anaerobic reactions of glycolysis release only about 5% of the available ATP, aerobic metabolism provides an

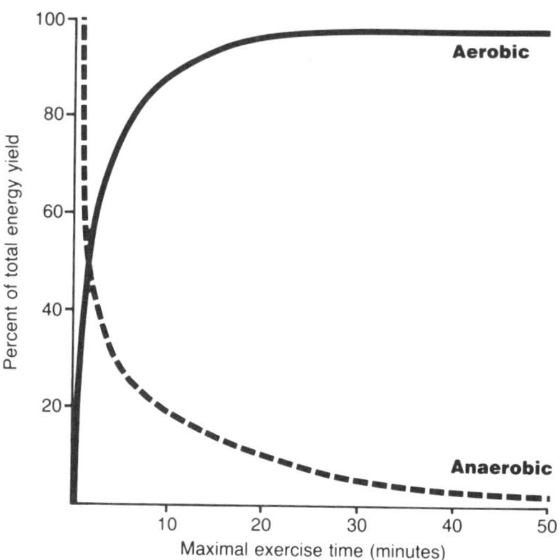

Figure 1.2. Relative contribution of aerobic and anaerobic metabolism during physical activity of increasing duration. In intense activities lasting 1½ to 2 minutes, the ATP-CP and lactic acid energy systems generate approximately 50% of the energy, while aerobic metabolism supplies the remainder. A marathoner, on the other hand, derives essentially 98% of his energy from aerobic metabolism during a 50-minute training run. (Adapted from Åstrand PO, Rodahl K: *Textbook of Work Physiology*. New York, McGraw-Hill Book Company, 1970, p 304.)

additional means for extracting energy from the glucose molecule. Pyruvic acid molecules are ultimately converted to acetyl Co-A, and carbon dioxide and hydrogen atoms are released in the process. Acetyl Co-A, which can also be formed by the degradation of fats or amino acids, then passes into the cell's mitochondria, where it is ultimately broken down in the presence of oxygen to carbon dioxide, water, and significant quantities of ATP. Indeed, over 90% of the total ATP production occurs via this pathway. This aspect of the chemical breakdown of acetyl Co-A is known as the Krebs citric acid cycle.

The aerobic system, which uses glycogen, fats, and proteins as energy substrates, provides large amounts of ATP for muscular energy (Table 1.1) (4). However, oxygen delivery to the cell is critical, and the capacity to provide it to the tissues usually determines the level of activity an individual can perform.

MUSCLE

Two distinct types of fibers have been identified in human skeletal muscle: red, slow-twitch fibers (type I) and white, fast-twitch fibers (type II); however, several subdivisions of the latter fiber type have been identified (II_a, II_{ab}, II_b) (Fig. 1.3) (5). Although most persons have a comparable number of slow- and fast-twitch fibers, there is enormous interindividual variability. The basic distribution of fiber types is probably determined genetically, and the contractile properties and glycolytic capacity are not normally modified by physical conditioning (6). In contrast, the oxidative capacity of both fiber types can be increased by chronic endurance exercise training (7).

Table 1.1.
Characteristics of the two mechanisms by which ATP is formed [a]

Mechanism	Food or Chemical Fuel	Oxygen Required?	Relative ATP Yield
I. Anaerobic			
1. Creatine phosphate	Creatine phosphate	No	Extremely limited
2. Glycolysis	Glycogen (glucose)	No	Extremely limited
II. Aerobic			
Krebs cycle and electron transport system	Glycogen, fats, proteins	Yes	Large

[a] Adapted from Mathews DK, Fox EL: The Physiological Basis of Physical Education and Athletics, ed. 2. Philadelphia, WB Saunders, 1976, p 14.

four fiber types		
I	slow oxidative	slow
IIa	fast oxidative	fast, fatigue resistant
IIab	fast, oxidative plus glycolytic	fast, intermediate fatigability
IIb	fast, glycolytic	fast, fatigable

Figure 1.3. Muscle structure, function, and control classification schemes.

Individuals with a higher ratio of slow-twitch (type I) to fast-twitch (type II) fibers generally perform better in endurance activities, which depend almost exclusively on the energy generated by aerobic metabolism. This is because slow-twitch fibers have a high concentration of myoglobin and mitochondria and low myofibrillar myosin ATPase activity, giving them a high oxidative capacity (8). Thus, the capacity of these fibers to generate ATP aerobically is much greater than that of the fast-twitch fibers. On the other hand, athletes with a higher ratio of type II to type I fibers are better suited for brief, high-intensity, sprint-type activities, which depend almost entirely on anaerobic metabolism for energy. The metabolic capabilities of these fibers are also important in stop-and-go and change-of-pace sports like basketball or football. In contrast to slow-twitch fibers, fast-twitch fibers possess a high capacity for the production of ATP during the initial stages of glycolysis. These fibers have high myosin ATPase activity, low myoglobin content, few mitochondria, low oxidative capacity, and high glycolytic capacity (8).

OXYGEN CONSUMPTION

A critical measure of metabolism and energy expenditure is the somatic oxygen consumption ($\dot{V}O_2$), expressed by a rearrangement of the Fick equation:

$$\dot{V}O_2 = HR \times SV \times (CaO_2 - C\bar{v}O_2)$$

where $\dot{V}O_2$ is oxygen consumption in milliliters per minute; HR is heart rate in beats per minute; SV is stroke volume in milliliters per beat; and $CaO_2 - C\bar{v}O_2$ is the arteriovenous oxygen difference in milliliters of oxygen per deciliter of blood. Thus, it is apparent that both central and peripheral regulatory mechanisms affect the magnitude of body oxygen consumption.

Oxygen Consumption at Rest: The "MET" Concept

Typical circulatory data at rest in a normal sedentary 30-year-old man are shown in Table 1.2. By dividing the absolute resting oxygen consumption (250 $ml \cdot min^{-1}$) by the man's body weight in kilograms (70 kg), one derives the energy requirement for basal homeostasis, termed one MET (metabolic equivalent), approximating 3.5 ml of oxygen per kilogram of body weight per minute ($ml \cdot kg^{-1} \cdot min^{-1}$). This expression of resting $\dot{V}O_2$, believed to originate from the work of Balke (9), is extremely important in exercise physiology, being independent of body weight and thus relatively constant for all persons. Furthermore, multiples of this value are often used to quantify relative levels of energy expenditure (10). Thus, it is useful in discussing energy costs with patients. For example, it is easier—and more meaningful—to explain to an individual that he has exercised at eight times his resting metabolic rate than to tell him he has consumed 28 $ml \cdot kg^{-1} \cdot min^{-1}$ of oxygen.

Oxygen Consumption During Exercise: Acute Cardiorespiratory Responses

Many cardiorespiratory mechanisms function collectively to support the increased metabolic demands on active muscle. The overall effect of these changes in heart rate, stroke volume, cardiac output, blood flow, blood pressure, arteriovenous oxygen difference, and pulmonary ventilation, is to deliver blood to the active tissues and provide oxygenation of that blood.

Heart Rate

Heart rate generally increases progressively as a function of exercise intensity: in other words, there is a roughly linear relationship between heart rate and workload or power output (11). Although heart rate will generally level off within 2 to 3 minutes at a given submaximal workload, at higher workloads it takes progressively longer to plateau or attain a "steady-state" rate. At even higher workloads a definable maximum heart rate is attained, which decreases with age. The equation, 220-age, provides an approximation of the maximal heart rate in normal healthy men and women, but the variance for any given age is considerable (standard deviation ~ ± 10 $beats \cdot min^{-1}$).

Stroke Volume

The stroke volume response to exercise is highly dependent on hydrostatic pressure effects. Stroke volume at rest in the erect position generally varies between 60 and 100 $ml \cdot beat^{-1}$ among healthy adults, while maximum stroke volume approximates 100 to 120 $ml \cdot beat^{-1}$. It appears that during exercise in the erect position, stroke

Table 1.2
Hemodynamic Determinants of Resting $\dot{V}O_2$ for a Normal Sedentary Man (70 kg)

	$\dot{V}O_2$	=	HR	×	SV	×	$(CaO_2 - C\bar{v}O_2)$
($ml \cdot kg^{-1} \cdot min^{-1}$)	($ml \cdot min^{-1}$)	(METs)	($beats \cdot min^{-1}$)		($ml \cdot beat^{-1}$)		($ml \cdot dl^{-1}$ blood)
3.5 [a]	250	1.0 [a]	70		70		5.1

[a] 3.5 $ml \cdot kg^{-1} \cdot min^{-1}$ = 1 MET (metabolic equivalent); average resting metabolic rate for all persons regardless of body weight.

volume will increase curvilinearly with the workload until it reaches a near-maximum value at approximately 50% of the individual's maximal capacity for exercise, increasing only slightly thereafter (12). Although it has been suggested that stroke volume may actually decrease at higher heart rates due to the disproportionate shortening in diastolic filling time (Fig. 1.4) (13, 14), this issue remains unsettled (15).

The reason for the increase in stroke volume with exercise was, for many years, believed to be due to the Frank-Starling mechanism. However, recent studies have shown that end-diastolic volume remains essentially unchanged or that it increases only slightly during exercise (16). Since only about 60% of the resting end-diastolic volume is ejected during ventricular systole (17), it appears that enhanced myocardial contractility, secondary to increased sympathetic stimulation and catecholamine output, results in a more complete emptying of the ventricle, thereby increasing stroke volume with exercise (16).

Cardiac Output

Cardiac output in healthy adults generally increases linearly with increases in workload, from a resting value of approximately 5 $l \cdot min^{-1}$ to a maximum of about 20 $l \cdot min^{-1}$ during upright exercise. However, maximum values of cardiac output are dependent upon many factors, the two most important being body size and the level of physical conditioning. At exercise levels up to 50% of a person's maximum capacity, the increase in cardiac output is accomplished through increases in both heart rate and stroke volume (12). At higher exercise intensities, the increase results almost solely from the continued rise in heart rate.

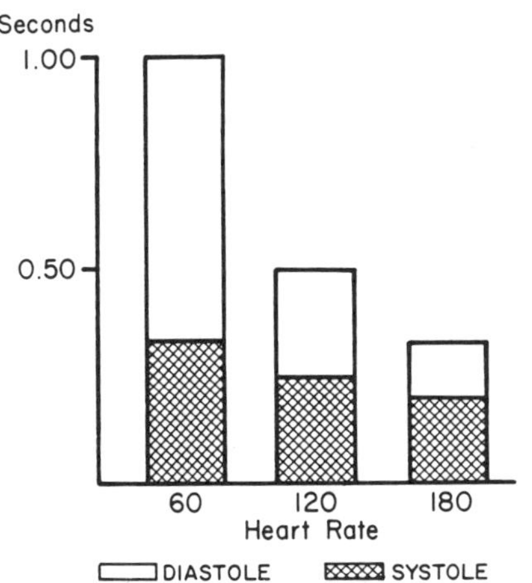

Figure 1.4. Relationship of systolic and diastolic time to heart rate. With increased heart rate, as during exercise, diastolic (filling) time is disproportionately shortened. (Adapted from Dehn MM, Mullins CB: Physiologic effects and importance of exercise in patients with coronary artery disease. *J Cardiovasc Med* 2:365–387, 1977.)

Arteriovenous Oxygen Difference

As the exercise intensity progresses from moderate to heavy loads, an increased extraction of oxygen from the available blood supply occurs at the muscle. The arterial and mixed venous oxygen content at rest are approximately 20 and 15 ml of oxygen per 100 ml (dl) of blood, respectively. However, as the workload approaches the point of exhaustion, the mixed venous oxygen content typically decreases to 5 $ml \cdot dl^{-1}$ blood or lower, thus widening the arteriovenous oxygen difference from 5 to 15 $ml \cdot dl^{-1}$ blood, corresponding to a threefold increase (12).

Blood Flow

At rest, only 15 to 20% of the cardiac output is distributed to the muscles; 80 to 85% goes to the visceral organs (stomach, liver, spleen, kidneys), the heart, and the brain (15). However, during exercise there is a shunting of blood so that the working muscles receive as much as 85 to 90% of the cardiac output, while blood flow to the visceral organs is decreased. Blood flow to the myocardium is increased in proportion to the increased metabolic activity of the heart, whereas that to the brain is maintained at resting levels (18).

During exercise, cutaneous blood flow is also greatly increased to facilitate heat dissipation. However, when maximal exertion is approached, the body sacrifices cutaneous circulation in order to meet the increasing metabolic requirements of working muscles, and consequently core temperature may quickly rise (19).

Blood Pressure

There is a linear increase in the systolic pressure with increasing levels of exercise, with maximal values typically reaching 190 to 220 mm Hg. Diastolic pressure changes little from rest to maximum exercise in the normal, healthy adult; thus, pulse pressure (i.e., systolic minus diastolic pressure) demonstrates a substantial increase in direct proportion to the intensity of exercise (20).

Pulmonary Ventilation

Pulmonary or minute ventilation ($\dot{V}E$), the volume of air inspired or expired per minute, increases from approximately 6 $l \cdot min^{-1}$ at rest to over 100 $l \cdot min^{-1}$ in the average sedentary adult male. This substantial increase in ventilation is accomplished through three- and fivefold increases in respiratory rate and tidal volume, respectively. For the most part, the increase in pulmonary ventilation is directly proportional to the increase in somatic oxygen consumed ($\dot{V}O_2$) and carbon dioxide produced ($\dot{V}CO_2$). However, at moderate to high levels of exercise, $\dot{V}E$ increases disproportionately relative to $\dot{V}O_2$, but not to $\dot{V}CO_2$. This suggests that pulmonary ventilation is perhaps regulated more by the need for carbon dioxide removal than oxygen consumption, and that ventilation is not normally a limiting factor to aerobic capacity ($\dot{V}O_2max$) (21).

MAXIMAL OXYGEN CONSUMPTION ($\dot{V}O_2max$)

Oxygen consumption increases in a linear fashion with increasing workloads. However, as the exercising subject approaches the point of exhaustion or fatigue, the capacity to take in oxygen reaches its limit and, despite further increases in workload, the oxygen consumption plateaus. This maximum value, referred to as the individual's maximal oxygen consumption ($\dot{V}O_2max$), serves as the most widely used and accepted criterion of cardiorespiratory endurance capacity or "physical fitness" (22, 23). The typical 10- to 12-fold increase in somatic oxygen transport and utilization achieved at maximal exercise is brought about by respective increases in the hemodynamic correlates of oxygen consumption, as shown in Table 1.3.

In reality, many sedentary normal adults and cardiac patients are unable to demonstrate the leveling off of oxygen consumption with increasing workloads. Most reach a level of fatigue and discomfort far below their physiologic maximum, precluding attainment of a "true" $\dot{V}O_2max$. This is why fatigue or symptom-limited peak performance, or $\dot{V}O_2$ peak, may differ considerably from the physiologic $\dot{V}O_2max$.

Measurement of the $\dot{V}O_2max$

Submaximal and maximal oxygen consumption ($\dot{V}O_2max$), fortunately, can be assessed noninvasively by measuring the volume and analyzing the oxygen content of expired air, corrected to standard temperature and pressure dry (STPD), using the equation (24):

$$\dot{V}O_2 = \dot{V}E\,(FIO_2 - FEO_2)$$

where $\dot{V}E$ is the expired measured volume per minute, FEO_2 is the directly measured concentration of oxygen in the expired air, FIO_2 is the concentration of oxygen in the inspired air, and normal room air is 0.2093.

Traditionally, maximal oxygen con-

Table 1.3
Mechanisms Responsible for the Increase in $\dot{V}O_2$ from Rest to Maximal Exercise [a]

Variable	Rest	Maximum Exercise	Increase
Heart rate	70 beats$\cdot min^{-1}$	190 beats$\cdot min^{-1}$	271%
Stroke volume	70 ml$\cdot beat^{-1}$	100 ml$\cdot beat^{-1}$	143%
CaO_2-$C\bar{v}O_2$	5.1 ml$\cdot dl^{-1}$ blood	15.8 ml$\cdot dl^{-1}$ blood	309%
$\dot{V}O_2$	250 ml$\cdot min^{-1}$	3000 ml$\cdot min^{-1}$	1200%
	3.5 ml$\cdot kg^{-1}\cdot min^{-1}$	43 ml$\cdot kg^{-1}\cdot min^{-1}$	
	1 MET	12 METs	

[a] **Typical values for a 30-year-old sedentary man (70 kg).**

sumption has been measured during the final minutes of exercise using an open circuit or Douglas bag technique (24). However, several automated systems are now available (Fig. 1.5).

Maximal oxygen consumption may be expressed on an absolute basis in liters per minute, reflecting total body energy output and caloric expenditure, where each liter of oxygen is equivalent to approximately 5 kcal. However, since large persons usually have a large absolute oxygen consumption simply by virtue of their large muscle mass, physiologists generally divide this value by body weight in kilograms to allow a more equitable comparison between individuals of different size. This variable, when expressed in milliliters of oxygen per kilogram per minute ($ml \cdot kg^{-1} \cdot min^{-1}$), is considered the best single index of physical work capacity or cardiorespiratory fitness (25).

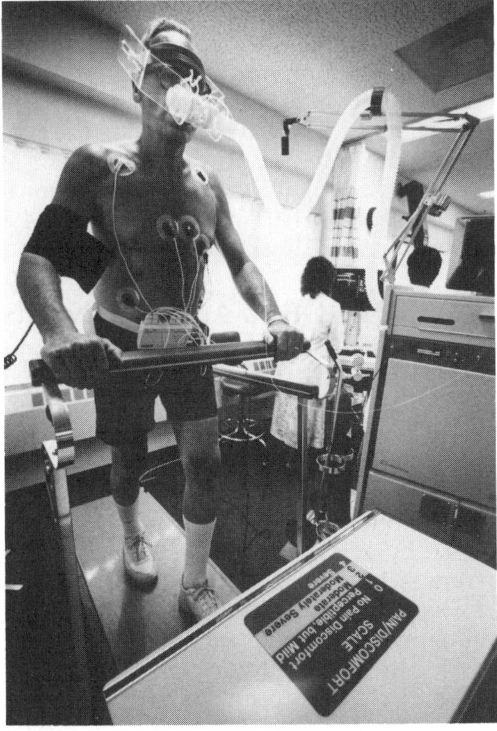

Figure 1.5. Determination of oxygen consumption during exercise testing using an automated metabolic measurement system (Medical Graphics 2001 CAD-Net).

Estimation of the $\dot{V}O_2max$

The equipment required for direct assessment of the $\dot{V}O_2max$ is expensive and requires technical expertise and frequent calibration; furthermore, collection of expired air inhibits verbal communication by the subject. Consequently, clinicians have increasingly sought other approaches to predict or estimate $\dot{V}O_2max$ during routine exercise testing.

Several investigators have proposed that the $\dot{V}O_2max$ can be predicted from the maximal exercise time or peak-attained workload when gas measurements cannot be conveniently made (26, 27). The rationale is that the mechanical efficiency of treadmill walking or cycle ergometry is relatively constant in healthy able-bodied persons. Thus, the oxygen requirement of a given workload can be estimated from published tables (28), nomograms (27), or formulas (26, 27, 29) based on the treadmill speed and grade, or the cycle ergometer workload or power output in kilogram meters per minute ($kg \cdot m \cdot min^{-1}$).

It is generally acknowledged that the treadmill or cycle ergometer workload, if performed for 2 or more minutes to attain a "steady-state," can be translated to an oxygen cost that will not differ significantly from one person to the next. It should be noted, however, that the oxygen cost of treadmill walking is weight-dependent, whereas the aerobic requirements of cycle ergometry are weight-independent. Thus, a given workload on the treadmill [e.g., 3.0 miles/hour ($mi \cdot h^{-1}$), 0% grade] requires approximately the same relative oxygen consumption, 3 METs or 10.5 $ml \cdot kg^{-1} \cdot min^{-1}$, for all persons, regardless of body weight. In contrast, a cycle ergometer workload of 900 $kg \cdot m \cdot min^{-1}$ requires an absolute oxygen consumption of approximately 2100 $ml \cdot min^{-1}$ for all persons, corresponding to 21 $ml \cdot kg^{-1} \cdot min^{-1}$ or 6 METs for the 100-kg man, and 28 $ml \cdot kg^{-1} \cdot min^{-1}$ or 8 METs for the 75-kg man (30).

Unfortunately, measured and estimated values of $\dot{V}O_2max$ often differ considerably. Froelicher and associates (31) reported a wide range of measured oxygen consumption for any particular maximal exercise time or workload. For example, at 11 minutes' exercise time in the Bruce (27) protocol, equivalent to a workload of 4.2 $mi \cdot h^{-1}$ at 16% grade, the mean measured oxygen uptake was approximately 44 $ml \cdot kg^{-1} \cdot min^{-1}$, but the range at the 95% limits of confidence was 32 to 58 $ml \cdot kg^{-1} \cdot min^{-1}$. Other investigators have shown that when the exercise time or peak workload is used to predict the $\dot{V}O_2max$, the aerobic capacity may be markedly overestimated (32, 33). Possible explanations for the disparity between measured and estimated $\dot{V}O_2max$ values include: population differences in energy expenditure, differences in level of physical fitness, inappropriate extrapolation of "steady-state" aerobic requirements to nonsteady-state work, variations in exercise intensity increments, and methodological variables (34).

What is a Normal $\dot{V}O_2max$? The Concept of Functional Aerobic Impairment (FAI)

It is important to express the $\dot{V}O_2max$ in $ml \cdot kg^{-1} \cdot min^{-1}$ as compared with average values. Bruce and coworkers (27) have developed the concept of functional aerobic impairment for this purpose. The FAI is the percentage difference between the patient's observed $\dot{V}O_2max$ and that predicted for a healthy person of the same age, sex, and habitual activity status. Subjects are classified as sedentary if they do not exert themselves at least once a week sufficiently to perspire. Average values of $\dot{V}O_2max$, expressed as $ml \cdot kg^{-1} \cdot min^{-1}$, expected in healthy men and women can be predicted from the following regressions (35):

Active men = 69.7–0.612 (age in years)
Sedentary men = 57.8–0.445 (age in years)
Active women = 42.9–0.312 (age in years)
Sedentary women = 42.3–0.356 (age in years)

FAI can be calculated from the following formula:

$$\%FAI = \frac{\text{Predicted } \dot{V}O_2max - \text{Observed } \dot{V}O_2max}{\text{Predicted } \dot{V}O_2max} \times 100$$

The normal value of the FAI is 0%; this indicates that the $\dot{V}O_2max$ is 100% of the age, sex-predicted value and that there is no functional impairment. Negative values for FAI indicate above-average fitness. For the sake of convention, the degree of FAI can be categorized as mild, moderate, marked, or extreme, which equals approximately 27 to 40%, 41 to 54%, 55 to 68%, and more than 68% FAI, respectively (35).

The concept of FAI is particularly useful in making serial evaluations of individuals as well as comparisons with peers. For example, a 46-year-old sedentary man with a $\dot{V}O_2max$ of 30.0 $ml \cdot kg^{-1} \cdot min^{-1}$ had an FAI of 19.6%: $[(37.3 - 30.0)/37.3] \times 100 = 19.6\%$. In other words, his aerobic capacity was only 80.4% of the average normal expected value. Four years later his $\dot{V}O_2max$ increased to 36.0 $ml \cdot kg^{-1} \cdot min^{-1}$ as a result of participating in a supervised physical conditioning program. Although the increase in $\dot{V}O_2max$ was 6.0 $ml \cdot kg^{-1} \cdot min^{-1}$, equivalent to 20% $(6.0/30.0 \times 100)$, the age-corrected FAI had improved from 19.6% to −1.0%. In other words, his functional aerobic capacity had increased from 80.4% at age 46, to 101% at age 50 years!

PHYSIOLOGIC VARIATIONS IN MAXIMAL OXYGEN CONSUMPTION ($\dot{V}O_2max$)

The functional reserve capacity of the cardiovascular and respiratory systems, largely reflected by the maximal oxygen consumption ($\dot{V}O_2max$), is adversely affected by aging, disuse, and disease. Differences in body size, muscle mass, age, sex, habitual level of activity, physical conditioning, and athletic training also account for much of the physiologic variation in $\dot{V}O_2max$ (12). Unfortunately, decreases in aerobic capacity may be subtle and are often not apparent; thus, it is possible for a large percentage of the $\dot{V}O_2max$ to be lost before the ability to perform daily activities becomes noticeably compromised (Fig. 1.6) (36).

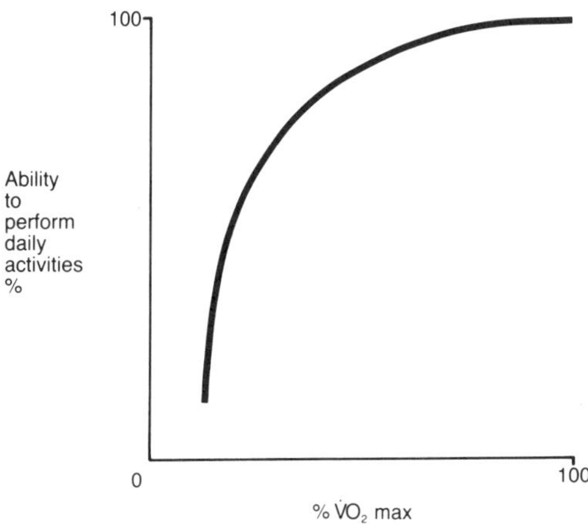

Figure 1.6. The reserve physiological capacity of the oxygen transport system is such that it is possible for much of the aerobic capacity ($\dot{V}O_2$max) to be lost before the demands of daily living become compromised. This appears to be particularly true among sedentary individuals. (Adapted from Jones NL, Campbell EJM: *Clinical Exercise Testing*. Philadelphia, WB Saunders 1981, p 2.)

Influence of Body Size and Muscle Mass

Numerous studies have examined the relationship between $\dot{V}O_2$max and body composition. Buskirk and Taylor (25) found that the correlation coefficients between absolute $\dot{V}O_2$max ($l \cdot min^{-1}$) and fat-free body weight and metabolically active tissue were 0.85 and 0.91, respectively. Similarly, Von Dobeln (37) reported a correlation of 0.75 between $\dot{V}O_2$max and lean body mass; in contrast to fat-free weight, the lean body mass contains a small percentage of essential fat. These findings suggest the $\dot{V}O_2$max, expressed in $l \cdot min^{-1}$, is highly dependent on the amount of lean tissue in the body. Since large persons usually have a large absolute $\dot{V}O_2$max simply as a result of their greater muscle mass, the $\dot{V}O_2$max is frequently expressed relative to body weight ($ml \cdot kg^{-1} \cdot min^{-1}$) or to lean body weight. This facilitates a more equitable comparison between persons of different size.

The maximal oxygen consumption can be augmented by increasing the mass of muscle employed in performing the task used to elicit the $\dot{V}O_2$max. For example, the classic study of Taylor and associates (22) showed that simultaneous running and arm cranking produced a significantly higher $\dot{V}O_2$max than running alone. Conversely, maximal oxygen consumption during arm cranking generally approximates only 64 to 80% of leg $\dot{V}O_2$max (38).

Relationship between Arm and Leg $\dot{V}O_2$max

Several investigators have examined the ability of leg $\dot{V}O_2$max to predict arm $\dot{V}O_2$max, and vice versa. Asmussen and Hemmingsen (39) showed that it was not possible to estimate leg $\dot{V}O_2$max from arm exercise testing. Similarly, Franklin and associates (40) reported a weak correlation ($r=0.32$) between $\dot{V}O_2$max during arm and leg exercise testing in healthy normal subjects (Fig. 1.7). Bar-Or and Zwiren (41) found that the correlation coefficient between arm and leg $\dot{V}O_2$max was only fair ($r=0.74$), similar to the correlation obtained by Bouchard et al. (42) who compared the $\dot{V}O_2$max determined by arm exercise testing in the standing position with the $\dot{V}O_2$max determined by four different leg exercise tests: cycling supine, cycling sitting, walking on a treadmill, and stepping on a bench. The former investigators (Bar-Or and Zwiren) speculated that re-

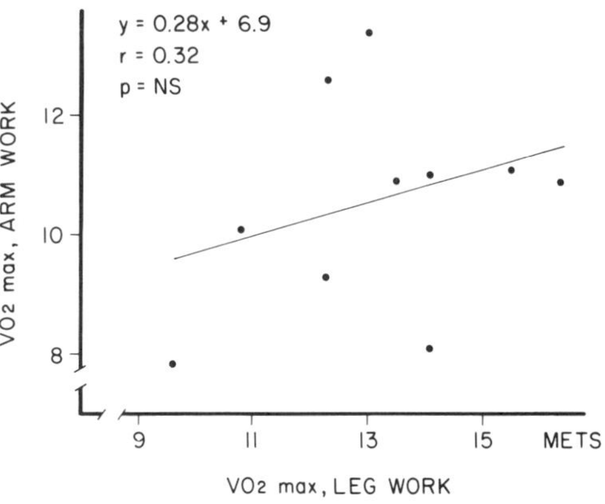

Figure 1.7. The relationship between $\dot{V}O_2$max (METs) during arm and leg ergometry is shown, using individual data. (From Franklin BA, Vander L, Wrisley D, Rubenfire M: Aerobic requirements of arm ergometry: Implications for exercise testing and training. *Phys Sportsmed* 11:81–90, 1983. Reproduced by permission.)

cruitment of trunk and leg muscles to different degrees in different subjects during the arm ergometer test lowered its validity as a predictor of leg $\dot{V}O_2max$.

In summary, the aforementioned studies indicate that leg and arm $\dot{V}O_2max$ generally provides a marginal estimate at best of reciprocal arm and leg aerobic capacity. Consequently, arm exercise testing appears to be the functional evaluation of choice for persons whose occupational and recreational physical activity is dominated by upper extremity efforts (Fig. 1.8) (28).

Influence of Age and Sex

The influence of age on maximal oxygen consumption in men and women is shown in Figure 1.9 (43). Although there is little difference in $\dot{V}O_2max$ among boys and girls between 6 and 12 years of age, considerable differences are apparent between the sexes following the onset of adolescence. $\dot{V}O_2max$ values for adult women average approximately 15 to 25% lower than for men. However, there is considerable debate as to whether these differences arise from cultural or biological factors. A change in the habitual level of physical activity at the time of puberty is most likely an important cultural or social factor. On the other hand, women have more body fat (and less "metabolically active" muscle mass) than men. The average concentration of hemoglobin is also lower among women, resulting in a reduced oxygen-carrying capacity of arterial blood.

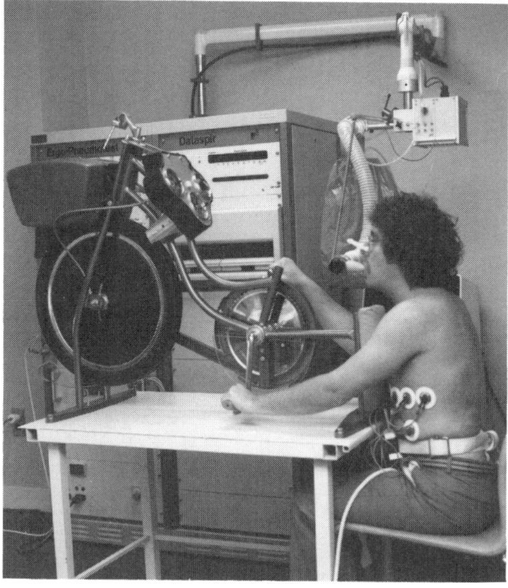

Figure 1.8. Schwinn model EX-2 cycle ergometer as modified for arm work. Removable bicycle handgrips have been fitted over the pedals. A padded breastplate helps to standardize arm position. Erich Jaeger Ergo-Pneumotest metabolic measurement system is shown in background.

Cross-sectional and longitudinal studies have revealed that beginning in the early 20s there is an average annual decrement in $\dot{V}O_2max$ of -0.28 ml·kg^{-1}·min^{-1} to -1.04 ml·kg^{-1}·min^{-1}, respectively (44). Part of this decline is the inevitable result of biological aging, with associated decreases in pulmonary and tissue gas exchange, maximum breathing capacity, maximum heart rate, and muscle mass; but part is probably also a consequence of increased sedentary living. Indeed, stratification of individuals according to habitual physical activity indicates that sedentary persons experience a threefold greater decline in $\dot{V}O_2max$ with age than do individuals who participate in regular weekly running (44).

Influence of Prolonged Bed Rest

Prolonged bed rest has been shown to result in physiologic deconditioning, including a marked reduction in $\dot{V}O_2max$. Saltin and associates (45) studied five young men before and after 3 weeks of bed rest and reported a significant 27% decrease in $\dot{V}O_2max$ (from 3.3 l·min^{-1} to 2.4 l·min^{-1}). The reduction in aerobic capacity was primarily the result of a 29% decrease in maximal stroke volume, from 104 ml before bed rest to 74 ml after bed rest; in contrast, maximal arteriovenous oxygen difference and heart rate remained essentially unchanged.

Although the diminution in $\dot{V}O_2max$ following prolonged bed rest has traditionally been attributed to the absence of daily physical activity, recent studies suggest that the reduction in oxygen transport capacity may simply reflect the lack of exposure to chronic orthostatic stress (46–48). Thus, it appears that the deterioration in $\dot{V}O_2max$ with prolonged bed rest may be lessened

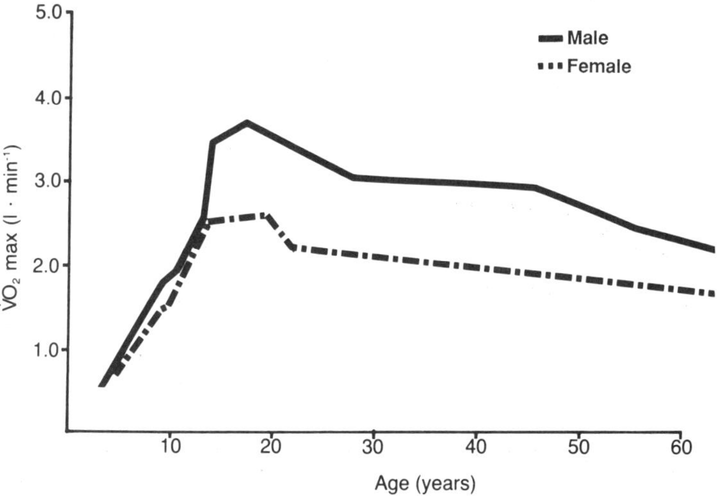

Figure 1.9. Influence of age on maximal oxygen consumption ($\dot{V}O_2$max) in males and females. Before the age of 12, the values for boys and girls are comparable. A peak in $\dot{V}O_2$max occurs between 15 and 20 years of age, followed by a gradual decline with advancing age. The average $\dot{V}O_2$max of a 60-year-old adult is approximately 70% of the mean value at the age of 20. (Adapted from Åstrand PO: *Health and Fitness*. Stockholm, Universaltryck, 1973, p 12.)

simply by regular exposure to gravitational stress, including intermittent sitting or standing (49).

Influence of Physical Conditioning/Athletic Training

Moderate endurance-type exercise training generally augments the $\dot{V}O_2$max by 10 to 25%, primarily due to an increase in the heart's stroke volume (6). Among previously sedentary middle-aged men and women, this may be extrapolated to nearly a 10-year functional rejuvenation (i.e., aerobic capacity approximates that of an untrained individual who is 10 years younger) (50). The extent of exercise-induced improvement in aerobic capacity generally shows an inverse relationship with age, habitual physical activity, and initial $\dot{V}O_2$max. Thus, young to middle-aged sedentary individuals (with low baseline $\dot{V}O_2$max) tend to show the greatest percentage increase in maximal oxygen consumption with physical conditioning. Improvement in $\dot{V}O_2$max with exercise training also shows a positive correlation with the conditioning frequency, intensity, and duration (Fig. 1.10) (51).

$\dot{V}O_2$max values (expressed relative to body weight) in elite and championship athletes vary from a high of 94 $ml{\cdot}kg^{-1}{\cdot}min^{-1}$, now reported in a cross-country skier, to values in the low-to-mid 40s for selected athletes participating in anaerobic-type sports (Fig. 1.11) (52). Virtually all world-class endurance athletes,

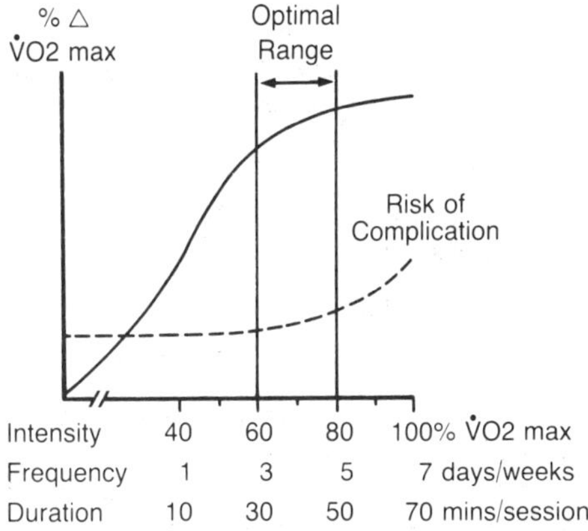

Figure 1.10. Relationship between training intensity, frequency, and duration and percent change in $\dot{V}O_2$max. (From Franklin BA, Wrisley D, Johnson S, Mitchell M, Rubenfire M: Chronic adaptations to physical conditioning in cardiac patients: Implications regarding exercise trainability. In Franklin BA, Rubenfire M (eds): *Cardiac Rehabilitation (Clinics in Sports Medicine)*. Philadelphia, WB Saunders, 1984, p 495. Reproduced by permission.)

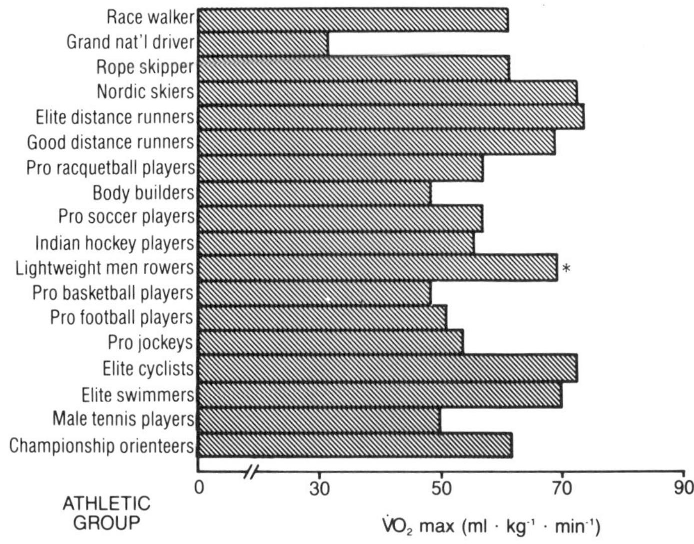

Figure 1.11. Average $\dot{V}O_2$max (ml·kg^{-1}·min^{-1}) values for various athletic groups. (Adapted from Franklin BA, Kaimal KP, Moir TW, Hellerstein HK: Characteristics of national-class race walkers. *Phys Sportsmed* 9:101–109, 1981.)

including elite distance runners and Nordic cross-country skiers, have a $\dot{V}O_2$max between 70 and 80 ml·kg^{-1}·min^{-1}, whereas many other championship athletes have a $\dot{V}O_2$max of 60 to 70 ml·kg^{-1}·min^{-1} (soccer players, cyclists, race walkers, elite swimmers, Alpine ski racers, rowers, orienteers, and ultra-marathoners). In contrast, the reported $\dot{V}O_2$max of masters athletes, professional bodybuilders, basketball players, national-class fencers (53), and volleyball players is between 40 and 50 ml·kg^{-1}·min^{-1}. Although strenuous physical training may produce a 25% or more increase in $\dot{V}O_2$max, it has become increasingly apparent that natural endowment (i.e., an exceptional genetic background), rather than training per se, plays the primary role in producing a gold medal winner in an Olympic endurance event.

Relationship Between Walk-Run Endurance Performance and Laboratory-Determined $\dot{V}O_2$max

The positive correlation between walk-run endurance performance and aerobic capacity was initially reported by Balke (26) when he suggested relating laboratory-determined $\dot{V}O_2$max either to the distance covered in a given time period or to the time required to run a given distance. Subsequently, Cooper (54) studied 115 U.S. Air Force male officers and airmen ($\bar{x}$ age = 22 years) who were evaluated by a 12-minute walk-run test for distance and a treadmill $\dot{V}O_2$max test. The correlation of the walk-run test data with the laboratory-determined $\dot{V}O_2$max was 0.897 (Fig. 1.12) (54). A regression equation was derived to predict laboratory-determined $\dot{V}O_2$max based on the distance covered in 12 minutes: walk-run distance (miles) = 0.3138 + 0.0278 $\dot{V}O_2$max (ml·kg^{-1}·min^{-1}). These findings indicate that walk-run performance testing can provide a good estimate of treadmill-determined $\dot{V}O_2$max in young, well-motivated subjects, and vice versa.

METABOLIC COST OF VARIOUS RECREATIONAL AND TRAINING ACTIVITIES

As a result of research in physiology laboratories and work classification clinics, the metabolic cost of many household, recre-

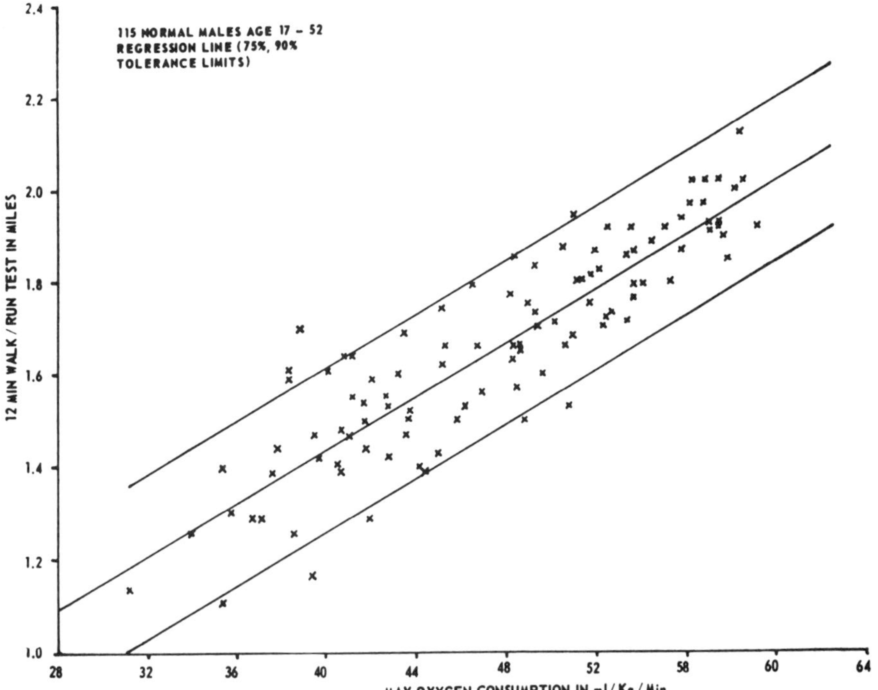

Correlation between maximal oxygen consumption and 12-minute walk-run performance in normal males. Within tolerance limits one is 75% confident that at least 95% of true maximal oxygen consumption can be found.

Figure 1.12. Correlation between maximal oxygen consumption and 12-minute walk-run performance in normal males. Within tolerance limits one is 75% confident that at least 95% of true maximal oxygen consumption can be found. (From Cooper KH: A means of assessing maximal oxygen intake: Correlation between field and treadmill testing. *JAMA* 203:201–204, 1968. Copyright 1968, American Medical Association.)

ational, and occupational activities has been defined in terms of oxygen uptake and caloric requirements (55). Table 1.4 provides the approximate metabolic cost of various recreational and exercise training activities. It should be emphasized, however, that these values represent "average" energy expenditures, and the metabolic cost of selected activities may vary considerably among individuals (56). The manner in which persons participate in activity varies widely in terms of energy expenditure, ranging from the lethargic to the energetic. Metabolic demands are also highly dependent on skill and efficiency. Activities that are little affected by skill include walking, jogging, and stationary cycling. On the other hand, the proficient tennis player may expend an average of 4 METs during singles tennis, whereas the amateur may be working at 9 METs; Table 1.4 lists singles tennis at 6 to 7 METs, equivalent to 21.0 to 25.0 $ml \cdot kg^{-1} \cdot min^{-1}$. Even other players may substantially alter the metabolic cost of recreational sports.

Walking versus Running versus Stationary Cycling: Estimation of Aerobic Requirements

Activities frequently employed in weight reduction and cardiovascular fitness programs include walking, running, and stationary cycle ergometry. Since these exercise modalities are least affected by variations in mechanical efficiency, equations have been derived to estimate the oxygen cost of a given activity during steady-state work (29). Although these formulas are equally

Table 1.4. Approximate Metabolic Cost of Various Recreational and Training Activities [a]

Activity	Metabolic Cost		
	$ml \cdot kg^{-1} \cdot min^{-1}$	METs	$kcal \cdot min^{-1}$ [b]
Walking ($1\ mi \cdot h^{-1}$)	4.0–7.0	1.5–2.0	2.0–2.5
Walking ($2\ mi \cdot h^{-1}$), bicycling ($5\ mi \cdot h^{-1}$), billiards, bowling, golf (power cart)	7.0–11.0	2.0–3.0	2.5–4.0
Walking ($3\ mi \cdot h^{-1}$), bicycling ($6\ mi \cdot h^{-1}$), volleyball, golf (pulling bag cart), archery, badminton (social doubles)	11.0–14.0	3.0–4.0	4.0–5.0
Walking ($3.5\ mi \cdot h^{-1}$), bicycling ($8\ mi \cdot h^{-1}$), table tennis, golf (carrying clubs), badminton (singles), tennis (doubles), many calisthenics	14.0–18.0	4.0–5.0	5.0–6.0
Walking ($4\ mi \cdot h^{-1}$), bicycling ($10\ mi \cdot h^{-1}$), ice skating, roller skating	18.0–21.0	5.0–6.0	6.0–7.0
Walking ($5\ mi \cdot h^{-1}$), bicycling ($11\ mi \cdot h^{-1}$), badminton (competitive), tennis (singles), square dancing, light downhill skiing, water skiing	21.0–25.0	6.0–7.0	7.0–8.0
Jogging ($5\ mi \cdot h^{-1}$), bicycling ($12\ mi \cdot h^{-1}$), vigorous downhill skiing, basketball, ice hockey, touch football, paddleball	25.0–28.0	7.0–8.0	8.0–10.0
Running ($5.5\ mi \cdot h^{-1}$), bicycling ($13\ mi \cdot h^{-1}$), squash racquets (social), handball (social), fencing, basketball (vigorous)	28.0–32.0	8.0–9.0	10.0–11.0
Running ($6.0\ mi \cdot h^{-1}$), handball (competitive), squash (competitive)	32.0 plus	10.0 plus	11.0 plus

[a] Adapted from Fox SM, Naughton JP, Gorman PA: Physical activity and cardiovascular health. III. The exercise prescription; frequency and type of activity. *Mod Concepts Cardiovasc Dis* 41:21–24, 1972.

[b] Represents gross caloric expenditure (i.e., includes the resting metabolic needs). Caloric requirements have been calculated for a 70-kg person and must be decreased or increased for lighter or heavier weights, respectively.

accurate for men and women when the activities are performed in neutral surroundings, environmental factors such as wind, snow, or sand may decrease mechanical efficiency and increase aerobic requirements.

Walking

The oxygen cost ($\dot{V}O_2$) of horizontal walking increases linearly and predictably for speeds between 50 and 100 $m \cdot min^{-1}$ (1.9 to 3.7 $mi \cdot h^{-1}$), and exponentially thereafter (29). Consequently, $\dot{V}O_2$ can be estimated with a reasonable degree of accuracy for walking speeds within this range. The oxygen cost of walking one $m \cdot min^{-1}$, equivalent to 0.1 $ml \cdot kg^{-1} \cdot min^{-1}$ per $m \cdot min^{-1}$, is added to a resting component of 3.5 $ml \cdot kg^{-1} \cdot min^{-1}$ or 1 MET, to obtain the total $\dot{V}O_2$ (57):

$$(ml \cdot kg^{-1} \cdot min^{-1}) = m \cdot min^{-1} \times \frac{0.1\ ml \cdot kg^{-1} \cdot min^{-1}}{m \cdot min^{-1}} + 3.5\ ml \cdot kg^{-1} \cdot min^{-1}$$

Example. Question: What is the $\dot{V}O_2$ in $ml \cdot kg^{-1} \cdot min^{-1}$ and METs of horizontal walking at 80 $m \cdot min^{-1}$ (3.0 $mi \cdot h^{-1}$)?

$$\begin{aligned} \dot{V}O_2 &= 80\ m \cdot min^{-1} \times \frac{0.1\ ml \cdot kg^{-1} \cdot min^{-1}}{m \cdot min^{-1}} + 3.5\ ml \cdot kg^{-1} \cdot min^{-1} \\ &= 11.5\ ml \cdot kg^{-1} \cdot min^{-1} \div 3.5\ ml \cdot kg^{-1} \cdot min^{-1} \\ &= 3.3\ \text{METs} \end{aligned}$$

Running

The $\dot{V}O_2$ for horizontal running increases in a linear and predictable manner for speeds greater than 134 $m \cdot min^{-1}$ (5 $mi \cdot h^{-1}$). However, for speeds between 100 $m \cdot min^{-1}$ and 134 $m \cdot min^{-1}$ (3.7 $mi \cdot h^{-1}$ to 5 $mi \cdot h^{-1}$) there is a "gray area" between fast walking and slow jogging that makes estimates of aerobic requirements tenuous at best (29). Since running is generally a less efficient activity than walking, the oxygen cost of running one $m \cdot min^{-1}$ approximates twice that for walking, i.e., 0.2 $ml \cdot kg^{-1} \cdot min^{-1}$ per $m \cdot min^{-1}$. This horizontal component is added to a resting component of 3.5 $ml \cdot kg^{-1} \cdot min^{-1}$ to obtain the gross $\dot{V}O_2$ (57, 58):

$$(ml \cdot kg^{-1} \cdot min^{-1}) = m \cdot min^{-1} \times \frac{0.2\ ml \cdot kg^{-1} \cdot min^{-1}}{m \cdot min^{-1}} + 3.5\ ml \cdot kg^{-1} \cdot min^{-1}$$

Example. Question: What is the $\dot{V}O_2$ in $ml \cdot kg^{-1} \cdot min^{-1}$ and METs to run on the flat at 200 $m \cdot min^{-1}$ (7.5 $mi \cdot h^{-1}$)?

$$\begin{aligned} \dot{V}O_2 &= 200\ m \cdot min^{-1} \times \frac{0.2\ ml \cdot kg^{-1} \cdot min^{-1}}{m \cdot min^{-1}} \\ &\quad + 3.5\ ml \cdot kg^{-1} \cdot min^{-1} \\ &= 43.5\ ml \cdot kg^{-1} \cdot min^{-1} \\ &\quad \div 3.5\ ml \cdot kg^{-1} \cdot min^{-1} \\ &= 12.4\ METs \end{aligned}$$

Leg Ergometry

The mechanical work rate or power output of stationary leg ergometry is determined by the product of the weight applied (kg), the distance (m) this weight moves per revolution ($m \cdot rev^{-1}$), and the number of revolutions per minute ($rev \cdot min^{-1}$), or $kg \cdot m \cdot min^{-1}$. Since the work rate is independent of body weight, the absolute $\dot{V}O_2$ (i.e., $ml \cdot min^{-1}$) at any power output is comparable among individuals of different size (29). However, a lighter individual would have a greater relative $\dot{V}O_2$ (i.e., in METs or $ml \cdot kg^{-1} \cdot min^{-1}$) than a heavier person when exercising at the same work rate.

$\dot{V}O_2$ on the stationary cycle ergometer can be estimated with reasonable accuracy for work rates between 300 and 1200 $kg \cdot m \cdot min^{-1}$ (29). The work associated with cycle ergometry is different from that of walking or jogging in that the horizontal component is eliminated because body weight is supported by a seat. However, the horizontal component is replaced by a vertical or resistive component where 1 $kg \cdot m \cdot min^{-1}$ approximates 2 $ml \cdot kg^{-1} \cdot m^{-1}$ (59, 60). The resting component of oxygen consumption (corrected for body weight) is again added to obtain the absolute $\dot{V}O_2$ (i.e., in $ml \cdot min^{-1}$):

$$(ml \cdot min^{-1}) = \frac{kg \cdot m}{min} \times \frac{2\ ml}{kg \cdot m} + (3.5\ ml \cdot kg^{-1} \cdot min^{-1} \times \text{body weight [kg]})$$

Example. Question: What is the absolute $\dot{V}O_2$ and MET level required to pedal at a work rate of 900 $kg \cdot m \cdot min^{-1}$ for a 90-kg person?

$$\begin{aligned} (ml \cdot min^{-1}) &= \frac{900\ kg \cdot m}{min} \times \frac{2\ ml}{kg \cdot m} \\ &\quad + (3.5\ ml \cdot kg^{-1} \cdot min^{-1} \times 90\ kg) \\ &= 2115\ ml \cdot min^{-1} \div 90\ kg \\ &= 23.5\ ml \cdot kg^{-1} \cdot min^{-1} \\ &= 6.7\ METs \end{aligned}$$

THE RESPIRATORY EXCHANGE RATIO (R)

As oxygen is utilized by the active tissues, carbon dioxide is produced and ultimately is expired via the lungs. The volume of carbon dioxide expired per minute ($\dot{V}CO_2$) divided by the volume of oxygen consumed during the same time interval ($\dot{V}O_2$) is referred to as the respiratory exchange ratio, $R = \dot{V}CO_2/\dot{V}O_2$. This is also known as the respiratory quotient (RQ) when measured at the cellular level.

R Value as an Index of Substrate Utilization

The R value is an important respiratory variable as it provides information regarding the proportion of energy derived from various foodstuffs at rest and during steady-state submaximal exercise. For example, an R value of 1.0 would signify that only carbohydrate was being burned; an R of 0.70, only fats; and any ratio between these two values would indicate the relative proportion of carbohydrate and fat being metabolized (61).

Carbohydrate

If carbohydrate is completely oxidized to CO_2 and H_2O, one volume of CO_2 is produced for each volume of O_2 consumed. Because of the molecular structure of sugar (two hydrogen atoms for every oxygen atom), all consumed oxygen can be used in the oxidation of carbon (62). The relationship can be described as follows:

$$C_6H_{12}O_6 + 6\ O_2 \rightarrow 6\ CO_2 + 6\ H_2O$$
(Sugar)
$$R = \dot{V}CO_2/\dot{V}O_2 = 6/6 = 1.0$$

Fat

Similarly when energy is derived from fat, oxygen combines both with carbon and hydrogen to form carbon dioxide and water, respectively (62). However, the volume of CO_2 production is necessarily different as shown below, and the R value would be expected to be less than one:

$$2\ C_{51}\ H_{98}\ O_6 + 145\ O_2 \rightarrow 102\ CO_2 + 98\ H_2O$$
$$R = \dot{V}CO_2/\dot{V}O_2 = 102/145 = 0.70$$

Although there are more than twice the number of kilocalories (kcal) in a gram of fat than carbohydrate, 9.45 versus 4.1 $kcal \cdot gm^{-1}$, it requires considerably more oxygen to release each calorie of energy. Consequently, although the body derives more energy when it uses a given amount of fat than when it metabolizes the same amount of carbohydrate, carbohydrate supplies a greater number of kcal per liter of oxygen consumed, 5.047 versus 4.686 kcal, respectively.

Protein

The R value for protein metabolism is estimated from known amino acids at approximately 0.80. However, since amino acids serve more of a regulatory function than a major energy source, protein is generally disregarded as a primary fuel for muscular work.

Substrate Utilization at Rest and During Exercise

When a person's energy is being derived from a mixed diet, the resting R value will approximate 0.83, signifying nearly equal utilization of fats and carbohydrates (Fig. 1.13) (63). During submaximal exercise, the selective utilization of fuel is related to the percentage of one's maximal oxygen uptake (% $\dot{V}O_2$max) that a workload represents. Carbohydrate utilization increases as a function of %$\dot{V}O_2$max, but free fatty acids remain a significant fuel source during mild-to-moderate intensity steady-state exercise (i.e., below 60% $\dot{V}O_2$max). Energy sources for maximal exercise, however, are exclusively from carbohydrate metabolism. As the body begins to rely increasingly on anaerobic processes, the buffering of lactic acid causes large quantities of CO_2 to be released. This results in a compensatory hyperventilation so that CO_2 production ($\dot{V}CO_2$) soon exceeds O_2 consumption ($\dot{V}O_2$), causing R to exceed unity (64). In this instance it is common to consider R as equal to 1.0, signifying carbohydrate as the primary fuel source.

R Value as an Index of Maximal Exertion

The R value is also an extremely helpful guide to the exercise test supervisor, indicating the ensuing attainment of exhaustion. Indeed, the R value may be used as a "lie detector" when the patient's request to stop exercise (presumably due to fatigue) seems incompatible with his or her overall degree of effort. R values that are less than 1.0 at peak exercise generally signify inadequate effort or poor motivation on the part of the patient. On the other hand, once the R exceeds unity, metabolism begins to rely chiefly on anaerobic processes, and the individual will not be able to continue ex-

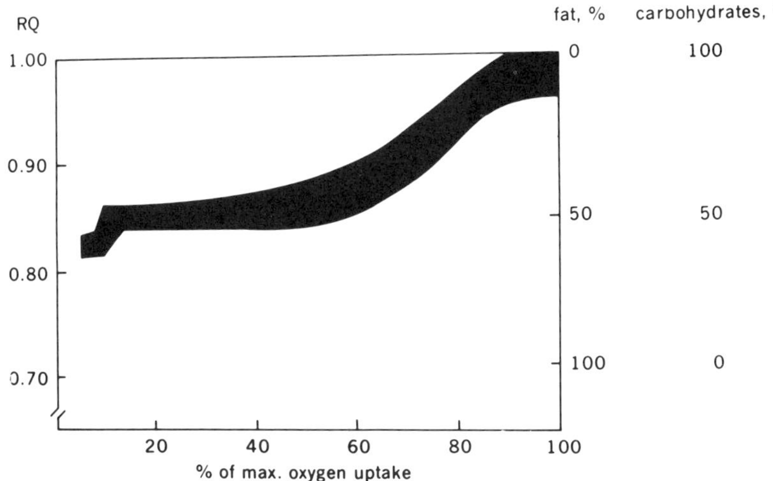

Figure 1.13. Relationship between respiratory quotient (RQ), substrate utilization, and percent of maximal oxygen uptake at rest and during exercise. (From Åstrand PO, Rodahl K: *Textbook of Work Physiology*. New York, McGraw-Hill Book Company, 1970, p 460. Reproduced by permission.)

ercising for much longer. During exhaustive exercise, it is common to find R values above 1.0 and as high as 2.1 (64). An R value of 1.15 to 1.20 during exercise has been suggested as subsidiary evidence that a "true" $\dot{V}O_2$max has been attained (65, 66). Some pulmonary patients, however, may reach exhaustion at R values below 1.0.

ANAEROBIC THRESHOLD

The anaerobic threshold (AT) has become a valuable measurement in the assessment of cardiovascular and pulmonary function, signifying the peak workload or oxygen consumption at which *oxygen demands exceed the circulation's ability to sustain aerobic metabolism*. At this point (the AT) energy release from anaerobic metabolism increases and a lactic acidemia results. Thus, the occurrence of the AT during a progressive exercise bout signifies insufficient oxygen delivery to the active muscles (67).

The physiology underlying the AT involves a temporary metabolic acidosis, which is compensated for by a respiratory alkalosis. As lactic acid is produced and buffered by bicarbonate in the blood, CO_2 is released in excess of that produced by energy metabolism. As a result of the increased CO_2 production ($\dot{V}CO_2$), the lowered pH of the blood, or both, minute ventilation ($\dot{V}E$) exhibits a break point in linearity. At that point (the anaerobic threshold), the values for $\dot{V}E$ and $\dot{V}CO_2$ increase out of proportion to the workload performed, that is, they increase more abruptly than expected (68).

Although the onset of metabolic acidosis during exercise has been traditionally determined by serial measurements of blood lactate, the abrupt increase in arterial lactate may now be determined by noninvasive methods from gas exchange (69, 70). Thus, the gas exchange anaerobic threshold can be measured by detecting the work rate or oxygen consumption just below the disproportionate increase in $\dot{V}E$ or $\dot{V}CO_2$ (Fig. 1.14) (69). This method correlates well with the lactate method and obviates the need to measure lactate in repeated blood samples. An increase in the ventilatory equivalent for oxygen ($\dot{V}E/\dot{V}O_2$) during exercise without a corresponding change in the ventilatory equivalent for CO_2 ($\dot{V}E/\dot{V}CO_2$) has also been reported to be a sensitive and reliable noninvasive technique for determining the anaerobic threshold (70). In contrast, although the respiratory exchange ratio increases as a function of exercise intensity, its inflection point identifying its increased slope at the AT is less pronounced than can be observed in other

25. Buskirk E, Taylor HL: Maximal oxygen intake and its relation to body composition, with special reference to chronic physical activity and obesity. *J Appl Physiol* 2:72–78, 1957.
26. Balke B, Ware RW: An experimental study of physical fitness of Air Force personnel. *US Armed Forces Med J* 10:675–688, 1959.
27. Bruce RA, Kusumi F, Hosmer D: Maximal oxygen intake and nomographic assessment of functional aerobic impairment in cardiovascular disease. *Am Heart J* 85:546–562, 1973.
28. Hellerstein HK, Franklin BA: Exercise testing and prescription. In Wenger NK, Hellerstein HK (eds): *Rehabilitation of the Coronary Patient*, ed 2. New York, John Wiley & Sons, 1984, p 201.
29. American College of Sports Medicine: *Guidelines for Graded Exercise Testing and Exercise Prescription*, ed 3. Philadelphia, Lea & Febiger, 1986, p 157.
30. Franklin BA, Insua JA: The "MET" concept in exercise testing and prescription. *Health Care Quarterly Rev* 1:14–16, 1982.
31. Froelicher VF, Thompson AJ, Noguera I et al: Prediction of maximal oxygen consumption: Comparison of the Bruce and Balke treadmill protocols. *Chest* 68:331–336, 1975.
32. Adams GE, Marlon AM, Quinn EJ: O_2 uptake in cardiac patients during treadmill testing. *CVP* 8:14–24, 1980.
33. Sullivan M, McKirnan MD: Errors in predicting functional capacity for postmyocardial infarction patients using a modified Bruce protocol. *Am Heart J* 107:486–492, 1984.
34. Franklin BA: Pitfalls in estimating aerobic capacity from exercise time or workload. *Appl Cardiol* 14:25–26, 1986.
35. Bruce RA: Principles of exercise testing. In Naughton JP, Hellerstein HK, Mohler IC (eds): *Exercise Testing and Exercise Training in Coronary Heart Disease*. New York, Academic Press, 1973, p 53.
36. Jones NL, Campbell EJM: *Clinical Exercise Testing*. Philadelphia, WB Saunders, 1981, p 2.
37. Von Dobeln W: Human standard and maximal metabolic rate in relation to fat-free body mass. *Acta Physiol Scand* 37:Suppl 126, 1956.
38. Franklin BA: Exercise testing, training and arm ergometry. *Sportsmed* 2:100–119, 1985.
39. Asmussen E, Hemmingsen I: Determination of maximum working capacity at different ages in work with the legs or with the arms. *Scand J Clin Lab Invest* 10:67–71, 1958.
40. Franklin BA, Vander L, Wrisley D et al: Aerobic requirements of arm ergometry: Implications for exercise testing and training. *Phys Sportsmed* 11:81–90, 1983.
41. Bar-Or O, Zwiren LD: Maximal oxygen consumption test during arm exercise—reliability and validity. *J Appl Physiol* 38:424–426, 1975.
42. Bouchard C, Godbout P, Mondor JC et al: Specificity of maximal aerobic power. *Eur J Appl Physiol* 40:85–93, 1979.
43. Åstrand PO: *Health and Fitness*. Stockholm, Universaltryck, 1973, p 12.
44. Dehn MM, Bruce RA: Longitudinal variations in maximal oxygen intake with age and activity. *J Appl Physiol* 33:805–807, 1972.
45. Saltin B, Blomqvist G, Mitchell JH et al: Response to exercise after bed rest and after training. *Circulation* 38[Suppl 7]:1–78, 1968.
46. Convertino VA, Hung J, Goldwater D et al: Cardiovascular responses to exercise in middle-aged men after 10 days of bed rest. *Circulation* 65:134–140, 1982.
47. Convertino VA, Sandler H, Webb P et al: Induced venous pooling and cardiorespiratory responses to exercise after bed rest. *J Appl Physiol* 52:1343–1348, 1982.
48. Hung J, Goldwater D, Convertino VA et al: Mechanisms for decreased exercise capacity after bed rest in normal middle-aged men. *Am J Cardiol* 51:344–348, 1983.
49. Convertino VA: Effect of orthostatic stress on exercise performance after bed rest: Relation to inhospital rehabilitation. *J Cardiac Rehabil* 3:660–663, 1983.
50. McDonough JR, Kusumi F, Bruce RA: Variations in maximal oxygen intake with physical activity in middle-aged men. *Circulation* 41:743–751, 1970.
51. Franklin BA, Wrisley D, Johnson S et al: Chronic adaptations to physical conditioning in cardiac patients: Implications regarding exercise trainability. In Franklin BA, Rubenfire M (eds): *Cardiac Rehabilitation (Clinics in Sports Medicine)*. Philadelphia, WB Saunders, 1984, p 495.
52. Franklin BA, Kaimal KP, Moir TW et al: Characteristics of national-class race walkers. *Phys Sportsmed* 9:101–109, 1981.
53. Vander LB, Franklin BA, Wrisley D et al: Physiological profile of national-class national collegiate athletic association fencers. *JAMA* 252:500–503, 1984.
54. Cooper KH: A means of assessing maximal oxygen intake: Correlation between field and treadmill testing. *JAMA* 203:201–204, 1968.
55. Fox SM, Naughton JP, Gorman PA: Physical activity and cardiovascular health. III. The exercise prescription; frequency and type of activity. *Mod Concepts Cardiovasc Dis* 41:21–24, 1972.
56. Franklin BA, Hellerstein HK: Realistic stress testing for activity prescription. *J Cardiovasc Med* 7:570–586, 1982.
57. Dill DB: Oxygen used in horizontal and grade walking and running on the treadmill. *J Appl Physiol* 20:19–22, 1965.
58. Margaria R, Cerretelli P, Aghemo P et al: Energy cost of running. *J Appl Physiol* 18:367–370, 1963.
59. Adams WC: Influence of age, sex, and body weight

on the energy expenditure of bicycle riding. *J Appl Physiol* 22:539–545, 1967.
60. Pugh LGCE: The relation of oxygen intake and speed in competitive cycling and comparative observations on the bicycle ergometer. *J Physiol* 241:795–808, 1974.
61. deVries HA: *Physiology of Exercise*, ed 3. Dubuque, William C. Brown Publishers, 1980, p 218.
62. Mathews DK, Fox EL: *The Physiological Basis of Physical Education and Athletics*, ed 2. Philadelphia, WB Saunders, 1976, p 52.
63. Åstrand PO, Rodahl K: *Textbook of Work Physiology*. New York, McGraw-Hill Book Company, 1970, p 460.
64. Issekutz B, Rodahl K: Respiratory quotient during exercise. *J Appl Physiol* 16:606–610, 1961.
65. Issekutz B, Birkhead NC, Rodahl K: Use of respiratory quotients in assessment of aerobic work capacity. *J Appl Physiol* 17:47–50, 1962.
66. Shephard RJ: *Endurance Fitness*. Toronto, University of Toronto Press, 1969, p 77.
67. Hollmann W: Historical remarks on the development of the aerobic-anaerobic threshold up to 1966. *Int J Sports Med* 6:109–116, 1985.
68. Wasserman K, Whipp BJ, Koyal SN et al: Anaerobic threshold and respiratory gas exchange during exercise. *J Appl Physiol* 35:236–243, 1973.
69. Davis JA, Vodak P, Wilmore JH et al: Anaerobic threshold and maximal aerobic power for three modes of exercise. *J Appl Physiol* 41:544–550, 1976.
70. Davis JA, Frank MH, Whipp BJ et al: Anaerobic threshold alterations caused by endurance training in middle-aged men. *J Appl Physiol: Respirat Environ Exercise Physiol* 46:1039–1046, 1979.
71. Costill DL: Physiology of marathon running. *JAMA* 221:1024–1029, 1972.
72. Costill DL, Fox EL: Energetics of marathon running. *Med Sci Sports* 1:81–86, 1969.
73. Costill DL, Thomason H, Roberts E: Fractional utilization of the aerobic capacity during distance running. *Med Sci Sports* 5:248–252, 1973.
74. Costill DL, Branam G, Eddy D et al: Determinants of marathon running success. *Int Z Angew Physiol* 29:249–254, 1971.
75. Rhodes EC, McKenzie DC: Predicting marathon time from anaerobic threshold measurements. *Phys Sportsmed* 12:95–98, 1984.
76. Ready AE, Quinney HA: Alterations in anaerobic threshold as the result of endurance training and detraining. *Med Sci Sports Exerc* 14:292–296, 1982.
77. Denis C, Fouquet R, Poty P et al: Effect of forty weeks of endurance training on the anaerobic threshold. *Int J Sports Med* 3:208–214, 1982.
78. Hellerstein HK, Franklin BA: Evaluating the cardiac patient for exercise therapy: Role of exercise testing. In Franklin BA, Rubenfire M (eds): *Cardiac Rehabilitation (Clinics in Sports Medicine)*. Philadelphia, WB Saunders, 1984, p 371.

CHAPTER 2

Healthy Adults

Larry W. Gibbons, M.D.
Steven N. Blair, P.E.D.

EXERCISE TESTING

The value of regular cardiovascular exercise in healthy adults has been established. Many physicians and other health care professionals have been leading advocates of exercise. Health care professionals are looked to for exercise advice on how much, how often, and how to get started. An exercise tolerance test and exercise prescription can help in this context. The American College of Sports Medicine recommends that apparently healthy adults have an exercise tolerance test at age 45 or above if they plan to begin a vigorous exercise program (1). For those who are already exercising, it may be beneficial to have an exercise test at age 45 if one has not been done earlier. There is, of course, some value in doing an exercise test at earlier ages for assessment of cardiovascular fitness. Repeat testing at a frequency that depends on individual factors is also of benefit.

Is an exercise test necessary in healthy adults who exercise or who desire to begin an exercise program? Though there are experts who believe that exercise testing is unnecessary in this group, the authors believe that it is advisable for at least three major reasons:

- A maximum exercise tolerance test does provide information on the presence of asymptomatic coronary disease. Coronary atherosclerosis does not produce symptoms early in the process. In as many as one-fourth or more of those who die from coronary atherosclerosis, sudden death is the first symptom. It is clear that individuals with far advanced multivessel coronary disease may be completely asymptomatic, and mild symptoms do not necessarily equate with mild disease.

Furthermore, it appears that approximately 30% of myocardial infarctions that do occur are silent.

In those infarctions that are *not* silent, a high percentage occurs in those who have had no prior warning. In a study of 577 consecutive patients who were treated in the emergency room with an acute myocardial infarction, 42% had no prior history of heart attack or *angina* (2).

Waiting for symptoms to occur prior to beginning an investigation for the presence of coronary disease is likely to identify the majority of patients only after the disease is far advanced and may have caused life-threatening complications.

Most of the coronary heart disease in the United States is still *asymptomatic* coronary disease and completely unknown to those in whom it resides. Is it worth finding out if coronary narrowing is present prior to the onset of symptoms? Most certainly it is. It has become clear that the prognosis of coronary disease can be altered significantly if risk factors are modified and the best medical tools are implemented. Prognosis can be altered even after extensive atherosclerosis has developed.

- A maximum exercise tolerance test can be a worthwhile means of assessing the level of cardiovascular fitness in a given patient prior to outlining an exercise prescription.

- An exercise tolerance test may be helpful in assessing the safety of exercise prior to beginning a vigorous exercise program. It has been demonstrated, for example, that complex ventricular irritability that occurs during maximum exercise testing increases the risk of sudden death (3).

Even though there is a higher incidence of false-positive tests in asymptomatic individuals than in those with chest pain, the abnormal test in an asymptomatic population still carries with it a five- to 15-fold increase in risk of developing future cardiovascular disease. A large number of studies have shown that an abnormal exercise electrocardiogram in asymptomatic subjects is still a valuable prognostic indicator of future coronary events (4, 5).

In addition to these three major uses of exercise testing in asymptomatic adults, it has become quite clear in the authors' experience that a maximal exercise test that results in a suboptimal rating of functional capacity can be a key stimulus to help an individual get started in an exercise program. In addition, a test that results in an excellent rating in cardiovascular fitness can be an important motivation in *keeping* individuals on a regular exercise program. In addition, Bruce and associates (6) have reported that a maximum exercise test can motivate individuals to change health behavior and coronary risk factors. In their survey conducted following participation in an exercise test, 63% of responders reported that as a result of testing, at least one health habit or coronary risk factor, such as cigarette smoking or taking antihypertensive medication, had been changed in a favorable direction.

Using a perceived exertion scale during exercise testing can help teach patients the level of exertion required to enjoy maximum benefit during their individual training sessions.

Maximal Testing

In testing apparently healthy adults, it is recommended that an exercise test be a maximal test. The maximal exercise test is more sensitive than a submaximal test in detecting any underlying cardiovascular abnormalities that might be present. Maximal testing also provides a more reliable and objective measure of cardiovascular fitness.

Fitness Categories

In assessing the level of cardiorespiratory fitness and discussing exercise prescription with an individual patient, it is often helpful to give the patient a frame of reference for where he or she stands in relationship to others of a similar age and sex. At The Cooper Clinic and Institute for Aerobics Research, fitness categories have been established for each sex and decade depending on total treadmill times. Percentile rankings of treadmill times are divided into fitness categories as follows:

Percentile Ranking	Fitness Category
0–14%	Very Poor
15–34%	Poor
35–64%	Fair
65–84%	Good
85–94%	Excellent
95% or greater	Superior

Based on more than 65,000 maximal exercise tests, the actual treadmill times that qualify for inclusion in each fitness category for males (Table 2.1) and females (Table 2.2) in each decade follow. The times are based on the Cooper Clinic modified Balke treadmill protocol: 3.3 $mi \cdot h^{-1}$, 0% elevation for first minute, 2% for second minute, +1% for each additional minute to 25%, then +0.2 $mi \cdot h^{-1}$ each minute until exhaustion.

The chart that follows allows conversion from Bruce, Ellestad, Naughton, and a sample cycle ergometer protocol to comparable Balke treadmill times (Table 2.3). This allows one to compute a comparative fitness level according to estimated oxygen consumption ($ml \cdot kg^{-1} \cdot min^{-1}$) or MET level, and classify an individual into a fitness category based on The Cooper Clinic and Institute for Aerobics Research population.

Evaluation Prior to Testing

Prior to undergoing an exercise test or beginning an exercise program, it is desir-

Table 2.1
Fitness Categories Males [a]

Fitness Category	Age Group (yr)				
	<30	30–39	40–49	50–59	60+
☐ Very poor	<14:59	<13:29	<11:59	<9:59	<6:59
☐ Poor	15:00–17:59	13:30–15:59	12:00–14:39	10:00–12:24	7:00–10:04
☐ Fair	18:00–21:09	16:00–19:59	14:40–17:59	12:25–15:59	10:05–13:42
☐ Good	21:10–24:59	20:00–23:29	18:00–21:58	16:00–19:29	13:43–17:14
☐ Excellent	25:00–27:59	23:30–26:29	21:59–24:59	19:30–22:59	17:15–20:59
☐ Superior	28:00 +	26:30 +	25:00 +	23:00 +	21:00 +

[a] **Based on the Cooper Clinic modified Balke treadmill protocol: 3.3 mi·h^{-1} (90 m·min^{-1}), 0% for 1st min, 2% for 2nd min, +1% for each additional min to 25%, then + 0.2 mi·h^{-1} each min until exhaustion.**

Table 2.2
Fitness Categories Females [a]

Fitness Category	Age Group (yr)				
	<30	30–39	40–49	50–59	60+
☐ Very Poor	<10:09	<8:59	<7:29	<5:59	<4:59
☐ Poor	10:10–12:52	9:00–11:29	7:30– 9:59	6:00– 7:59	5:00– 6:29
☐ Fair	12:53–15:59	11:30–14:59	10:00–12:59	8:00–10:38	6:30– 9:16
☐ Good	16:00–19:59	15:00–17:39	13:00–15:59	10:39–13:14	9:17–11:59
☐ Excellent	20:00–23:01	17:40–20:30	16:00–18:29	13:15–15:55	12:00–15:33
☐ Superior	23:02 +	20:31 +	18:30 +	15:56 +	15:34 +

[a] **Based on the Cooper Clinic modified Balke treadmill protocol: 3.3 mi·h^{-1} (90 m·min^{-1}), 0% for 1st min, 2% for 2nd min, + 1% for each additional min to 25%, then + 0.2 mi·h^{-1} each min until exhaustion.**

able for an individual to have a physical examination. If a physical examination is not practical, a cardiac exam is required. A medical history may be the most vital part of this evaluation and should include, of course, questions on signs and symptoms of cardiovascular, pulmonary, metabolic, and orthopedic disease as well as family history, exercise history, and a risk factor profile. Laboratory studies are valuable to assess coronary risk and should include a complete lipid profile with HDL and LDL cholesterol levels, triglycerides, and serum glucose.

An evaluation prior to exercise testing is important because an exercise test can only be interpreted properly when one knows the clinical background of a given patient. In addition, the information learned may significantly affect the exercise prescription. Also, the time when an individual is preparing to start an exercise program provides an ideal opportunity to measure selected parameters such as percent body fat or cholesterol, which might otherwise go unevaluated. As an individual initiates an exercise program, he or she is often motivated at the same time to lose weight or change the diet or stop smoking or work on improving other cardiovascular risk factors.

If one is making recommendations for the population as a whole, it is impossible to suggest that every *healthy* American man and woman age 45 or above have an exercise tolerance test. There are simply not facilities available for such screening, and the associated health care costs would be

Table 2.3
Comparative Fitness Level Computation[a]

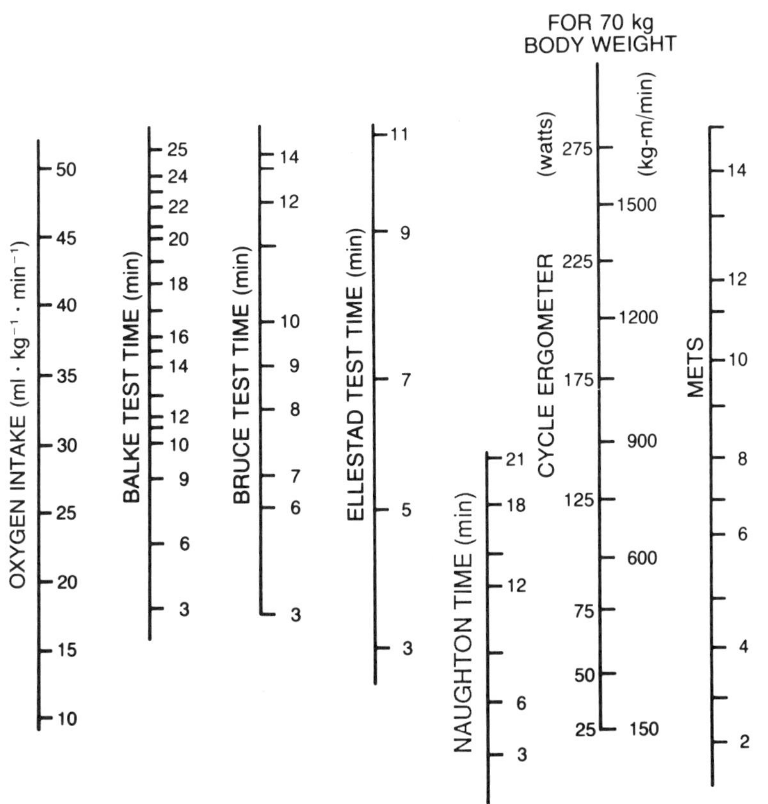

[a] Exercise intensity equivalents can be estimated by drawing a horizontal line from the time on a given treadmill or cycle ergometer protocol to oxygen uptake (on the left) or MET level (on the right). From American College of Sports Medicine: Guidelines for Exercise Testing and Prescription, ed 3. Philadelphia, Lea & Febiger, 1986, p 26.

prohibitive. A public health recommendation for universal exercise testing, therefore, is not practical. However, in the individual case where funds and facilities are available, much can be gained from a properly administered maximal exercise test.

Interpreting Abnormal Tests

Some physicians hesitate to recommend exercise testing in asymptomatic adults because of fear of a false-positive result, which might lead to mental anguish and unnecessary expense and risk (albeit small) while follow-up tests are done to decide whether or not an abnormal test in an asymptomatic individual is a true- or false-positive.

The exercise tolerance test is, of course, neither 100% sensitive nor 100% specific. Sensitivity refers to the likelihood that disease present in an individual will be detected with a given testing procedure. Specificity refers to the likelihood that an individual who is disease-free will be correctly identified by having a negative result with a given testing procedure. False-negative and false-positive tests occur in asymptomatic adults as well as others. A normal test does not necessarily mean that coronary disease is absent. An abnormal test does not necessarily mean that disease is present or will develop in the future. The true sensitivity and specificity of maximal exercise testing in presumably healthy adults are unclear. Most research places the sensitivity of an optimally administered exercise test in an asymptomatic population somewhere between 50–85% depending on the number of vessels involved. The specificity appears to be somewhere between 80–90%, using 50–70% narrowing of at least one coronary artery on coronary angiography as the diagnostic standard.

Factors that increase the sensitivity of exercise testing in asymptomatic adults are:

1. Maximal testing to exhaustion or other exercise-limiting symptoms.
2. Use of 12–15 electrodes on the chest.
3. Using all available data from an exercise test, such as heart rate and blood pressure response, rather than just ST-segment depression.
4. Using a very broad criterion for defining an abnormal test (i.e., 0.5 mm of ST depression). However, this is not recommended since it also decreases the specificity greatly and adds significantly to the number of false-positive tests.

How does one interpret an exercise test in asymptomatic individuals and recommend appropriate follow-up without creating a cardiac neurosis and without missing potentially lethal disease?

It is the opinion of the authors that an abnormal exercise test in an asymptomatic individual is best viewed as a risk factor rather than a diagnosis. As mentioned previously, in the asymptomatic population not everyone with an abnormal exercise test has coronary disease or will develop coronary disease. But even in this population those with an abnormal response have a five- to 15-fold increased relative risk of developing complications of coronary disease as opposed to those with a normal test. Not everyone with an elevated cholesterol level has coronary disease or will develop coronary disease. However, this does not prevent us from measuring cholesterol levels in healthy individuals in an effort to assess risk and decide upon the appropriate measures to lower cholesterol in those in whom there is enough elevation to present a risk. An abnormal exercise test in an asymptomatic individual is a much more powerful risk factor than serum cholesterol, cigarette smoking, family history, or hypertension.

Not every murmur heard with the practitioner's stethoscope is an indication of valvular or muscular heart disease. Most murmurs are quite innocent, especially in those who are asymptomatic. This, however, does not prevent the practitioner from putting a stethoscope on the patient's chest for fear he will find a murmur that he will not be able to explain to the patient as most likely an innocent murmur, thus creating undue fear in the mind of the patient. Physicians are quite competent in explaining heart murmurs that seem to be innocent. In the same way, thoughtful and careful physicians can explain to patients who have no risk factors and are unlikely to have coronary narrowing, but who are found to have abnormal exercise tolerance tests, that the abnormal test is likely a false-positive.

Of course, there is much we do not understand concerning an exercise test that shows significant ST-segment depression when a subsequent coronary angiogram is completely normal. Perhaps the abnormal test is an indication of a cardiovascular abnormality other than coronary disease. Another possibility is that the abnormal exercise test result might signify small vessel coronary disease that cannot be easily identified with the angiogram. Coronary angiography is also, of course, not an infallible test to detect the presence or absence of disease.

Pre- and Posttest Probabilities

False-positive exercise tests are not uncommon in asymptomatic populations. These false-positive tests may be due to identifiable factors such as ventricular hypertrophy or hypokalemia or vasoregulatory causes, etc. (Comprehensive lists of causes for false-positive and false-negative exercise tests have been published elsewhere.) In many instances, no specific cause can be identified. In the asymptomatic population a false-positive test should be interpreted utilizing knowledge regarding the prevalence of disease in that population. Bayes' theorem states that the likelihood that a positive test represents true disease is directly related to the prevalence of disease in the population being tested. This means that in populations in which the actual prevalence of coronary disease is low, for example in asymptomatic individuals with no risk factors, an abnormal (positive) test is much more likely to be a false-positive test than is an abnormal test in a population with a high prevalence of disease (e.g., older men with multiple risk factors).

It is important, thus, to remember that the pretest likelihood of having coronary disease based on such factors as age, sex, presence or absence of symptoms, smoking status, and serum cholesterol profile governs how one interprets the test after it has been completed.

In clinical practice the critical decision to be made is whether or not an abnormal exercise test in an asymptomatic individual truly is an indication of disease or whether it is a false-positive. This can be expressed as a "probability" or a "likelihood" that a positive test is a true-positive.

Froelicher, for example, using Bayes' theorem and a hypothetical test sensitivity of 70% and a specificity of 90%, calculates the probability that an abnormal test truly represents disease and the probability that a normal test truly represents absence of disease (7). He makes these calculations for four different populations: those with typical angina, those with atypical angina, those with nonangina-like chest pain, and those who are asymptomatic in order to show how the pretest likelihood of disease influences the posttest probability of disease once the test has been completed (Table 2.4).

It can be seen in this example that even with a negative test, an individual with typical angina still has a high likelihood of having coronary disease whereas a negative test in an asymptomatic individual carries with it a very strong probability that no disease is present. This latter fact means that a clinician who finds a normal maximal exercise test in an asymptomatic individual can provide very convincing and solid reassurance that in fact no disease is present. On the other hand, the example clearly illustrates that an abnormal test in an asymptomatic individual is much less likely to

Table 2.4
Probability of Coronary Disease [a]

Population Type	Test Result	Posttest Probability of Disease (%)
Angina	Abnormal	98
	Normal	75
Atypical Angina	Abnormal	88
	Normal	25
Nonanginal Chest pain	Abnormal	44
	Normal	4
Asymptomatic	Abnormal	27
	Normal	2

[a] From Froelicher VF: *Exercise Testing and Training.* New York, Le Jacq, 1983, p 83.

represent a true-positive test than the same abnormality in a person with any type of chest pain.

The degree of abnormality of the test also influences the posttest probability of disease as is illustrated by the following graph (Figure 2.1), which relates the pretest likelihood of disease with the posttest likelihood of disease depending on the magnitude of ST-segment depression (8).

Bayes' theorem and the related concepts and examples just discussed are of value but are still abstract and theoretical. Nothing can substitute for sound clinical judgment after a careful review of all the data assembled during the history, the physical examination, and the test procedure.

In addition to the application of Bayes' theorem as illustrated by these examples, there are a number of recently published schemes or formulas using data collected during the testing procedure itself to enhance the accuracy of interpreting abnormal exercise test results and deciding which positive tests are true-positive. These formulas use such variables as maximum heart rate achieved, duration of exercise, changes in ST slope related to heart rate, etc. (9, 10). These new formulas introduce worthwhile concepts into the difficult arena of exercise test interpretation, but it may be somewhat confusing to decide which of the new formulas to use. Perhaps it would be most practical at this

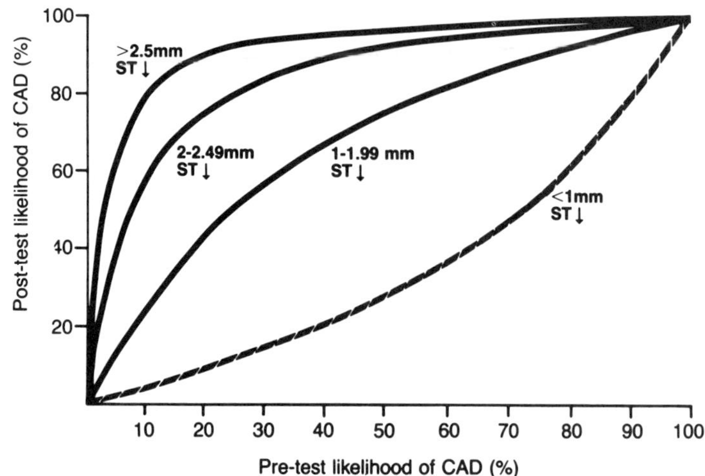

Figure 2.1. Pre- and posttest likelihood of coronary artery disease (CAD) according to the degree of ST depression present. For example, if the pretest likelihood of disease is high, less ST depression is needed for a high posttest likelihood of CAD. (From Epstein SE: Implications of probability analysis on the strategy used for noninvasive detection of coronary artery disease. *Am J Cardiol* 46:491–499, 1980.)

time in concluding the discussion of false-positive test results to simply include a list of the factors known to increase the likelihood that an abnormal test in an asymptomatic individual is a true abnormal test and not a false-positive (Table 2.5):

Follow-Up

If one considers an abnormal exercise test in an asymptomatic adult to be a risk factor rather than a diagnosis, the question still remains: "What is the appropriate fol-

Table 2.5
Factors That Increase the Likelihood That an Abnormal Exercise Test in an Asymptomatic Individual Is a True-Positive Test

1. Male Sex
2. Age over 50
3. ST-segment depression of 2 mm or more
4. Cigarette smoking
5. High blood pressure
6. Total cholesterol/HDL ratio over 5.0
7. ST-segment depression that occurs at low workloads
8. Failure to reach 85% of one's predicted maximal heart rate
9. Chest pain during the treadmill test
10. Ventricular irritability that accompanies ST-segment depression during a treadmill test
11. Horizontal or downsloping ST-segments (as opposed to upsloping ST-segments)
12. ST-segments that are depressed both in exercise and recovery
13. An abnormal test in a patient who has had a previous normal test
14. Limited functional capacity as demonstrated on the exercise test
15. Flat or dropping systolic blood pressure during the exercise test
16. Marked increase in R wave amplitude at maximal exertion
17. Prolongation of QT interval with exercise or widening of the QRS complex with exercise
18. ST-segment depression of a given magnitude is more likely to be diagnostic of disease if the QRS voltage is low rather than high (ST-depression magnitude is strongly influenced by the magnitude of QRS voltage)

low-up for a newly detected abnormal exercise test in an asymptomatic individual?"

The level of follow-up depends, of course, on the pretest likelihood of disease based on the number of other risk factors present, including age and sex of the patient, and the extent of the abnormality manifest during testing. One possible scheme for following up abnormal exercise tolerance tests in asymptomatic adults is outlined in Table 2.6.

Women

The incidence of false-positive tests is higher in women than in men. This is especially true in asymptomatic populations. Ellestad reports that exercise-induced ST-segment depression in normal women under age 45 is four times more common in women than in men (11). At The Cooper Clinic, in more than 10,000 maximal exercise tests conducted on women, only 8.6% had an equivocal result and only 3.8% were abnormal. The average age of these women was approximately 40. Even in women, it is still usually possible using the above criteria to differentiate between a true-positive test and a false-positive test without doing coronary angiography. The same principles used in differentiating a true abnormal test from a false-positive test apply in women as in men.

Safety

Exercise testing in asymptomatic adults is quite safe. Reported complication rates vary widely but more recent studies show rates generally between 0 and 4 complications (serious arrhythmia, myocardial infarction, or death) per 10,000 tests (12). Deaths in asymptomatic adults during exercise testing are extremely rare. In 15 years of maximal exercise testing at The Cooper Clinic, for example, in more than 65,000 exercise tests done in a population in which less than 10% have previously known coronary disease, there have been no immediate deaths and only six complications (myocardial infarctions or serious arrhythmias requiring intervention).

Musculoskeletal Testing

If more comprehensive exercise testing is desirable and practical, it may be advisable to include tests of musculoskeletal strength and endurance and flexibility as well as the cardiovascular tests already discussed.

Lack of abdominal muscle strength may

Table 2.6
Recommended Follow-up for Abnormal Exercise Tests in Healthy, Asymptomatic Adults

		Magnitude of ST-Segment Depression	
		1.0 to 1.9 mm ST-segment depression [b]	2.0 mm ST-segment depression or more [b]
Number of major [a] risk factors present	0	A	B
	1	A	B or C
	2	B	C
	3	C	D

[a] **Major risk factors:**
1. **History of high blood pressure (above 145/95)**
2. **Elevated total cholesterol/high density lipoprotein cholesterol ratio (above 5)**
3. **Cigarette smoking**
4. **Abnormal resting ECG**
5. **Family history of coronary or other atherosclerotic disease prior to age 50**
6. **Diabetes mellitus**
7. **Age over 50**

[b] **Follow-up Recommendations**
A. **Retest in 1 year—modify risk factors (if present)**
B. **Retest in 3–4 months—modify risk factors**
C. **Radionuclide study (i.e., Thallium scan)**
D. **Coronary angiogram**

be an important factor in the development of low back pain, for example. Evaluating abdominal strength can be done with a 1-minute timed sit-up test. Standards obtained from a population of healthy adults are available in Nieman's comprehensive reference manual (13).

Hand strength may be important in many activities of daily living and in the prevention of upper extremity injury. A useful test of hand strength is the grip strength test with a hand dynamometer. Established norms for this test are available in the same source listed above (14).

Muscle strength may be evaluated by measuring the greatest weight that can be lifted only once with each muscle group. Obviously precautions are very important in this testing to prevent musculoskeletal injury. Protocols for testing muscle strength are available in a number of different reference materials (15).

A sample test of muscular endurance would use a fixed percentage of the individual's body weight or a fixed percentage (for example 70%) of the maximum muscle strength as measured above. The subject would lift this weight as many times as possible. The YMCA bench press is an example of this type of muscular endurance test. The protocol can be obtained in the references cited (16).

Tests of leg strength can be performed using Cybex or similar equipment if such equipment is available. Generally this type of leg strength evaluation using more expensive equipment is available only in large fitness centers and is not practical in the individual physician's office.

Flexibility measurements could be done quite easily with a sit-and-reach test. A protocol for doing such a test is included in Nieman's publication cited above (17).

EXERCISE PRESCRIPTION

Even in the healthy adult, it is important to give specific exercise recommendations. Specific rather than general exercise prescription helps to give the patient reassurance that he or she is proceeding properly, may help to avoid injury from early overuse, and gives one a goal as to how much is necessary to achieve the anticipated benefits.

An exercise prescribed by a physician or other health professional should ideally be both pleasant and practical for the individual. The practical aspects, however, are most important. It is useless to prescribe racquetball or swimming, for example, even though the patient may enjoy both immensely, if such facilities are not easily accessible.

Walking

Walking is a practical activity for most adults, especially those who are just beginning to exercise. Walking can be done almost anywhere and requires no special equipment. In cold climates it is often possible to find some type of indoor facility, such as a shopping mall, where one can walk year-round. The only major disadvantage of walking is the time required. To get full benefit from walking, three miles is the recommended distance. Most individuals can eventually work up to a speed of 15 min/mile or faster. Here is a sample walking program for someone who is just beginning. Such a program would be appropriate for a 40- to 60-year-old patient with no cardiac or orthopedic problems.

Walking Program

Week	Distance (miles)	Time (min)	Freq/Week (times)
1	1.0	18:00	5
2	1.0	16:00	5
3	1.5	24:00	5
4	1.5	23:00	5
5	2.0	32:00	5
6	2.0	30:00	5
7	2.5	37:30	5
8	2.5	36:30	5
9	3.0	45:00	5
10	3.0	< 45:00	5

Stationary Cycling

Stationary cycling is another practical activity especially for the homemaker or busy executive. Moreover, it is an attractive alternative to outdoor exercise during certain times of the year. It is possible for most individuals to read while they use the stationary cycle if a magazine rack is attached to the handle bars. In addition, almost any family can find a place for a stationary cycle in front of a television, where time passes quickly. Stereo headphones can also be attached to help make the exercise more pleasant. Here is a sample program for a 30- to 50-year-old with no cardiac or orthopedic problems.

Stationary Cycling Program

Week	Speed (mph)	Duration (min)	PR* after Exercise	Freq/Week (times)
1	15	5:00	120	5
2	15	7:30	130	5
3	15	10:00	130	5
4	15	16:00	130	5
5	15	18:00	130	5
6	17.5	21:00	140	5
7	20	21:00	140	5
8	20	24:00	140	5
9	20	27:00	140	5
10	20	30:00	140	5

*Pulse Rate

Note: Add enough resistance so that the pulse rate, counted for 10 seconds immediately after exercise and multiplied by 6, equals the number specified. If it is higher, lower the resistance before cycling again, and if it is lower, increase the resistance. However, these pulse rate guidelines may not be appropriate for all individuals. As a general rule, the exercise intensity should feel "somewhat hard."

Running

Running is practical and easy for most individuals who do not have orthopedic problems. Nonetheless, there are some common misconceptions among many new and long-time runners.

Misconception 1: Speed is essential to get the benefits.

Fact. Exercise need not be exhaustive to be beneficial. Many healthy adults feel they must strain to near exhaustion in order to achieve benefits. Recent evidence confirms that moderate exercise provides all of the significant health benefits. The cardiovascular benefits of running do not depend on speed. Even the slowest jog confers the vast majority of health-related benefits that come from running. These benefits occur at a pace of 10 minutes per mile or even slower as long as distance and regularity are maintained.

Misconception 2: One must be a long-distance runner in order to get the benefits.

Fact. Although a precise dose-response curve for running and other forms of exercise as they relate to health benefits has yet to be defined, it appears that the major changes in cardiovascular risk and improvement in maximum oxygen consumption occur within the first *15 miles* of running per week (18).

Misconception 3: Women cannot or should not run.

Fact. Years of practical experience have shown that there is no special risk for women who run vigorously. There is no evidence that orthopedic problems are significantly more common in women who run, or that any loss of feminine figure occurs. Only those women with stress incontinence should in most cases avoid running.

Here is a progressive walk-jog program for a middle-aged runner (35–55 years of age) who is just starting out, assuming no orthopedic or cardiac problems.

Jogging Program

Week	Activity	Distance (miles)	Time (min)	Freq/Week (times)
1	Walk/Jog	1.0	13:00	5
2	Walk/Jog	1.0	12:00	5
3	Walk/Jog	1.0	11:30	5
4	Walk/Jog	1.0	11:00	5
5	Walk/Jog	1.5	18:00	5
6	Walk/Jog	1.5	17:00	5
7	Walk/Jog	1.75	21:00	5
8	Walk/Jog	1.75	20:00	5
9	Jog	2.0	22:00	5
10	Jog	2.0	21:00	5
11	Jog	2.0	20:30	5
12	Jog	2.0	< 20:00	5

Outdoor Bicycling

Bicycling, in theory, is excellent cardiovascular exercise. In practice, it is difficult for many individuals to find an area where bicycling can be continuous without stopping for traffic, stoplights, etc. Bicycling also carries a greater danger than most other types of exercise because of the exposure to traffic. Weather also presents a problem in some areas. If one does have a safe and suitable place to bicycle, here is an acceptable program, again assuming no medical contraindications.

Cycling Program

Week	Distance (miles)	Time (min)	Freq/Week (times)
1	2.0	12:30	5
2	2.0	11:00	5
3	2.0	9:45	5
4	3.0	16:00	5
5	3.0	14:30	5
6	4.0	18:30	5
7	5.0	22:00	5
8	6.0	25:30	5
9	7.0	29:00	5
10	8.0	33:00	5

Swimming

Swimming has some advantages over other types of cardiovascular exercise because it is nonweight bearing and gives one some additional upper extremity strengthening. For those adults who have not developed the skill to swim, swimming classes can be arranged in most areas. Swimming seems to be especially valuable for those with a history of lower back problems. Here is a sample program for a 30- to 50-year-old man or woman who is healthy, but who has been sedentary.

Swimming Program

Week	Distance (yards)	Time (min)	Freq/Week (times)
1	300	10:00	5
2	350	11:00	5
3	400	12:00	5
4	450	13:00	5
5	500	14:00	5
6	550	15:00	5
7	600	16:00	5
8	650	18:00	5
9	700	19:00	5
10	750	20:00	5
11	800	21:00	5
12	850	22:00	5
13	900	23:00	5

Other Exercises

There is evidence that vigorous competitive sports that involve movement of large muscle groups over a long period of time can be just as effective in improving cardiovascular fitness as running, swimming, and other individual exercises. However, participation in vigorous competitive sports should be discouraged for individuals who are just starting an exercise program. It is much better to begin with an initial 6- to 10-week conditioning program involving walking, running, or swimming before one begins participation in more vigorous competitive sports.

One and one-half hours of singles tennis, 45–60 minutes of racquetball, 45–60 minutes of basketball, soccer, squash, or handball will suffice as a satisfactory exercise session that will provide the majority of health-related exercise benefits.

Some have found the minitrampoline to be a useful device for those who must exercise indoors. Because the elasticity of the minitrampoline lessens the work of running, in our experience it requires approximately one and one-half to two times the duration required in standard running to enjoy equal benefits. Or, if one desires a workout of equal intensity and duration to running, a heart rate 10–15 beats per minute higher must be maintained on the minitrampoline.

Aerobic dancing has a significant cardiovascular benefit. Approximately 45 minutes of a suitable aerobics dance class will provide an adequate workout as long as it is done regularly. The ideal surface for aerobic dancing is a hardwood floor suspended on some type of absorbent material. A concrete floor with a vigorous bouncing aerobics class presents considerable hazard for musculoskeletal injury. A good aerobics dance program will offer separate classes for beginning, intermediate, and advanced students. Dancing lightly and making an effort to glide rather than bounce vigorously should help decrease the risk of musculoskeletal injury.

Choosing the Right Exercise

Dr. Ken Cooper rates cross-country skiing as the best cardiovascular exercise of all because it uses several major muscle groups and, in studies done around the world, seems to have produced the athletes with the highest maximum oxygen consumption ($\dot{V}O_2max$) (19). The cross-country ski machine may be a way of getting similar benefits inside the home for those who are not able to ski outdoors or for those who want the benefits of cross-country skiing year-round. He recommends swimming and jogging as the second and third best aerobic exercises, respectively, again largely because they require the use of many major muscle groups. Swimming also seems to be a particularly safe exercise both from a musculoskeletal and cardiovascular standpoint.

Recent studies suggest that even low levels of physical activity may have substantial benefits. Most of the population who exercise probably do not perform enough physical activity on a sufficiently regular basis to reach optimal levels of relative maximum oxygen consumption but may still enjoy health benefits.

Low-Level Exercise

Large epidemiologic studies have shown that the risk of coronary heart disease can be lowered by even light or moderate exercise as long as it is performed regularly. Heavy exercise may further decrease the risk, but substantial benefit is obtained by even light or moderate work (20).

A recent study in young men showed that a group trained at low intensity (45% of $\dot{V}O_2max$) increased aerobic capacity more slowly than a similar group trained at high intensity, but that after 12–18 weeks the overall gain in maximum oxygen consumption was not significantly different in the two groups (21).

There are some advantages in participating in a variety of exercises rather than limiting activity to one exercise alone. It appears that most individuals prefer to limit their activity to one exercise, but a variety of different exercises may add to the pleasure and enjoyment of exercise and decrease the risk of injury. Variety probably also contributes to overall fitness by involving a greater number of muscle groups. It may also help adherence.

Even though cardiovascular benefits are usually considered the most important priority, there are other important benefits from regular exercise, such as help in weight control, for example. The chart that follows is a useful summary of some of the most popular types of exercise and the relative value of cardiovascular, muscular, and weight control benefits provided (Table 2.7) (22).

One should encourage adults who have not exercised previously to progress slowly. Those who are motivated to begin exercise will have the tendency to overexert the first few weeks. Gradual progress is important for the following reasons:

1. It helps to prevent injury.
2. The benefits of exercise are long term, not short term. Taking a few more weeks to build up to the desired level of activity does not set anyone back over the long run.
3. Individuals who exercise too strenuously may find the activity so unpleasant that they will find many reasons to stop.

It is important not to assume that individuals know how to manage an exercise

Table 2.7
Exercise and Energy Expenditure Chart [a]

	Aerobic Benefits	Muscle Strength	Weight Control	$Kcal \cdot h^{-1}$
Jogging	4[b]	3	4	600
Bicycling	4	3	3	500
Swimming	4	4	4	600
Handball, squash, racquetball	4	3	3	420
Cross-country skiing	4	4	4	600
Downhill skiing	2	3	2	410
Basketball	4	3	3	420
Tennis (singles)	3	3	3	410
Calisthenics	1	4	2	320
Walking	3	2	3	320
Golf (no carts)	1	1	1	320
Softball and baseball	1	1	1	264
Bowling	1	1	1	270

[a] From Pamphlet, *Fitness 3,* Roach Drug Company, P.O. Box 203, Wood Ridge, NJ.
[b] 4 = very good; 3 = good; 2 = fair; 1 = poor.

program. Even though there is now much more information available in the media to the public about appropriate guidelines for exercise, it is better to prepare a standard set of instructions to give to all patients so that problems do not occur because of misinformation. Here are some guidelines that might be appropriate.

1. Regularity is the most important element of a program. Try to maintain a frequency of four or five workouts per week.
2. If you walk or run, be sure to obtain a good pair of shoes such as those made by Nike, New Balance, Adidas, Saucony, Etonic or Brooks. A number of excellent shoes are available in addition to those listed.
3. If one is just beginning, start slowly and comfortably. This may help to prevent muscle and joint injuries. Also, workouts should be reduced following any injury, illness, or after any other period of inactivity.
4. Appropriate warm-up and cool-down are also important. Never sit or lie down immediately after exercise or go directly to the whirlpool, steam room, or shower. A gradual cool-down for about 5 minutes will allow for adequate readjustment of the cardiovascular system.
5. Adequate fluid replacement is a problem among many who exercise. It is especially important during the warm weather months that about 10 to 12 ounces of fluid be consumed approximately 60 minutes before exercise. One should then drink 10 to 12 ounces of fluid for every 10 to 15 minutes of exercise. The tendency is to not drink enough fluid. The recommended form of fluid is plain, cool water.
6. Problems and setbacks will undoubtedly occur. Plan for how you will deal with them in order to get back on schedule.
7. It may be helpful to keep a record of your exercise. The Aerobics Points System has proved worthwhile for many (23).

Is there a "best time" of day to exercise? Morning exercise may be associated with fewer interruptions. This is an important advantage. Noontime is also an excellent time to exercise. For most people exercise produces a temporary decrease in appetite and this keeps one from eating as much at the noontime meal. One can then return to work without the sleepiness often associated with eating a heavy lunch and enjoy more vigor and alertness during the afternoon work hours.

There is now a considerable body of evidence that regular exercise has benefit in controlling anxiety or stress. For those who are troubled with anxiety and stress, exercising in the evening just before supper may have considerable benefit. The theory is that exercise at this time will help to relieve the anxiety produced by a stressful day's activities. There has been a preliminary report that exercising in the morning may increase the risk of cardiovascular complications, but this does not appear to be a major concern. In quantitating the cardiovascular benefit that comes from exercise, there is no evidence that the time of day when one exercises makes any difference.

Strength and Flexibility Exercises

Even though the types of exercises discussed to this point, which are primarily cardiovascular, are associated with the most important health benefits that come from regular exercise, strength and flexibility exercises are also important. It would be useful for the physician or health professional to prescribe a strength and flexibility program along with endurance exercise recommendations.

There is considerable logic though little hard evidence to suggest that musculoskeletal exercise for strength and flexibility may decrease the incidence and/or severity of some of the common musculoskeletal and degenerative diseases, such as osteoarthritis and low back pain. Certainly it has become clear that Williams' low back exercises help to decrease the frequency and severity of recurrences in individuals with a low back pain syndrome. Although data are lacking, it also appears very plausible that strength training, stretching, and calisthenics will make many of the activities of daily living, such as carrying in the groceries or carrying a heavy briefcase, easier and less likely to produce musculoskeletal injury.

Here are sample upper body exercises that one may use with a set of hand dumbbells. A beginning weight of 3 to 5 pounds is suggested with gradual progression to 10 pounds or higher if well tolerated (Table 2.8).

Nautilus, Eagle, and other similar equipment is now widely available and can be used to develop significant musculoskeletal strength and endurance. There is as yet no convincing evidence that participating in this type of exercise improves cardiovascular fitness significantly.

To obtain the maximal benefit from such machines, it is essential that correct procedures be followed. Merely having access to strength-training equipment does not insure a good result. The following guidelines are appropriate:

1. Start each session by working from the large muscle groups to the small muscle groups.
2. Perform one set of 8–12 repetitions, with no more than 12 exercises in any workout.
3. Each exercise should be continued until fatigue causes cessation. Once 12 repetitions are performed, increase the weight by approximately 5%.
4. It is recommended to train no more than 3 times a week, unless upper and lower body workouts are performed on opposite days.
5. Always concentrate on flexibility by slowly stretching during the first three repetitions of each exercise.
6. It is always recommended to move slower, never faster, if in doubt about the speed of movement.
7. Workout routines should be changed often to prevent staleness.

Flexibility exercises are widely available and should be incorporated in a complete exercise prescription. Stretching the Achilles tendons, calf muscles, hamstrings, back, and trunk is most important. The best time to perform these stretching exercises is probably after a brief, low-level warm-up and prior to the most intensive part of the cardiovascular exercise session or after the cardiovascular workout itself.

Table 2.8
Dumbbell Exercises

These strength exercises can be performed almost anywhere. Proper breathing is important, as this will allow for maximal muscle effort. When lifting the weight, exhale; when returning the weight to starting position, inhale. It is important to maintain a smooth rhythm throughout the exercise. Usually 1 to 3 sets of 10 repetitions (light weight) are recommended.

Dumbbell swing: (standing)

Hold one dumbbell overhead and grip with both hands, knees slightly flexed and feet shoulder width apart. Swing the dumbbell down between the legs and return to starting position (keep the arms straight throughout the movement). Major muscles exercised: (quadriceps, gluteus maximus, hamstring, erector spinae).

Dumbbell press: (standing or sitting)

Press the dumbbells alternately overhead and in a vertical movement, over the shoulders, and return them to shoulder height (deltoids, triceps, trapezius).

Dumbbell curls:

Curl the dumbbell with the arm by bending the elbow toward you. This can be performed by alternating weights or by continuous repetitions (biceps, brachioradialis, radial flexors).

Lateral raise:

Raise both arms out to the side to shoulder height then return to your side. Throughout the exercise, keep the arms as straight as possible and avoid unnecessary body swing (deltoids, trapezius, rhomboids, serratus anterior).

CHRONIC ADAPTATIONS TO TRAINING

How the body adapts to exercise training will vary significantly from individual to individual because of genetic differences. This occurs even in individuals who are given identical exercise prescriptions. Nonetheless, there are common responses, which are observable and measurable. Some of the central (circulatory) and peripheral adaptations to regular exercise are apparent within a few weeks of physical conditioning. Other effects may not be fully evident for a number of months.

Perhaps the most well known adaptation to cardiovascular exercise in apparently healthy adults is an increase in the $\dot{V}O_2max$, expressed in milliliters of oxygen per kilogram per minute. Assuming there are no orthopedic or cardiovascular limitations, the $\dot{V}O_2max$ may increase in healthy adults as much as 20–30% in 6 months of an aerobic conditioning program if one starts in a deconditioned state.

Perhaps the most useful benefit of endurance exercise, however, is an improvement in work capacity. Work capacity most certainly in part is related to $\dot{V}O_2max$, but probably relates more to the efficiency of submaximal oxygen utilization. It is clear that a number of other factors, which are outlined in subsequent paragraphs, are also involved. These increases in maximal and submaximal work capacity undoubtedly account for much of the increase in energy, vigor and stamina that are reported by those who exercise regularly.

Coronary Risk Factors

Much evidence has now been accumulated that demonstrates a favorable change in a number of coronary risk factors in response to a regular exercise program. Regular cardiovascular exercise will increase HDL cholesterol. Some early changes in HDL may occur in 3 months, but Williams et al. (24) have reported that it takes at least 9 months to significantly raise HDL cholesterol with exercise. It appears that the increase in HDL cholesterol is a result of less catabolism of HDL rather than more production. It also appears that much of the increase in HDL cholesterol that occurs in association with exercise is a result of an increase in the HDL_2 fraction, which appears to be the fraction primarily associated with the protective effect in heart disease. The increase in HDL cholesterol with habitual high-level aerobic exercise is more prominent in men than in women. Whether or not the increase in HDL cholesterol that accompanies increased aerobic activity brings with it a reduction in subsequent coronary events has not as yet been firmly established though some evidence has begun to appear.

In addition to the beneficial increase in HDL cholesterol, there are now both cross-sectional and longitudinal data documenting a lowering of serum triglycerides, a lowering of total cholesterol/HDL ratio, and a decrease in systolic and diastolic blood pressure in response to regular exercise (25–27). The drop in blood pressure is modest, especially in those who are normotensive to begin with. In individuals who have elevated blood pressures, the drop in systolic and diastolic blood pressure will likely be more significant. These changes in blood pressure may occur with as little as 3 to 6 months of a conditioning program.

Recent evidence has been published that fitness also confers relative protection against the future development of hypertension (28).

There is some evidence that exercise through some as yet unknown mechanism may help those who smoke to quit. Evidence for this association is still inconclusive, however.

Changes in coronary risk factors are presumably at least part of the reason for the decreased incidence of coronary disease in those who exercise. Other evidence has been accumulated that exercise reduces coronary disease risk independent of changes in risk factors (29).

Endurance training and musculoskeletal training both result in a decrease in percent body fat. Exercise burns calories acutely, of course, but also may result in some extended increase in the resting metabolic rate. Those who combine exercise with calorie restriction preserve lean body mass and preferentially lose adipose tissue. With the myriad of health problems associated with being overweight, the long-term effect of regular exercise in lowering body weight and percent body fat has far-reaching significance.

Changes in the Circulatory System

Perhaps the most easily measured adaptation of the circulatory system itself to chronic exercise is a drop in the resting heart rate. It is not unusual for an endurance-trained 50-year-old to have a heart rate in the 40s. It is very common for 60- to 69-year-olds to have heart rates of 50 beats per minute. There is, of course, some genetic influence in how low the resting heart rate goes in response to conditioning.

As the resting heart rate drops, stroke volume increases and thus cardiac output is maintained. In addition to the increase in stroke volume, other changes in the heart itself have been documented in response to regular physical conditioning. There is good evidence that chronic exercise increases left ventricular end-diastolic volume (30). There is less evidence to suggest an increase in left ventricular wall thickness in response to exercise but it does seem that some increase in wall thickness does occur in those who participate extensively in aerobic exercise over long periods of time (31). Increases in wall thickness are more likely to occur, and increases that occur are more likely to be significant, in individuals who engage in heavy musculoskeletal exercise such as weightlifting for long periods of time.

The increases in ventricular diameter and end-diastolic volume are significant when compared with controls, but still are rarely outside normal limits. Even in highly conditioned, world-class endurance athletes, measurements are almost never in the range to be confused with pathologic dilation or hypertrophy (30). In lean, highly conditioned athletes, voltage on scaler ECG recordings may be very large indeed, but this seems to be more a function of leanness than conditioning, and the large voltages are not generally mirrored by abnormal echocardiographic measurements of wall thickness or chamber size (30). Competitive weight lifters may increase wall thickness beyond normal limits, but again the abnormalities generally are slight.

It does not appear that the increase in end-diastolic volume, which occurs in highly conditioned athletes, has any harmful physiologic effect. It is less clear whether or not the increase in wall thickness that occurs in such athletes as weight lifters may have adverse effects over time.

There is some evidence in animals that vigorous cardiovascular exercise may increase the lumen size of coronary arteries (32). This may have important implications in evaluating the role of exercise in the prevention and treatment of coronary disease.

Other Chronic Effects of Exercise

Other central and peripheral changes reported to occur in response to long-term exercise are as follows:

1. A decrease in myocardial catecholamine concentrations. This could raise the threshold to ventricular fibrillation.
2. A greater total blood volume (both plasma and red cells).
3. An increased number of capillaries per skeletal muscle cell.
4. An increase in vital capacity.
5. An increase in lung ventilation and lung diffusion capacity.
6. An increase in the anaerobic threshold allowing one to exercise for a longer period of time and at higher intensity before there is significant lactic acid buildup.
7. An increase in blood flow to the working muscle with constriction of blood flow to those areas that are inactive (e.g., abdominal organs).
8. An increased ability to supply blood flow to the skin for cooling.
9. Partial heat acclimatization even when exercise is not performed in hot climates. Sweat increases in amount, starts faster, and contains less salt.
10. An increase in the concentration of some oxidative enzymes.
11. An increase in muscle glycogen stores.
12. An increased release of free fatty acids.
13. An increased ability to metabolize fat for energy by exercising muscle.

14. An increase in the number of slow-twitch muscle fibers.
15. An increase in the number of mitochondria in individual skeletal muscle cells.
16. A more efficient oxygen extraction from blood at the tissues.
17. An increased strength of bones, ligaments, and tendons, with an increase in the cartilage thickness in certain joints.
18. An increase in insulin sensitivity and glucose tolerance.
19. A decrease in recovery heart rate.

Psychological Changes

Via mechanisms that have not as yet been fully elucidated, there is evidence that chronic exercise training decreases levels of anxiety and tension in individuals who participate consistently (33). Exercise has been used effectively in treating anxiety states and mild-to-moderate depression (34). Whether or not these changes occur as a result of biochemical alterations in the central nervous system or simply as a result of the increase in confidence and self-esteem as fitness improves, is unclear.

There is some evidence that regular exercise can help individuals deal with stress and stressful events in their lives. It is clear that an increase in self-esteem occurs in those who exercise. There is also some evidence that exercise can be helpful in altering Type A behavior patterns. Whether or not the reduction in Type A behavior has any effect in reducing any "Type A"-associated risk of coronary disease is not clear.

There is also some evidence that exercise may help extend the period of useful living in the elderly. Dr. Roy Shephard estimates that at least 15–16 ml/kg of oxygen consumption may be necessary to sustain independent living (35). By maintaining this level of $\dot{V}O_2max$ through regular cardiovascular exercise training, he estimates that training may extend the period of independent living as long as 8–14 years (35).

Paffenbarger has recently reported evidence that for the first time suggests that exercise may also extend the quantity of years and not simply the quality (36).

And finally, in a field in which only preliminary investigation has been completed, there are reports that chronic exercise may stimulate immunologic resistance to infection (37).

PRECAUTIONS, LIMITATIONS, AND PROBLEMS

Musculoskeletal Injuries

Exercise in healthy adults is, on the whole, quite safe. Minor injuries in adults who begin exercise programs are not uncommon, but serious injuries are rare. The most common sites of musculoskeletal injury in adult runners age 30–60 are listed in order as follows: knee, foot, ankle, lower leg, shin, upper leg, back, and hip. In separate studies reported by Koplan and Blair, self-reported injury rates were as high as 24% to 37% per year in middle-aged runners completing 10–25 miles per week (38–39). If the definition of injury is restricted to a problem that leads to a physician visit, the rates are, of course, much lower. Using this definition of injury, even the most common site of injury (knee) had injury rates below 2% per year in a study recently reported in a large group of middle-aged male runners (39). One interesting finding in this latter data is that nonrunners also reported a reasonably high level of musculoskeletal injuries each year. It seems clear, thus, that studies that do not include a control group may attribute spuriously high rates of injury to the exercise.

Aerobic dance injuries have been reported at very high levels in some studies. Richie and associates reported injury rates of 76% for instructors and 43% for students in an 18-month study (40). The definition of injury in this study, however, seems unduly broad. When the definition is clarified as causing one to stop dancing, rates in aerobic dancing were reported at 10–20% per year. Injury rates for walking are very low as are rates in swimming and stationary cycling. Outdoor bicycling, however, is much more dangerous. There is a considerable risk of accidental collision with automobiles or other bicycles. Slippery pavement, objects in the road, or potholes may cause a fall with serious consequences. Dogs are a hazard not peculiar to bicycling alone but seem to be a special problem to bicyclers. It is essential to wear a sturdy helmet and to have a rear view mirror. Because of these and other hazards of outdoor bicycling, stationary cycling has some obvious advantages in safety. Injury rates are lower in bicyclers than in runners but the potential for disabling or life-threatening injury is much higher in those who bicycle.

Not surprisingly, there are data documenting an increased incidence of exercise injury with an increase in exercise frequency. Pollock, for example, found that a 5-day per week training program versus a 3-day per week program in beginning runners led to injury rates of 39% versus 12%, respectively (41). As expected, there is also considerable data showing an increase in injury rates as total mileage increases. Pollock, again, reported an increase in the injury rate from 22% to 54% in his beginning runners if the running time was increased from 15 to 45 minutes (41). Surprisingly, there are at this time no good data to support an association of running injury with age, gender, years of running, speed, stretching, terrain, surface, or time of day, though it seems logical that such factors have an effect.

A great deal of concern has arisen over the potential of long-term weight-bearing exercise, especially running, to damage joints in the lower extremities. This concern has been allayed in part by two recent studies that failed to show any significant association between long-distance running and an increase in the incidence of degenerative joint disease (42, 43).

Marathon running may provide significant psychological and personal rewards but, in the author's opinion, the medical disadvantages of marathon running (i.e., the risk of musculoskeletal injury) outweigh the medical advantages.

Precautions

Despite the absence of data, clinical experience and common sense suggest the following precautions:

1. In any weight-bearing exercise, obtaining shoes with proper support is essential. With running, the foot carries 2–3 times the body weight as it hits the ground. If a person runs 30 miles per week, there are one million foot-strikes per year. It does not make sense to wear shoes that are not designed for the particular activity in which one is participating.
2. It appears that a gradual warm-up will reduce the incidence of injury. It seems logical that stretching also should decrease the incidence of exercise injury. Several minutes of slow aerobic activity is the best warm-up. Flexibility exercises should not be engaged in before the muscles are warm. It seems most sensible to stretch immediately after this slow aerobic warm-up prior to the more vigorous cardiovascular phase or, just after the cool-down, or both.
3. Concrete is much harder than asphalt. A smooth dirt track or cinder track is probably the best surface for running, but a smooth asphalt running surface is not bad. Grass, because it is usually uneven and may hide small holes or other uneven areas, is not an ideal running surface unless one has a well-groomed area. The ideal surface for aerobic dancing is a hardwood floor suspended on an absorbent material.
4. It also seems sensible and fits with clinical experience that sudden increases in mileage or speed or other abrupt changes in an exercise routine are dangerous and may cause injury. Although there are no well designed studies to test this hypothesis, many experts believe that most training injuries occur because of high mileage, high intensity, or too rapid changes in mileage or intensity.
5. Beginning runners seem to be more prone to musculoskeletal injury than seasoned runners at similar mileage.
6. Running style can be important. One should run with neck and arms as loose and free-moving as possible. It is also best to run flat-footed or with a heel-to-toe movement. One should never run long distances on the balls of one's feet.
7. Heat-related injuries are a significant

risk. Once one begins vigorous exercise, it is almost impossible to keep up with the loss of fluid. Guidelines on fluid replacement have been outlined previously in this chapter. Those most susceptible to heat injury are the young and the elderly, the obese, those on drugs, those with a past history of heat problems, and those who are unacclimatized. It is best to wear light loose clothing that allows air circulation. It is also advisable to allow two weeks to become acclimatized to exercising in hot weather regardless of the individual's initial level of conditioning. Plastic sweat suits should be strictly avoided. Plain water is probably the best replacement fluid. Hypertonic beverages containing salt should be avoided. Salt tablets should never be used.

8. Competition should be avoided in the early weeks of any exercise program. Competition may stimulate an inappropriately high intensity level.
9. Running and walking surfaces should not only be smooth and soft, but level from side to side. Running on the slant may produce knee or foot problems. When using a banked indoor track, the running direction should be alternated from day to day to help reduce this possibility.
10. It is important to stay alert during vigorous exercise. Nieman summarizes this principle as follows: "Personal safety during running and cycling involves several principles. Run on the left side of the road facing traffic. Avoid high traffic areas and run defensively. Obey pedestrian laws. Try to avoid running at night. Know your route well. Avoid all provocation. Try to always run with a partner. Cyclers should obey all traffic laws and ride defensively, keeping right with the flow of traffic." (44)
11. There is some evidence suggesting that exercise in the inner city environment may increase the blood levels of carboxyhemoglobin. In a study done by Nicholson and Case reported in March 1983, there was a significant increase in carboxyhemoglobin in subjects running one-half hour along a busy highway (45). These levels were transiently the same as those sometimes found in chronic cigarette smokers. Standing in the same area, however, produced similar increases in carboxyhemoglobin. It appears living in automobile-infested urban areas is the major hazard rather than exercising in those environments. Even so, it seems prudent to avoid busy roadways when exercising out of doors.

Cardiovascular Risks

Serious cardiovascular complications in association with vigorous exercise are very rare. Vander and associates (46) have reported in a large survey that adults participating in recreational physical activity experience one nonfatal cardiac event for every 1,124,400 hours of activity, and one fatal event for every 887,526 hours. In data compiled at The Aerobics Center in Dallas, Texas, there have been three cardiac events, including one death, in more than 5,000,000 miles of running and walking and a total of 1,250,000 hours of vigorous activity in middle-aged adults (Gibbons, LW: unpublished data).

Individuals who die or who have serious cardiovascular complications in association with vigorous exercise almost invariably have coronary disease or other significant cardiovascular disease. Those without disease simply do not have cardiovascular problems as a result of vigorous exercise. Because of the increased demands exercise puts on the cardiovascular system, it does increase the risk of a cardiac event transiently. However, exercise seems to be the trigger for the event, not the underlying cause.

Here are the factors that appear to affect exercise safety:

1. Any risk factor associated with coronary disease (i.e., high cholesterol, high blood pressure, etc.).
2. Age.
3. Smoking.
4. Frequency of exercise. In those who ex-

ercise irregularly, the benefits of exercise in protecting against coronary disease appear to be outweighed by the transient increase in risk during the exercise session itself (47).

5. Competition in those unprepared for the increase in intensity.
6. Heat.
7. Improper cool-down. Dimsdale and associates (48) reported a tenfold increase in norepinephrine levels during the early recovery period in individuals who stopped exercise suddenly rather than cooling down gradually. Their report suggests that the worst possible strategy for exercise cessation would be to have the patient abruptly stop exercising and stand. The best strategy would be for the workload to be diminished gradually.

Other Risks

Another less commonly known and more poorly documented risk of vigorous exercise is negative addiction. In individuals who become addicted to vigorous exercise, the activity becomes so compelling that the individual exercises to excess and the exercise itself may begin to detract from life rather than add to it. A hard-core exercise addict must run daily, manifests withdrawal symptoms if deprived of exercise, and runs even when his physician says he shouldn't, according to Dr. Bill Morgan (49). These individuals feel guilty if they do not run and have a constant urge to increase mileage and pace. The time commitment for these expanding exercise sessions becomes a significant problem, and these are often individuals who experience injury after injury, which they refuse to let heal properly before returning to their vigorous exercise regimen.

SUMMARY

Even in asymptomatic adults, exercise testing can aid in identifying coronary atherosclerosis before it causes symptoms. In addition, exercise testing is useful in assessing cardiovascular fitness and can help establish the safety of vigorous exercise prior to starting an exercise program.

It is helpful to conduct a limited medical evaluation including a medical history and a brief cardiovascular examination prior to giving an exercise prescription. An exercise test can only be interpreted properly when one knows the clinical background of a given patient. Knowing this pretest likelihood of disease is essential in interpreting the results of the exercise tolerance test. The significance of an abnormal test is directly related to the prevalence of disease in the population being tested.

A percentage of the abnormal test results in asymptomatic individuals will be false-positive. Using all available clinical information and all information that can be obtained from the exercise test itself, it is generally possible to identify those individuals in whom further diagnostic testing should be carried out. In only a small percentage of asymptomatic patients who are found to have an abnormal exercise tolerance test is coronary angiography necessary. Characteristics of the ST-segment depression itself, such as time of occurrence, slope, and depth of depression, as well as maximal heart rate achieved during the test and functional capacity, can be of great help in assessing the significance of an abnormal test in an asymptomatic individual.

There is benefit to be derived from testing muscle strength and flexibility in addition to cardiovascular fitness, if sufficient time and resources are available.

It is important to give specific rather than general exercise prescriptions. A prescribed exercise must be both pleasant and practical if it is to be followed consistently. Walking, stationary cycling, and running are three of the most practical types of exercise for adults. It appears from recent research that even low-level physical activity may provide considerable benefit.

Evidence is now substantial that consistent cardiovascular exercise beneficially affects a number of important coronary risk factors. There is now cross-sectional and longitudinal evidence that exercise raises HDL cholesterol, lowers the total cholesterol/HDL ratio, lowers triglycerides, and lowers both systolic and diastolic blood pressure. There is also epidemiologic evidence that cardiovascular exercise will help protect against the future development of high blood pressure.

Exercise causes significant changes in the circulatory system and in other parts of the body. Stroke volume is increased and resting heart rate is decreased. There is an increase in left ventricular volume and wall thickness, though these changes are minor and are unlikely to be outside normal limits except in those who exercise for long periods of time over many years.

Several peripheral adaptations also occur as part of the body's chronic response to exercise, including an increased number of capillaries per muscle cell, an increase in the concentration of certain oxidative enzymes in the mitochondria, more efficient oxygen extraction from tissues, an increase in insulin sensitivity and glucose tolerance, and an increased ability to metabolize fat for energy.

A regular exercise program may help extend the period of useful living in the elderly. It is possible that regular exercise may extend the period of independent living as long as 8–14 years.

Minor musculoskeletal injuries are common as a result of a vigorous exercise program in adults. One must be careful, however, not to attribute all musculoskeletal problems to the exercise itself. Musculoskeletal injuries also occur in nonexercising adults.

It appears that an increase in the mileage and an increase in frequency of exercise are both significantly related to the risk of injury. There are no convincing data to support an association of running injury with age, gender, years of running, speed, stretching, terrain, surface, or time of day. Much more research is needed to confirm risk factors for exercise injuries.

One of the greatest dangers inherent in vigorous exercise is heat injury. Appropriate fluid replacement is essential, especially when exercising in hot weather, high humidity, or both. Generally, with special regard to fluid replacement, heat-related injuries are preventable.

Serious cardiovascular complications in association with vigorous exercise are extremely rare. Those who die or have cardiac complications in association with vigorous exercise are almost always those with preexisting significant heart disease. Factors that appear to affect exercise safety include the presence of any coronary risk factor, frequency of exercise, competition, heat, and improper cool-down.

REFERENCES

1. American College of Sports Medicine: *Guidelines for Exercise Testing and Prescription*, ed 3. Philadelphia, Lea & Febiger, 1986, p 2.
2. Harper RW, Kennedy G, DeSanctis RW, et al: The incidence and pattern of angina prior to acute myocardial infarction: a study of 577 cases. *Am Heart J* 97:178–183, 1979.
3. Lown B: Sudden cardiac death: the major challenge confronting contemporary cardiology. *Am J Cardiol* 43:318–328, 1979.
4. Giagnoni E, Secchi MB, Wu SC, et al: Prognostic value of exercise EKG testing in asymptomatic normotensive subjects. *N Engl J Med* 309:1085–1089, 1983.
5. Ellestad M: *Stress Testing*, ed 3. Philadelphia, F.A. Davis Company, 1986, p 316.
6. Bruce RA, DeRouen TA, Hossack KF: The value of maximal exercise tests in risk assessment of primary coronary heart disease events in healthy men. *Am J Cardiol* 46:371–378, 1980.
7. Froelicher VF: *Exercise Testing and Training*, New York, Le Jacq, 1983, p 83.
8. Epstein SE: Implications of probability analysis on the strategy used for noninvasive detection of coronary artery disease. *Am J Cardiol* 46:491–499, 1980.
9. Okin PM, Kligfield P, Ameisen O, et al: Improved accuracy of the exercise electrocardiogram: identification of three vessel coronary disease in stable angina pectoris by analysis of peak rate-related changes in ST-segments. *Am J Cardiol* 55:271–276, 1985.
10. Hollenberg M, Zoltick JM, Go M, et al: Comparison of a quantitative treadmill exercise score with standard electrocardiographic criteria in screening asymptomatic young men for coronary heart disease. *N Engl J Med* 313:600–606, 1985.
11. Ellestad M: *Stress Testing*, ed 3. Philadelphia, F.A. Davis Company, 1986, p 340.
12. Ellestad M: *Stress Testing*, ed 3. Philadelphia, F.A. Davis Company, 1986, p 124.
13. Nieman DC: *The Sports Medicine Fitness Course*, Palo Alto, Bull, 1986, p 366.
14. Nieman DC: *The Sports Medicine Fitness Course*, Palo Alto, Bull, 1986, p 369.
15. Nieman DC: *The Sports Medicine Fitness Course*, Palo Alto, Bull, 1986, p 122.

16. Nieman DC: *The Sports Medicine Fitness Course*, Palo Alto, Bull, 1986, p 122.
17. Nieman DC: *The Sports Medicine Fitness Course*, Palo Alto, Bull, 1986, p 368.
18. Cooper KH: *Aerobics Program for Total Well-Being*, Toronto, Bantam Books, 1982, p 119.
19. Cooper KH: *Running Without Fear*, New York, M. Evans, 1985, p 113.
20. Paffenbarger RS, Hyde RT, Wing AL, et al: The natural history of athleticism and cardiovascular health. *JAMA* 252:491–495, 1984.
21. Gaesser GA, Rich RG: Effects of high and low intensity exercise training on aerobic capacity and blood lipids. *Med Sci Sports Exerc* 16:269–274, 1984.
22. Pamphlet, *Fitness 3*, Roach Drug Company, P.O. Box 203, Wood Ridge, NJ.
23. Cooper KH: *Aerobics*, New York, Bantam Books, 1968, p 145.
24. Williams PT, Wood PD, Haskell WL, et al: The effects of running mileage and duration on plasma lipoprotein levels. *JAMA* 247:2674–2678, 1982.
25. Cooper KH, Pollock ML, Martin RP, et al: Physical fitness level versus selected coronary risk factors. *JAMA* 236:166–169, 1976.
26. Gibbons LW, Blair SN, Cooper KH, et al: Association between coronary heart disease risk factors and physical fitness in healthy adult women. *Circulation* 67:977–983, 1983.
27. Blair SN, Cooper KH, Gibbons LW, et al: Changes in coronary heart disease risk factors associated with increased treadmill time in 753 men. *Am J Epidemiol* 118:352–359, 1983.
28. Blair SN, Goodyear N, Gibbons LW, et al: Physical fitness and incidence of hypertension in healthy normotensive men and women. *JAMA* 252:487–490, 1984.
29. Paffenbarger RS, Wing AL, Hyde RT: Physical activity as an index of heart attack risk in college alumni. *Am J Epidemiol* 108:161–175, 1978.
30. Gibbons LW, Cooper KH, Martin RP, et al: Medical examination and electrocardiographic analysis of elite distance runners. *Ann NY Acad Sci* 301:283–296, 1977.
31. Landry F, Bouchard C, Dumesnil J: Cardiac dimension changes with endurance training. *JAMA* 254:77–83, 1985.
32. Kramsch DM, Aspen AJ, Abramowitz A, et al: Reduction of coronary atherosclerosis by moderate conditioning exercise in monkeys on an atherogenic diet. *N Engl J Med* 305:1484–1489, 1981.
33. Buffone GW: Running and depression. In Sachs ML, Buffone GW (eds): *Running as Therapy*. Lincoln, NB, and London, University of Nebraska Press, 1984, p 6.
34. Burger BG: Running away from anxiety and depression: a female as well as male race. In Sachs ML, Buffone GW (eds): *Running as Therapy*. Lincoln, NB, and London, University of Nebraska Press, 1984, p 138.
35. Shephard RJ: Physical training for the elderly. *Clin Sports Med* 5:515–533, 1986.
36. Paffenbarger RS, Hyde RT, Wing AL, et al: Physical activity, all cause mortality, and longevity of college alumni. *N Engl J Med* 314:605–613, 1986.
37. Simon H: Immunology of exercise. *JAMA* 252:2735–2738, 1984.
38. Koplan JP, Powell KW, Sikes RK: An epidemiologic study of the benefits and risks of running. *JAMA* 248:3118–3121, 1982.
39. Blair SN, Kohl HW, Goodyear N: Rates and risks for running and exercise injury. *Research Quarterly For Exercise and Sports* 58:221–228, 1987.
40. Richie DH, Kelso SF, Bellucci PA: Aerobic dance injuries: a retrospective study of instructors and participants. *Phys Sportsmed* 13:130–140, 1985.
41. Pollock ML, Gettman LR, Milesis CA, et al: Effects of frequency and duration of training on attrition and incidence of injury. *Med Sci Sports Exerc* 9:31–36, 1977.
42. Panush RS, Schmidt C, Caldwell JR, et al: Is running associated with degenerative joint disease? *JAMA* 255:1152–1154, 1986.
43. Lane NE, Bloch DA, Jones HH, et al: Long distance running, bone density, and osteoarthritis. *JAMA* 255:1147–1151, 1986.
44. Nieman DC: *The Sports Medicine Fitness Course*. Palo Alto, Bull, 1986, p 231.
45. Nicholson JP, Case DV: Carboxyhemoglobin levels in New York City runners. *Phys Sportsmed* 11:135–138, 1983.
46. Vander L, Franklin B, Rubenfire M: Cardiovascular complications of recreational physical activity. *Phys Sportsmed* 10:89–98, 1982.
47. Siscovick DS, Weiss NS, Fletcher RH, et al: The incidence of primary cardiac arrest during vigorous exercise. *N Engl J Med* 311:874–877, 1984.
48. Dimsdale JE, Hartley H, Guiney T, et al: Post exercise peril. *JAMA* 251:630–632, 1984.
49. Morgan WP: Negative addiction in runners. *Phys Sportsmed* 7:57–70, 1979.

CHAPTER 3

Cardiac Patients

Barry A. Franklin, Ph.D.
Herman K. Hellerstein, M.D.
Seymour Gordon, M.D.
Gerald C. Timmis, M.D.

Exercise testing of the cardiac patient provides quantitation of cardiorespiratory function, from the initial manifestations of the acute event (via predischarge exercise testing) to convalescence and recovery (1). Exercise tests have immediate value in assessing functional capacity and the safety of physical exertion as well as long-term prognostic significance in regard to morbidity and mortality. In addition, the results may be used to determine the effects of interventions such as coronary artery bypass surgery, percutaneous transluminal coronary angioplasty, medications, or physical conditioning.

The objective of exercise tests is to evaluate quantitatively the following variables: aerobic capacity of the body, that is, the peak or maximal oxygen uptake ($\dot{V}O_2max$); hemodynamics, assessed by the heart rate and systolic/diastolic blood pressure responses; limiting clinical signs or symptoms (e.g., angina pectoris); and associated changes in electrical functions of the heart, especially supraventricular and ventricular arrhythmias and ST-segment displacement (2).

Clinical variables that should be monitored include blood pressure (cuff method), heart rate, and multiple lead electrocardiograms, which increase sensitivity but may reduce specificity. Although the monitoring of 12 or more leads is recommended by some clinicians, we have found that recording three leads is adequate for most clinical situations and favor the precordial leads V_1 or V_2, V_5 or CM_5, and aVF—an approximate orthogonal lead system, equivalent to Z, X, and Y vector leads, respectively. However, a single lead (V_5 or CM_5) will reveal ST-segment depression in about 80% of all instances that have been detected with a multiple lead system (3). Other informative variables include perceived exertion ratings (4), ventricular systolic time intervals, and the direct measurement of expired gases for submaximal and maximal oxygen uptake and anaerobic threshold determinations.

Informed consent prior to the test, safety precautions, trained personnel, a defibrillator and emergency equipment are essential prerequisites when evaluating the cardiac patient.

CONVENTIONAL EXERCISE TESTING OF THE LOWER EXTREMITIES

Standard lower extremity exercise tests, employing either the treadmill or cycle ergometer, have the advantage of reproducibility and quantitation of physiologic responses to known external workloads.

Treadmill Testing Versus Leg Cycle Ergometry

Both treadmill exercise and cycle ergometry have advantages and disadvantages in evaluating patients with heart disease. The cycle ergometer has the advantage of requiring less space, making less noise, and generally costing less than the treadmill. It also minimizes movement of the thorax and arms, which facilitates better quality electrocardiographic (ECG) recordings and blood pressure measurements (5). In addition, body weight does not significantly affect absolute aerobic requirements (i.e., $l \cdot min^{-1}$) and caloric expenditure at a given power output (6). Its main disadvantage is that it is an unfamiliar method of exercise for many Americans, often resulting in limiting localized muscle fatigue (7). Treadmill testing, on the other hand, provides a more common form of physiologic stress (i.e., walking) in which subjects are more likely to attain a slightly higher $\dot{V}O_2max$ and peak heart rate.

Despite the potential of treadmill exercise to elicit a higher $\dot{V}O_2max$ and peak heart rate than cycle ergometry, it remains unclear whether there is a clinically significant difference between the two modalities in evoking ischemic signs or symptoms. Ford and associates (8) found that chest pain and ischemic ST-segment depression occur less frequently with cycle ergometer exercise than with treadmill exercise despite a significantly higher rate-pressure product with the former. However, Wicks and coworkers (9) reported a close relationship between the magnitude of ST-segment changes induced by maximal exercise testing with treadmill and cycle ergometry in postmyocardial infarction patients. Foster et al. (10) demonstrated a consistent relationship between aerobic capacity on the treadmill and cycle ergometer and have suggested a method for predicting treadmill aerobic capacity (METs; 1 MET = 3.5 $ml \cdot kg^{-1} \cdot min^{-1}$) from cycle ergometer functional capacity using the following equation: Treadmill METs = 0.98 (cycle ergometer METs) + 1.85.

Methods and Protocols

Figure 3.1 shows several commonly used multistage treadmill and cycle ergometer exercise protocols (2). Exercise stages are progressive in intensity, and the duration at each stage, 2 or more minutes, insures that most cardiorespiratory variables reach a relatively constant or "steady-state" value. The major differences among protocols involve the magnitudes of the increments in aerobic requirements for each stage and the methods by which they are produced. The latter include increases in speed or grade, or both, in treadmill testing, and increases in external load (kilograms) and/or pedaling speed in cycle ergometer testing.

The conventional Bruce test (11) is perhaps the most familiar and widely employed because it offers a rapid and safe exercise progression for which normative values for heart rate, blood pressure, and oxygen uptake have been established. The protocol, however, has several limitations. The initial workload (stage I), corresponding to 1.7 $mi \cdot h^{-1}$, 10% grade, has an aerobic requirement of 4 to 5 METs, equivalent to an oxygen uptake of 14.0–17.5 $ml \cdot kg^{-1} \cdot min^{-1}$, which exceeds the aerobic capacity of many cardiac patients. Since the workload progression requires simultaneous increases in both speed and grade, it is sometimes difficult for patients to adapt to the large work increments between stages, typically 2.5–3.0 METs. Consequently, patients often fail to attain a leveling off or plateauing of physiologic responses, and delineation of the precise MET level at the ischemic or anginal threshold is therefore difficult. In addition, the Bruce protocol is a walk-jog test with a variable transition point from walking to jogging at stage IV (9th to 12th minute), resulting in a variety of mechanical efficiencies at this stage with varying oxygen costs. Finally, the ECG may be distorted by artifact caused by muscle movement and foot impact during jogging.

Consideration of these limitations, particularly in deconditioned patients, has resulted in the development of a "modified" Bruce protocol consisting of one or two preliminary 3-minute stages at 1.7 $mi \cdot h^{-1}$, 0% grade, and/or 1.7 $mi \cdot h^{-1}$, 5% grade. A recent comparison of the Naughton and modified Bruce treadmill protocols (Fig. 3.1) for postmyocardial infarction exercise testing revealed no significant differences in maximum heart rate, rate-pressure product, or workload achieved (12). Although the Naughton protocol resulted in a significantly longer mean maximal exercise duration, 17.3 ± 5.0 versus 14.8 ± 2.8 minutes, the protocols were equally effective in detecting ischemic responses 6 weeks after myocardial infarction.

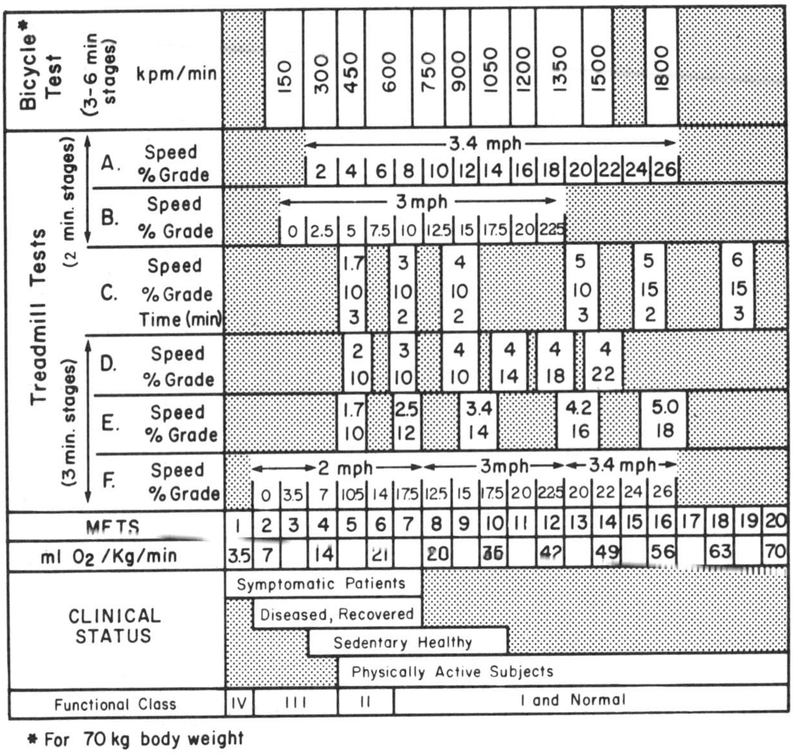

Bicycle Test* (3–6 min stages)	kpm/min	150, 300, 450, 600, 750, 900, 1050, 1200, 1350, 1500, 1800
Treadmill Tests (2 min. stages) A.	Speed	3.4 mph
	% Grade	2, 4, 6, 8, 10, 12, 14, 16, 18, 20, 22, 24, 26
B.	Speed	3 mph
	% Grade	0, 2.5, 5, 7.5, 10, 12.5, 15, 17.5, 20, 22.5
C.	Speed	1.7, 3, 4, 5, 5, 6
	% Grade	10, 10, 10, 10, 15, 15
	Time (min)	3, 2, 2, 3, 2, 3
Treadmill Tests (3 min. stages) D.	Speed	2, 3, 4, 4, 4, 4
	% Grade	10, 10, 10, 14, 18, 22
E.	Speed	1.7, 2.5, 3.4, 4.2, 5.0
	% Grade	10, 12, 14, 16, 18
F.	Speed	2 mph; 3 mph; 3.4 mph
	% Grade	0, 3.5, 7, 10.5, 14, 17.5 (2 mph); 12.5, 15, 17.5, 20, 22.5 (3 mph); 20, 22, 24, 26 (3.4 mph)
METS		1, 2, 3, 4, 5, 6, 7, 8, 9, 10, 11, 12, 13, 14, 15, 16, 17, 18, 19, 20
ml O_2/Kg/min		3.5, 7, 14, 21, 20, 36, 42, 49, 56, 63, 70
CLINICAL STATUS		Symptomatic Patients; Diseased, Recovered; Sedentary Healthy; Physically Active Subjects
Functional Class		IV, III, II, I and Normal

* For 70 kg body weight

Figure 3.1. Estimated oxygen and MET requirements of commonly used treadmill and cycle ergometer exercise protocols are shown. Methods: A and B, Balke; C, Ellestad; D, Kattus; E, Bruce; F, National Exercise and Heart Disease Project. (From Hellerstein HK, Franklin BA: Exercise testing and prescription. In Wenger NK, Hellerstein HK (eds), *Rehabilitation of the Coronary Patient.* ed 2. New York, John Wiley & Sons, Inc., 1984, p 201. Reproduced by permission.)

Figure 3.2 illustrates a treadmill walking protocol that is useful for both diagnostic exercise testing and for exercise prescription for persons with or without heart disease (13). The protocol, which has been used safely in over 40,000 tests since 1960, offers normative data on oxygen consumption ($\dot{V}O_2$) so that aerobic capacity may be estimated from the workload attained. Since the protocol is limited to walking only, $\dot{V}O_2$ values increase in a linear fashion, rising approximately 1.0 MET per stage from about 4.0 METs at 1.5 mi·h^{-1}, 10% grade, to 9.0 METs at 4.0 mi·h^{-1}, 10% grade. Zohman and associates (13) reported that the maximal walking speed attained at 10% grade on the treadmill, when achieved on level ground, often yields the appropriate target heart rate zone for cardiovascular conditioning, regardless of whether the patient was taking β-blockers.

Aerobic Requirements of Leg Ergometry

Aerobic requirements at a given external workload, expressed as ml·kg^{-1}·min^{-1} or METs, may be estimated from the treadmill speed and percent grade or the cycle ergometer power output (kg·m·min^{-1}), corrected for body weight (Fig. 3.1). It should be emphasized, however, that the cardiac patient's oxygen uptake may be markedly overestimated when it is predicted from exercise time or workload (2). Several explanations have been offered to account for this phenomenon (14). The $\dot{V}O_2$ values presented in Figure 3.1 were obtained from

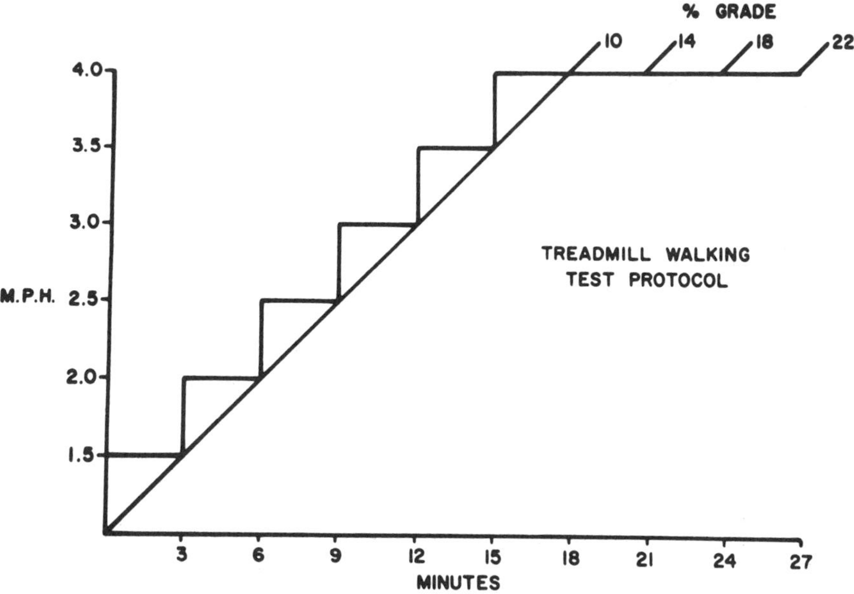

Figure 3.2. Treadmill walking test protocol. M.P.H. = miles per hour, speed of the treadmill; minutes = duration of exercise; % grade = inclination of treadmill. MET level at 10% grade, 1.5 mph = 4.3; 2.0 mph = 5.1; 2.5 mph = 5.9; 3.0 mph = 6.9; 3.5 mph = 8.0; 4.0 mph = 9.4. MET levels then increase to approximately 12, 14 and 15 at 14%, 18%, and 22% grade, respectively. (From Zohman LR, Young JL, Kattus AA: Treadmill walking protocol for the diagnostic evaluation and exercise programming of cardiac patients. *Am J Cardiol* 51:1081–1086, 1983. Reproduced by permission).

healthy young adults and apply only when the subject has achieved steady-state conditions (i.e., completed the stage) without holding the handrails. It has also been suggested that myocardial damage may slow oxygen uptake kinetics, perhaps accounting for the fact that cardiac patients often demonstrate lower submaximal and maximal oxygen uptake values and a larger oxygen debt for standard workloads (2,15). Finally, β-adrenergic blocking medications have been shown to result in a slower adaptation of oxygen consumption to steady-state submaximal workloads (16).

Achievement of Maximal Oxygen Consumption

There is considerable debate concerning the ability of the patient who is limited by angina to exercise maximally, that is, to demonstrate a true physiologic maximal oxygen consumption, because it is argued that the onset of chest pain or discomfort prevents achieving a plateau in $\dot{V}O_2$ at peak exercise. However, Eldridge and associates (17) recently found that many patients with coronary artery disease (CAD) can achieve a plateau in $\dot{V}O_2$ at maximal effort during a continuous treadmill protocol. Eighty percent of patients limited by angina achieved a plateau in $\dot{V}O_2$ over the final 90 seconds of exercise, compared with 77% of normal subjects. These results indicate that symptoms limiting exercise, even angina pectoris, do not influence the ability of many cardiac patients to exercise maximally.

ARM EXERCISE TESTING

Dynamic arm exercise testing provides a reproducible noninvasive method to evaluate cardiovascular function in subjects with neurologic, vascular, or orthopedic impairment of the lower extremities (18). In addition, arm exercise testing appears to be the functional evaluation of choice for persons whose occupational and recreational physical activity is dominated by upper extremity efforts, since leg exercise testing suboptimally predicts arm performance capacity (19–22).

Arm-crank ergometry has been shown to offer a satisfactory, but perhaps not equivalent, alternative to leg exercise testing for the ECG detection of myocardial ischemia or the provocation of angina pectoris, or both. Several investigators have examined the ischemic response to arm versus leg exercise; however, the results are conflicting. Schwade et al. (20) noted no difference in the sensitivity of arm compared with leg exercise in eliciting myocardial ischemia in 33 men with CAD. Similarly, Shaw and associates (23) found no difference in the ischemic response to arm ergometry versus treadmill testing. In contrast, Balady and coworkers (24) recently reported that arm exercise testing was less sensitive than leg exercise in detecting CAD. Of 30 symptomatic patients with angiographically proven CAD, only 12 (40%) developed ST-segment depression or angina during symptom-limited arm ergometry, compared with 26 (86%) during maximal treadmill testing, despite a comparable peak rate-pressure product for both tests.

Equipment: Wheelchair Versus Arm-Crank Ergometers

Equipment suitable for arm exercise testing includes wheelchair or arm-cycle ergometers, the latter either mechanically or electrically braked. Although a comparison of the physiologic responses to wheelchair and arm-cycle ergometry revealed a significantly lower physical work capacity (by 36%) and maximal heart rate (by 7%) for the former, $\dot{V}O_2$ max was comparable for both exercise modes (25). Since both types of ergometry yielded similar $\dot{V}O_2$ max values, it was concluded that clinical exercise testing using arm-cycle ergometry would probably provide a valid estimate of an individual's aerobic potential for wheelchair-type activity.

One commercially available ergometer, the Schwinn Air-Dyne, offers quantified exercise for the arms, using only the arm levers; the legs, using only the pedals; or the upper and lower extremities combined, using the levers and pedals simultaneously. The ergometer wheel, based on a unique air displacement principle, is driven by the pedals, the arm levers, or both. The faster the wheel is turned, the greater the volume and resistance of air moved and the greater the workload performed [range: 150–2100 kg·m·min^{-1} (25–340 watts, W)].

Methods and Protocols

In our studies of cardiac patients, we have modified a conventional leg cycle ergometer (Schwinn Bio-Dyne) for arm cranking. The arm ergometer is mounted on a table at a height of 68 to 70 cm so that the subject can arm crank seated upright with the feet flat on the floor (Fig. 3.3). During cranking, the arms are alternately extended at right angles to the body, allowing for a slight bend at the elbow at maximal reach, analogous to the lower limb extension in leg cycling.

Selection of an initial workload and workload increments per stage must consider the disparity in cardiorespiratory and hemodynamic responses to arm versus leg exercise, as well as the subject's physical status. At a given submaximal workload, arm exercise is performed at a greater physiologic cost than is leg exercise, but maximal responses are generally lower during arm exercise. Therefore, chronotropic and aerobic reserves, relative to incremental loading, are attenuated for arm exercise as compared with leg exercise. In addition, since most cardiac patients are not physically conditioned for sustained upper extremity exercise, there is a tendency for early fatigue. Consequently, low initial work loads and small workload increments per stage should be employed when testing cardiac patients.

A review of progressive multistage arm-cycle ergometer exercise testing protocols for patients with CAD is provided in Table 3.1, with specific reference to initial workload and workload increments per stage, duration of discontinuous or continuous stages, cranking rate, and test end points (18). Exercise stages were 2–3 minutes in duration, and discontinuous protocols typ-

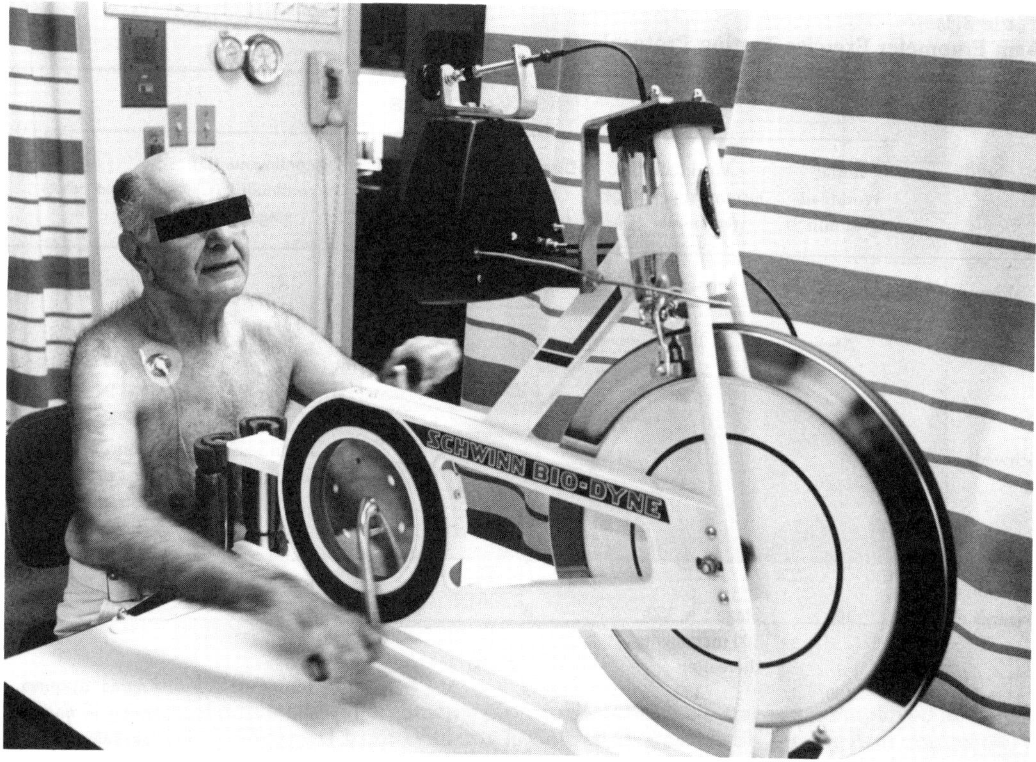

Figure 3.3. The Schwinn Bio-Dyne cycle ergometer as adapted for arm exercise is shown. Bicycle handgrips have been fitted over the pedals, clamps secure the ergometer to a sturdy metal table, and a padded breastplate helps to standardize arm position.

ically allowed 1–2 minutes of rest between stages, during which high quality ECG tracings and blood pressure measurements were obtained (27). The initial workload (warm-up) generally consisted of arm cranking at power outputs of 200 $kg{\cdot}m{\cdot}min^{-1}$ (33 W) or less. Workload increments per stage averaged 100–150 $kg{\cdot}m{\cdot}min^{-1}$, with cranking rates of 40 to 60 revolutions per minute ($rev{\cdot}min^{-1}$). Peak effort was generally defined as the power output at which the subject was no longer able to maintain the designated pedal speed, notwithstanding encouragement, or the workload at which significant clinical signs or symptoms developed.

In contrast to the standard arm exercise testing protocols summarized in Table 3.1, Williams and coworkers (30) designed a unique arm ergometer protocol in which the initial and incremental workloads are individually determined, based on the subject's body weight (Fig. 3.4). The protocol is conceptually analogous to several of the conventional treadmill exercise testing protocols illustrated in Figure 3.1, in that the aerobic requirements at each stage can be quantified in terms of METs, with 1 MET increments per stage.

Aerobic Requirements of Arm Ergometry

Our previous studies (22) showed that the regression of oxygen uptake ($\dot{V}O_2$) on power output during arm ergometry was $y = 3.06\ x + 191$ ($y = \dot{V}O_2$ in $ml{\cdot}min^{-1}$; x = power output in $kg{\cdot}m{\cdot}min^{-1}$), where $r = 0.91$ and $Sy{\cdot}x = 191.6$. Since absolute arm $\dot{V}O_2$ ($ml{\cdot}min^{-1}$) at a given workload demonstrated the least variability between

generally begin with a lower exercise intensity (e.g., ≤ 2.5 METs), proceed with smaller increments of work per stage, and employ reduced peak workloads. Fastidious recording methods, supervision procedures, and safety precautions are essential. The attenuated protocol is designed to simulate and slightly exceed the somatic and myocardial aerobic requirements of activities that will be encountered at home during convalescence. For this reason, early postinfarction tests (3–14 days) typically impose peak workloads of up to 5 METs, equal to a body oxygen uptake of 17.5 $ml \cdot kg^{-1} \cdot min^{-1}$; however, in the absence of signs and symptoms, a test may be carried safely to higher workloads (34, 35).

Whether the predischarge exercise test should be symptom-limited or stopped when an arbitrary "submaximal" heart rate or workload is achieved is still controversial. DeBusk and Haskell (36) compared protocols limited by heart rate or symptoms and found them to be equally safe and effective for eliciting both ischemia and arrhythmias soon after an uncomplicated myocardial infarction. On the other hand, Starling and associates (37) found that the symptom-limited exercise test was superior, yielding a higher frequency of ischemic ST-segment depression or angina without increasing the risk of the test.

Figure 3.5 presents several protocols commonly used for predischarge exercise testing (2). The two most commonly used treadmill protocols are the modified Bruce (38) and Naughton (39), starting at 1.7 $mi \cdot h^{-1}$, 0% grade, and 2.0 $mi \cdot h^{-1}$, 0% grade, respectively. Both tests employ a constant treadmill speed and increase grade or incline every 3 minutes. The cycle ergometer protocol consists of pedaling at 50 or 60 $rev \cdot m^{-1}$ for 3–4 minutes at each of two or three progressive loads, adjusted for body weight to impose peak loads of up to 5 METs.

Guidelines for Stopping the Postinfarction Predischarge Exercise Test

The criteria for discontinuing a predischarge exercise test are often more conservative than those for terminating fatigue-limited or symptom-limited exercise tests. Accordingly, one of three "submaximal" end points may be employed: (a) heart rate; (b) workload; or (c) perceived exertion rating. Such tests are generally terminated once a predetermined heart rate response (usually 70–75% of the age-predicted maximal heart rate, a heart rate of 120–140 $beats \cdot min^{-1}$, or a peak rate ≥ 30 $beats \cdot min^{-1}$ above rest), workload (usually up to 5 METs), or perceived exertion rating (usually "somewhat hard" to "hard") is attained (5, 40). In contrast, tests limited by symptoms or physical signs are stopped because of the development of mild-to-moderate angina, severe dyspnea or fatigue, dizziness, ataxia, 2 mm or more of ischemic ST-segment depression, threatening ventricular arrhythmias (e.g., three or more consecutive PVCs), a fall in the systolic blood pressure of 20 mm Hg or more, or a hypertensive blood pressure response (systolic of 230 mm Hg or more, or diastolic of 110 mm Hg or more) (41). Exercise-induced ST-segment elevation *with angina* may reflect transmural ischemic injury and should also be used as a stopping point (31).

Interpretation of Results

The responses to predischarge exercise testing provide objective information about the patient's functional capacity, need for additional diagnostic studies (angiograms, nuclear studies), and therapeutic strategies (including medications, interventional techniques, or surgery). Delaying discharge from the hospital or retesting after administration of cardiac medications may be indicated for patients who demonstrate significant arrhythmias, ischemic ST-segment depression, or angina.

Certain responses to predischarge exercise testing have been shown to be prognostically useful. *The presence of exercise-induced ST-segment depression appears to be the most reliable prognostic indicator, identifying patients at increased risk for sudden cardiac death and recurrent infarction* (5, 31, 40). Exercise-induced angina pectoris (42), even without concomitant ST-segment depression, is also prognostically valuable, while ventricular arrhythmias, exertional hypo-

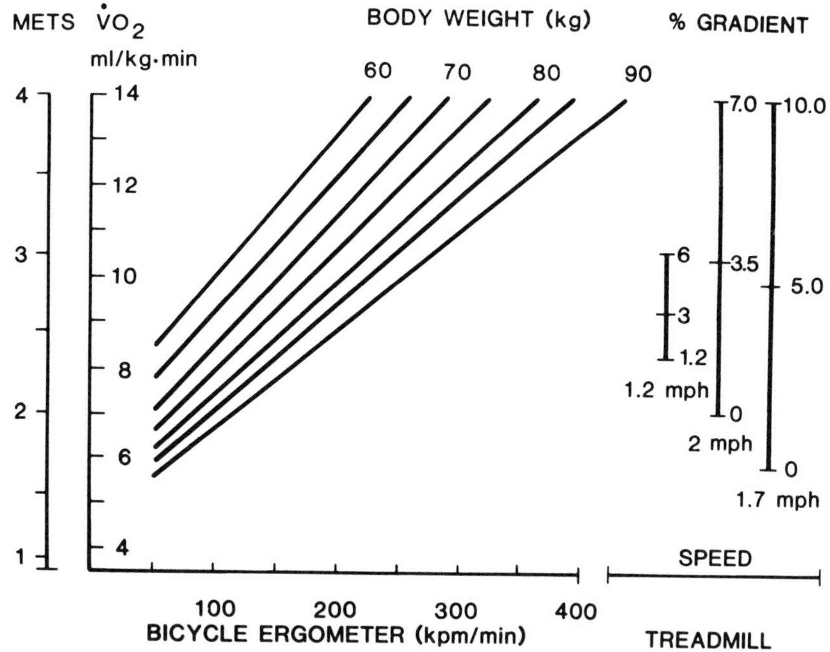

Figure 3.5. Estimated oxygen and MET requirements are shown for four low-level exercise protocols suitable for testing patients with acute myocardial infarction prior to discharge from the hospital. (From Hellerstein HK, Franklin BA: Exercise testing and prescription. In Wenger NK, Hellerstein HK (eds): *Rehabilitation of the Coronary Patient.* ed 2. New York, John Wiley & Sons, Inc. 1984, p 219. Reproduced by permission).

tension (a relatively common response), and poor exercise capacity have been reported as inconsistent predictors of posthospital mortality (43, 44). Precordial ST-segment elevation is associated with anterior myocardial infarction and a decreased left ventricular ejection fraction. As an isolated or independent finding, however, it does not portend a poor prognosis (7).

EXERCISE TESTING FOR RISK STRATIFICATION

Identification of patients soon after myocardial infarction who are at increased risk for subsequent cardiac events offers two major benefits: (a) patients at moderate-to-high risk can be evaluated for more intensive pharmacotherapy, interventional cardiac catheterization, or surgery, and (b) patients at low risk can be spared immediate cardiac catheterization and unwarranted restriction of their vocational and recreational activities (31).

DeBusk and associates (45) emphasized in their risk stratification algorithm (Fig. 3.6) that it is the degree of left ventricular dysfunction and residual resting or exercise-induced myocardial ischemia that determines the risk of future cardiac events. In this algorithm, by 3 weeks after hospitalization, 100 survivors of documented acute myocardial infarction were distributed as follows: 50 patients were in the low-risk group (less than 2% annual mortality) because of an absence of severe resting or exercise-induced myocardial ischemia and of severe left ventricular dysfunction; 30 patients were at moderate-to-high risk (10–25% first-year mortality) because of severe resting or exercise-induced ischemia in the presence of moderate-to-good left ventricular function; and 20 patients were at high risk (> 25% first-year mortality) because of clinically evident severe pump failure or severe left ventricular dysfunction.

Although nearly one-half the patients who will have a reinfarction or die within the year after acute myocardial infarction can be identified on the basis of severe is-

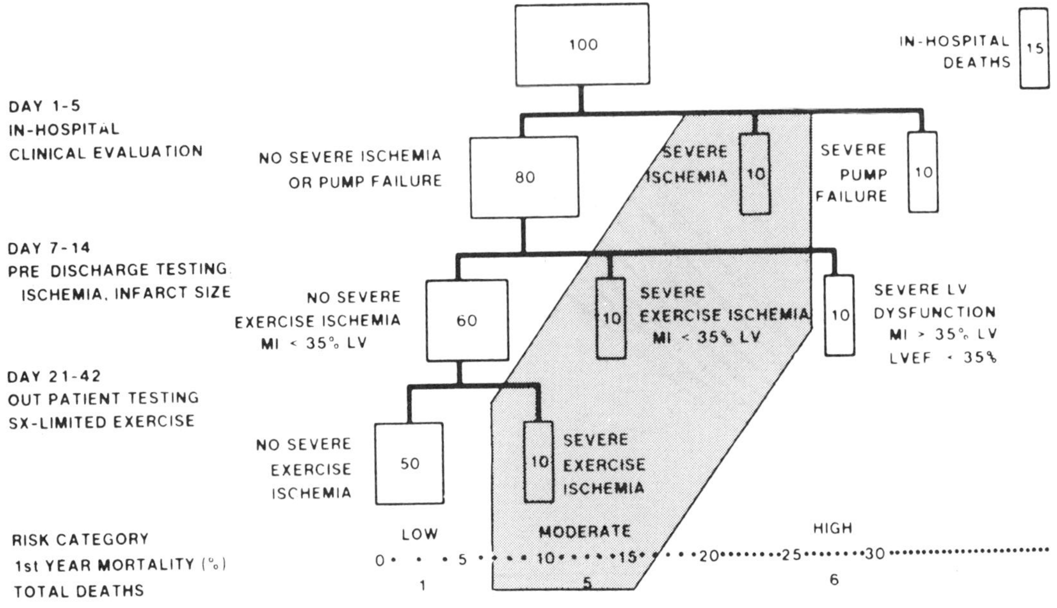

Figure 3.6. The size of each patient subset (number in boxes) in the algorithm is approximate and will vary according to the patient population. Stratification of patients into the three main risk categories (low, moderate, and high) is based on the extent of myocardial ischemia (MI) and left ventricular (LV) dysfunction. A variety of clinical observations and tests may be used to detect these abnormalities at various times after acute myocardial infarction. Patients in the shaded area are those most likely to experience a reduction in mortality from coronary revascularization. LVEF denotes left ventricular ejection fraction, and SX signifies symptom-limited. (From DeBusk RF, Blomqvist CG, Kouchoukos NT, et al.: Identification and treatment of low-risk patients after acute myocardial infarction and coronary-artery bypass graft surgery. *N Engl J Med* 314:161–166, 1986.)

chemia or pump failure during the first 5 days of hospitalization, there is a need to identify patients at increased risk who do not demonstrate these abnormalities. Exercise testing soon after myocardial infarction provides a means of detecting residual myocardial ischemia. Abnormal findings suggest that additional areas of myocardium are served by stenosed coronary vessels and are still in jeopardy. According to the above risk stratification algorithm, approximately 30% of all survivors of acute myocardial infarction will demonstrate resting or exercise-induced ST-segment depression, angina pectoris, or both, signifying a cohort of patients who are at moderate-to-high risk for a future cardiac event. Such individuals are considered appropriate candidates for coronary arteriography and, possibly, angioplasty or revascularization surgery (45).

Prognostic Value of Multiple Exercise Variables

McNeer and associates (46) demonstrated that the ST-segment response, duration of exercise (a correlate of fitness or aerobic capacity), and the maximal heart rate identified low- and high-risk subgroups more accurately than coronary artery anatomy alone. Nearly one-half of their cohort of 1472 patients were taking β-blockers at the time of testing, yet the significance of these findings remained valid. Over 97% of their patients who showed ≥ 1 mm ST-segment depression at relatively low workloads (i.e., Bruce Stages I or II) had significant CAD. Of these patients, more than 60% had three-vessel disease, and over 25% had significant stenosis (≥ 50%) of the left main coronary artery. A more recent report from the Coronary Artery Surgery Study confirmed these findings (47).

Bruce and DeRouen (48) analyzed multiple hemodynamic and clinical variables and found three non-ECG parameters that were related to increased mortality in cardiac patients. These were: cardiomegaly, a systolic blood pressure less than 130 mm Hg at peak exercise, and an exercise duration under 3 minutes (Bruce protocol), corresponding to an aerobic capacity below 5 METs.

ELECTROCARDIOGRAPHIC RESPONSES TO EXERCISE TESTING

Electrocardiographic responses to exercise tests should be interpreted according to the type and degree of ST-segment displacement and the presence of supraventricular and ventricular arrhythmias. Such information is useful in evaluating selected clinical interventions—for example, coronary artery bypass surgery, percutaneous transluminal coronary angioplasty, medications, or physical conditioning.

ST-Segment Depression

The interpretation of exercise-induced myocardial ischemia has historically relied on the presence of three types of ST-segment depression: horizontal, downsloping, and slowly upsloping. However, negative tests are often considered "inconclusive" when the peak heart rate achieved is not 85% or more of the predicted maximum, because of inadequate cardiac stress (5).

Current consensus considers an abnormal electrocardiographic response as 1.0 mm or more of horizontal or downsloping ST-segment depression at 80 msec beyond the J-point, although some clinicians argue for more stringent criteria (i.e., 2.0 mm rather than 1.0 mm), which would increase specificity but decrease sensitivity (5). In contrast, slowly upsloping ST-segment depression is considered a weaker indicator of myocardial ischemia and may be classified as normal or abnormal according to the ST-segment index (McHenry index) (49).

Measuring the ST-Segment Index

To determine the ST-segment index, which is the algebraic sum of the STJ depression in millimeters (mm) and the ST slope in millivolts per second (mV/sec), a baseline ECG is first established from three consecutive QRS complexes in which the PR interval falls on the same isoelectric line (49). The ST slope and depression can be calculated by hand using the transparent overlay shown in Figure 3.7 (50). ST-segment depression is the distance in mm from the baseline to the J-point. The ST slope is measured by forming a tangent from two points: (a) J-point, and (b) 80 msec past the J-point. The tangent is extended 2.5 cm (1 second) from the intersect and the slope is read in mV/sec. An ST-segment index of zero or less is considered to be abnormal, assuming that the magnitude of the ST depression is at least 1.0 mm (Fig. 3.8) (49).

Characteristics of Exercise-Induced ST-Segment Depression that Increase the Likelihood of Disease

The degree and type of ST-segment depression, as well as its time of onset and persistence, all appear to have diagnostic value. In general, the more pronounced the exercise-induced ST-segment depression, the greater the likelihood of significant CAD. Moreover, downsloping ST depression is associated with a higher incidence of subsequent coronary events than either the horizontal or upsloping pattern. A graver prognosis is also seen when the ST depression evolves into a downsloping pattern in recovery as compared to the ST abnormality becoming upsloping. Significant ST-segment depression that occurs early in a protocol (i.e., Bruce Stages I or II), at relatively low heart rates (e.g., less than 130 beats·min^{-1}), and/or that persists several minutes into recovery is also sugges-

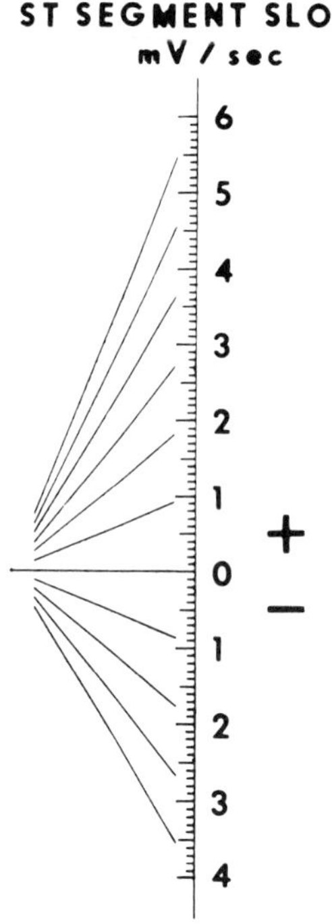

Figure 3.7. Transparent overlay used to quantitate ST-segment slope (mV/sec) and depression (millimeters). (Adapted from Lester FM, Sheffield LT, Reeves TJ: Electrocardiographic changes in clinically normal older men following near maximal and maximal exercise. *Circulation* 36:5–14. 1967.)

tive of severe disease and an unfavorable prognosis (46, 51).

Relating ST-Segment Depression to Heart Rate

Although simple measurement of the magnitude of exercise-induced ST-segment depression has been the traditional diagnostic benchmark, several recent studies have shown that the ST-segment/heart rate (ST/HR) slope, a method that normalizes the degree of exercise-induced ST-segment depression for corresponding increases in heart rate, more accurately reflects the balance between myocardial oxygen supply and demand (52). This physiologic approach seems justified in that there is little reason why 1.0 mm of ST-segment depression in a patient who exercises to a peak rate of 150 beats·min^{-1} should be taken as a reflection of more ischemia than 0.5 mm ST depression occurring in another patient who achieves a peak rate of only 75 beats·min^{-1}.

Analysis of the rate-related change in exercise-induced ST-segment depression, the ST/HR slope, has been shown to significantly improve the accuracy of the exercise ECG. Kligfield and associates (52), using an ST/HR slope value of 11 mm/bpm/1000 (1.1 μV/bpm) as an upper limit of normal, improved the exercise test sensitivity from 57% to 91% in patients with stable angina, while preserving the specificity of the test at > 90%. In addition, an ST/HR slope value of 60 mm/bpm/1000 (6.0 μV/bpm) was found to partition patients with and without three-vessel CAD with a sensitivity of 78%, specificity of 97%, a positive predictive value of 93%, and an overall test accuracy of 90%. However, the method was less accurate (i.e., reduced sensitivity and positive predictive value) in predischarge testing after recent myocardial infarction (53). These data suggest that the ST/HR slope can markedly improve the accuracy of exercise electrocardiography in patients with remote infarction by analysis of the maximum rate-related change in ST-segment depression that occurs during effort.

Uninterpretable ST-Segment Depression

In the presence of digitalis, substantial ST-segment depression at rest, left ventricular hypertrophy, left bundle-branch block, or the pre-excitation (Wolff-Parkinson-White [WPW]) syndrome, ST-segment abnormalities that develop during exercise are uninterpretable with respect to evidence of myocardial ischemia (41, 54). Although exercise-induced ST changes in the inferior and right precordial leads are difficult to interpret in the presence of right branch block, the lateral precordial leads (V_{4-6}) may be read as a reliable indicator of myocardial ischemia (55). Additional factors that may contribute to spurious ST-segment depression are anemia, hypokalemia, alkalosis, mitral valve prolapse, and

ABNORMAL ECG RESPONSE
UPSLOPING ST-SEGMENT DEPRESSION

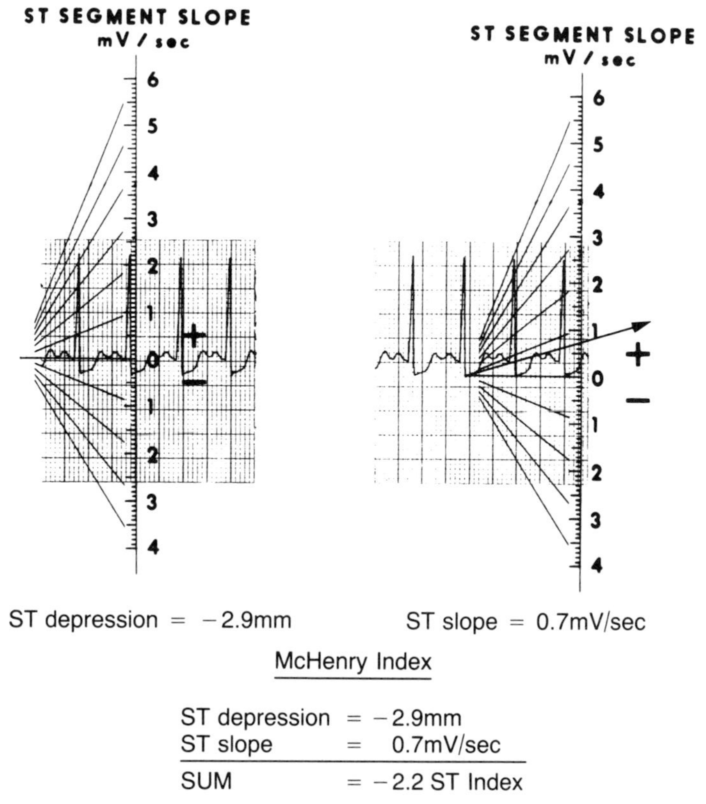

Figure 3.8. Example showing calculation of McHenry index using transparent overlay to determine ST-segment slope and depression.

certain other valvular and congenital heart diseases (56). Diuretics, by virtue of their potential to cause hypokalemia (57), digitalis preparations (58), and estrogen therapy (59) may also cause "positive tests" in the absence of significant CAD.

Influence of Medications

Beta-blockers often prevent the patient from attaining the desired level of cardiac stress, resulting in a reduced peak rate-pressure product and a higher prevalence of false-negative responses (60). However, it is generally recommended that a β-blocking agent not be withdrawn before a diagnostic exercise test is performed, particularly in patients with advanced CAD.

Calcium antagonists (61) and nitrates (62) may increase the exercise duration or work load required to elicit abnormal ST-segment depression or angina and, in some cases, may prevent the appearance of these signs/symptoms. If the purpose of the test is to establish a diagnosis of ischemic heart disease, these drugs should be withheld, if clinically feasible, for at least 12 hours.

In patients taking digoxin, it is best to discontinue the drug for at least 10–14 days before "diagnostic" testing, provided there are no strong clinical contraindications (41).

ST-Segment Elevation

Exercise-induced ST-segment elevation in leads displaying a previous Q wave infarction almost always reflects an aneurysm or a wall motion abnormality (63). In the absence of significant Q waves or Prinzmetal's angina, exercise-induced ST-segment elevation is often associated with a fixed, high-grade coronary stenosis corresponding to the site of ischemia seen electrocardiographically (5). In addition, there is evidence that this finding represents more severe ischemia than ST depression, reflecting transmural as opposed to subendocardial ischemia (64).

Supraventricular and Ventricular Arrhythmias

Isolated atrial or ventricular ectopic beats and short runs of supraventricular tachycardia commonly occur during exercise testing and do not seem to have any diagnostic or prognostic significance for CAD. However, the prognostic significance of exercise-induced ventricular ectopic rhythms is confusing. Ventricular arrhythmias during exercise increase simply as a function of age (from 15–35% of men below 35 years of age have such rhythms as compared with 50–60% of men between 45 and 55 years of age) (65). Recent studies indicate that the suppression of resting ventricular arrhythmias during exercise does not exclude the presence of underlying CAD; conversely, premature ventricular beats that increase in frequency, complexity, or both, do not necessarily signify underlying ischemic heart disease (66). On the other hand, it is widely acknowledged that frequent paired or multiform ventricular premature beats, salvos, or ventricular tachycardia occurs more commonly in cardiac patients and at significantly lower heart rates than in persons without heart disease (67). *Such threatening forms of ventricular ectopy are even more likely to be associated with significant CAD and a poor prognosis if they occur in the presence of ischemic ST-segment depression* (5, 51). Since these ventricular arrhythmias may be the harbingers of ventricular fibrillation, exercise should be terminated, and antiarrhythmic therapy should be considered.

HEMODYNAMIC RESPONSES

Although the ST-segment response has been the primary, and often sole, criterion for assessing effort-induced myocardial ischemia, the evaluation of hemodynamic responses (i.e., heart rate and blood pressure) during exercise has now been shown to enhance the predictive value of exercise testing (7).

Heart Rate

The "normal" heart rate response to progressive exercise is a relatively linear increase, corresponding to 8–12 beats·MET^{-1} for sedentary subjects (68). A patient with a markedly blunted heart rate response to exercise is said to have "chronotropic incompetence" or "sustained relative bradycardia," identified by a peak exercise heart rate that is two standard deviations or greater below the age-predicted maximal heart rate for normal subjects (69–71). This finding during exercise, even in the absence of significant ST-segment depression, has been related to left ventricular dysfunction, multivessel CAD, and a higher incidence of subsequent cardiac events (72).

The age-predicted maximal heart rate can be estimated in one of the following two ways: 220 minus age in years or 215 minus (0.66 × age in years) (11). Since the maximal heart rate normally decreases with age, impairment of chronotropic capacity due to heart disease and/or medications can be calculated by the following formula:

$$\text{Percentage chronotropic impairment} = \frac{a-b}{a} \times 100$$

where a = age-predicted maximal heart rate, b = heart rate attained at peak or maximal effort.

Blood Pressure

The "normal" hemodynamic response to exercise is a progressive increase in systolic blood pressure, typically 8–12 mm Hg·MET^{-1} with a possible plateau at peak exercise (68). Diastolic pressure usually falls slightly or remains unchanged. An exercise-induced increase of more than 15 mm Hg in diastolic pressure is considered a sign of severe CAD even in the absence of ischemic ST-segment depression (73).

The peak systolic blood pressure achieved during exercise appears to be prognostically significant. In a cohort of 1586 cardiac men, Irving and associates (74) showed a negative correlation between the maximal systolic blood pressure during exercise and the annual rate of sudden cardiac death (Table 3.3). Accordingly, exertional hypotension, defined as an exercise-induced drop in systolic blood pressure (≥ 10 mm Hg) or a failure of systolic pressure to rise above 130 mm Hg, is associated with severe ischemic heart disease and an increased mortality in patients with CAD (75).

The postexercise systolic blood pressure response may also be used as a diagnostic tool. Amon and coworkers (76) reported that some cardiac patients have recovery values of systolic blood pressure that exceed those measured at peak exercise. Patients who exhibited this phenomenon often had severe angiographically documented CAD. These investigators concluded that ratios of early recovery systolic blood pressure to the peak exercise systolic blood pressure are more sensitive than exercise-induced ST-segment depression and angina for identifying patients with CAD.

SYMPTOMS

It is critical for the clinician to note all symptoms that occur during and after the exercise test. Especially important are symptoms that may represent classic angina pectoris, such as substernal pressure radiating across the chest and/or down the left arm, back, jaw, or stomach, or lower neck pain or discomfort. Such symptoms can be subjectively rated by the patient on a scale of 1 to 4: 1 = perceptible but mild; 2 = moderate; 3 = moderately severe; and 4 = severe. Ratings of more than "2" should generally be used as end points for exercise testing.

Although patients with marked ST-segment abnormalities are often asymptomatic, when angina pectoris occurs in conjunction with ST-segment displacement the likelihood of electrocardiographic changes being due to CAD is significantly increased (77). Moreover, exercise-induced angina pectoris alone is now considered an "independent" variable that identifies a subset of patients at higher risk of subsequent coronary events (42).

Table 3.3. Correlation between maximal exercise systolic pressure and annual rate of sudden cardiac death[a]

Maximal systolic pressure, mm Hg	Annual rate of sudden death, per 1,000
< 140	97.0
140–199	25.3
> 200	6.6

[a] From Irving et al.[74]

SAFETY OF EXERCISE TESTING

In the widely quoted Rochmis and Blackburn study (78), involving 170,000 exercise tests from 73 medical centers, the mortality rate of exercise testing was found to be 1 death/10,000 (0.01%), and the combined morbidity/mortality to be 4/10,000 (0.04%). A more recent survey of 518,448 exercise stress tests conducted in 1,375 centers revealed a 50% lower mortality rate, 0.5 deaths/10,000 tests (0.005%), but a higher combined complication rate, 8.86/10,000 tests (0.09%) (79). Although the complications associated with exercise testing appear to be relatively low, the ability to maintain a high degree of safety depends on knowing when not to perform the test, when to terminate the test, and being prepared for any emergency that might arise (5).

Young and associates (80) reviewed exercise-related complications in 263 patients with *worrisome ventricular arrhythmias* who underwent a total of 1377 maximal treadmill tests. Complications occurred in 24 patients (9%) during 32 tests; however, there were no deaths or myocardial infarctions. Clinical variables previously considered to confer increased risk during exercise, such as poor left ventricular function, high-grade ventricular arrhythmias (Lown grade 4A or 4B), exertional hypotension, and ST-segment depression, were not predictive of complications. It was concluded that maximal exercise testing can be safely conducted in patients with malignant arrhythmias.

EXERCISE PRESCRIPTION

Exercise training is widely recognized as an important component in developing rehabilitation strategies for patients with CAD, including those with residual left ventricular dysfunction or exertion-induced myocardial ischemia, and for patients who have undergone coronary artery bypass graft surgery or angioplasty (81). The physician who prescribes exercise for such patients must consider the patient's age, sex, clinical status, related medical problems, habitual physical activity, musculoskeletal integrity, and most important, the information derived from a multistage exercise-tolerance test.

This section reviews the physiologic and clinical bases for the prescription of exercise in the cardiac patient, with specific reference to early outpatient cardiac rehabilitation (phase II) and home- or gymnasium-based exercise training programs (phase III) (82, 83). Extensive guidelines for exercise prescription for the inpatient (phase I) are available elsewhere (84).

COMPONENTS OF THE EXERCISE SESSION

Exercise training sessions should include a preliminary warm-up (10 minutes), a conditioning phase (30–50 minutes), a cool-down (5 minutes), and ideally, an optional recreational game (10–15 minutes).

Warm-up

Warm-up exercises facilitate the transition from rest to the conditioning phase, stretching postural muscles and increasing blood flow. More important, a gradual warm-up may reduce the potential for exercise-induced ischemic responses. Barnard and associates (85, 86) found that sudden strenuous exertion without prior warm-up elicited ST-segment depression in 60–70% of healthy men with normal ECG responses to maximal steady-state exercise testing. These abnormalities were generally reversed by prior warm-up exercise (i.e., jogging in place) and appeared to be related to an unfavorable ratio of the systolic tension time to the diastolic pressure time index. Similarly, Foster and coworkers (87, 88) observed abnormalities of left ventricular function (decreased left ventricular ejection fraction and diffusely hypokinetic wall motion) during sudden strenuous exercise in healthy men who had previously demonstrated normal left ventricular performance during incremental exercise. The deterioration in myocardial function was partially ameliorated by a preliminary warm-up, supporting Barnard's hypothesis that subendocardial ischemia is an important mechanism in the response to sudden strenuous exertion (88). In contrast, Stein et al. (89) failed to observe either ST-segment depression or left ventricular dysfunction during sudden strenuous exercise in postmyocardial infarction patients taking β-adrenergic blocking agents. The mechanism by which these drugs may serve to protect ventricular function in this setting is not clear.

The warm-up should include a musculoskeletal and cardiorespiratory component. Calisthenic exercises should precede activities that involve total body movement to increase the heart rate to within 20 beats·min^{-1} of the heart rate prescribed for endurance training. *Our experience suggests that the best warm-up for any aerobic activity is the prescribed activity performed at a lower intensity* (81). Thus, patients who use jogging during the conditioning phase should warm up with brisk walking; for participants who use the stationary cycle ergometer, "zero" load or mild tension cycling serves as an ideal warm-up.

Cool-down

Cool-down activities such as slow walking or mild tension pedaling permit a return of the heart rate and blood pressure to near preexercise values. Continued movement after vigorous exercise also enhances venous return, thereby reducing the potential for hypotension and related consequences; promotes the dissipation of body heat; facilitates more rapid removal of lactic acid than stationary recovery (90); and ameliorates the potential, deleterious effects of the postexercise rise in plasma catecholamines (91).

Omission of a cool-down immediately after vigorous exercise may result in a transient decrease in venous return, possibly reducing coronary blood flow when heart rate and myocardial oxygen demands may still be high. Sequelae may include angina pectoris, ischemic ST-segment depression, or significant ventricular dysrhythmias. Of 61 cardiovascular complications reported during the exercise training of cardiac patients, at least 44 (72%) occurred during either the warm-up or cool-down phases (92).

Recreational Games

The inclusion of enjoyable recreational games after the conditioning phase often enhances compliance (93). However, game rules should be modified to decrease the energy cost and heart rate response to play (2). Modifications should minimize skill requirements and competition, and should maximize the potential for successful participation. For example, a volleyball game that allows one or more bounces of the ball per side facilitates longer rallies, provides additional fun, and reduces the skill required to play. Through such modifications, the exercise leader is better able to emphasize the primary objective of the activity, which is enjoyment of the game itself (94).

Conditioning Phase

The conditioning phase should include aerobic endurance exercise and, for selected patients, muscular strength and endurance training (95, 96). Regular aerobic exercise improves the patient's hemodynamic and cardiorespiratory responses to submaximal and maximal exercise; it should, however, be prescribed in specific terms of intensity, duration, frequency, and type of activity.

INTENSITY

The prescribed exercise intensity should be above a minimal level required to induce a "training effect," yet below the metabolic load that evokes abnormal clinical signs or symptoms (2). For most cardiac patients, the threshold intensity for exercise training probably lies between 40% and 60% $\dot{V}O_2max$ (6); moreover, considerable evidence suggests that it increases in direct proportion to the pretraining $\dot{V}O_2max$ or the level of habitual activity (97).

The optimal intensity for aerobic-exercise training probably occurs between 57% and 78% $\dot{V}O_2max$, as indicated by two physiologic variables that signify increasing reliance on anaerobic metabolism: the respiratory exchange ratio ($\dot{V}CO_2/\dot{V}O_2$) as it approaches unity, and blood lactate when it increases abruptly (Fig. 3.9)—acute responses associated with favorable long-term adaptation and improvement in oxygen transport capacity (2).

Improvement in $\dot{V}O_2max$ increases curvilinearly with increasing intensities of exercise to a peak of about 78% $\dot{V}O_2max$, with little additional cardiorespiratory benefit thereafter (2). Although higher intensity training (i.e., up to 90% $\dot{V}O_2max$) (98–100) may provide "direct" cardiac benefits such as an improvement in left ventricular ejection fraction, such regimens are generally proscribed because of the increased risk of orthopedic (101) and cardiovascular complications (102, 103).

The "sliding scale" method, as recommended by the American College of Sports Medicine (6), empirically estimates a relative exercise training intensity that increases in direct proportion to the initial peak or symptom-limited aerobic capacity ($\dot{V}O_2max$). The baseline intensity, set at 60% $\dot{V}O_2max$, is added to the $\dot{V}O_2max$, expressed as METs, to obtain the percentage of $\dot{V}O_2max$ that should be used for physical conditioning. For example, a patient with a 5 MET capacity would train at 65% of his $\dot{V}O_2max$ (60 plus 5), corresponding to an average training intensity of 3.25 METs. Accordingly, Figure 3.10 shows the recommended training intensity (METs) for cardiac patients with aerobic capacities ranging from 2–12 METs.

Heart Rate

To attain a desired metabolic load for exercise training, one must either measure the oxygen uptake directly or have an

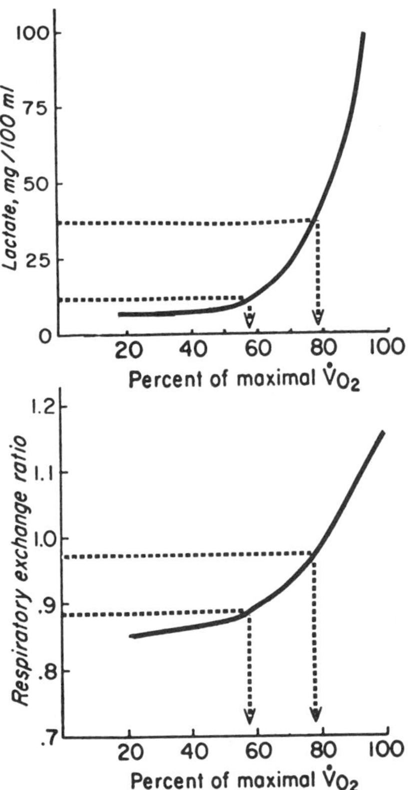

Figure 3.9. Relationship between intensity of exercise expressed as per cent maximal oxygen uptake ($\dot{V}O_2$max) and changes in respiratory exchange ratio (R) and serum lactate (mg/100 ml). Between the range of 57% and 78% $\dot{V}O_2$max (which corresponds to 70–85% of maximal heart rate), a disproportionate increase occurs in serum lactate, and R approaches unity. (From Hellerstein HK, Franklin BA: Exercise testing and prescription. In Wenger NK, Hellerstein HK (eds): *Rehabilitation of the Coronary Patient.* ed 2. New York, John Wiley & Sons, Inc. 1984, p 238. Reproduced by permission.)

equivalent index thereof. Since heart rate and oxygen uptake are linearly related during dynamic exercise involving large-muscle groups, a predetermined training or target heart rate (THR) has become widely adopted as an indicator of exercise intensity (104).

One of the most commonly employed methods of establishing the THR is the maximal heart rate reserve method of Karvonen and associates (105), in which THR = (maximal heart rate minus resting heart rate) × 60% to 80% plus resting heart rate. A given percentage of the maximal heart rate reserve in healthy young men has been shown to be nearly identical to the same percentage of $\dot{V}O_2$max used during graded exercise testing (106). On the other hand, it appears this method may overestimate the desired aerobic training intensity in early cardiac rehabilitation, since it fails to correct for a nonlinear heart rate-oxygen uptake relationship (107).

Another method that is widely used to compute the THR is to estimate per cent of $\dot{V}O_2$max from relative submaximal heart rate (% HRmax) using a fixed percentage (i.e., 70–85%) of the measured maximal heart rate (HRmax) (108, 109). This method has been shown to yield remarkably similar regressions of per cent $\dot{V}O_2$max on per cent HRmax (i.e., 60–80% $\dot{V}O_2$max ≈ 70–85% HRmax) (110), regardless of the subject's age or sex, the presence or absence of CAD, $\dot{V}O_2$max, body weight, per cent body fatness, muscle groups involved, exercise testing mode, or cardiac medications, including propranolol (111) and diltiazem (112). However, limitations of the method include the underestimation of the THR for a given MET load, adjusted by adding a correction factor of 15% to the calculated THR (6); considerable individual variability in the relationship between per cent HRmax and per cent $\dot{V}O_2$max (113, 114); and wide interindividual variability in metabolic acidosis at a given per cent HRmax, using ventilatory anaerobic threshold as the reference criterion (115).

Using Exercise Respiratory Measurements to Compare Methods of Exercise Prescription

Coplan and coworkers (116) compared several methods for determining exercise intensity, using heart rate at the ventilatory (anaerobic) threshold and at 50% $\dot{V}O_2$max as the recommended upper and lower limits for training. Exercise prescription based on either 80% HRmax or the heart rate corresponding to 70% $\dot{V}O_2$max yielded the greatest number of subjects falling within this range. Nevertheless, even these methods yielded an exercise intensity that exceeded the ventilatory threshold 15–20%

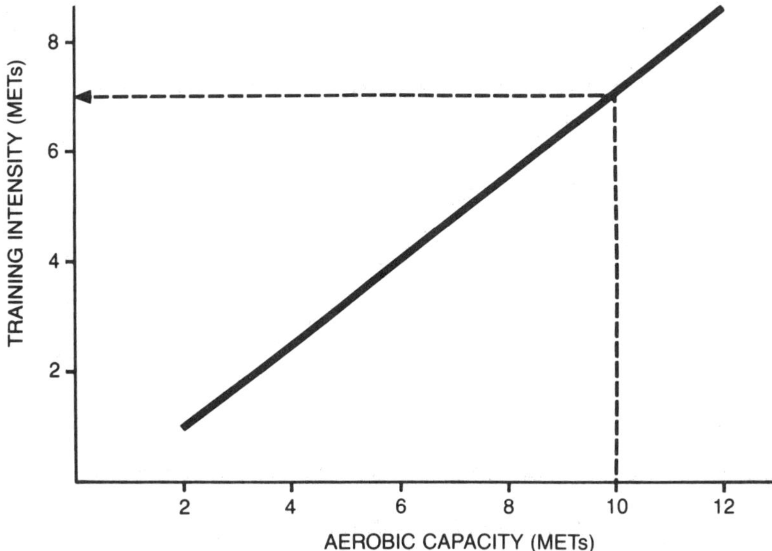

Figure 3.10. "Sliding scale" method for estimating relative exercise-training intensity (METs) from the peak or symptom-limited aerobic capacity (METs). For example, a cardiac patient with an aerobic capacity of 10 METs would use a training intensity of 7 METs.

of the time. It was concluded that exercise prescriptions should be based on direct assessment of the ventilatory threshold. The preferred method to use when respiratory measurements are not available is an exercise intensity based on 80% HRmax.

Rating of Perceived Exertion

The rating of perceived exertion (RPE) is a useful and important adjunct to heart rate as an intensity guide for exercise training. The RPE scale, first introduced by Borg (4), consists of 15 grades from 6 to 20, as shown in Figure 3.11.

Exercise rated as 12 to 13 (somewhat hard) generally corresponds to the upper limit of prescribed training heart rates during the early stages of outpatient cardiac rehabilitation (phase II) (117). Later, for higher levels of training (i.e., phase III), ratings of 13 to 15 are appropriate, corresponding to 70–85% of the HRmax, which is equivalent to 57–78% $\dot{V}O_2$max (2, 118). The anaerobic or ventilatory threshold generally occurs within this range, with an average RPE of 13.5 and 14.2 for subjects with and without CAD, respectively (2).

The concept of perceived exertion appears to be valid even for patients whose

6

7 very, very light

8

9 very light

10

11 fairly light

12

13 somewhat hard

14

15 hard

16

17 very hard

18

19 very, very hard

20

Figure 3.11. Rating of perceived exertion (RPE) scale, which includes fifteen progressive numerical levels, ranging from 6 to 20, with descriptive "effort ratings" at every odd number. Among healthy young individuals, the RPE often approximates one-tenth of the heart rate response to exercise. (From Borg G: Perceived exertion as an indicator of somatic stress. *Scand J Rehabil Med* 2:92–98, 1970.)

heart rates are attenuated by propranolol, since similar RPEs are obtained at a given percentage of maximum heart rate reserve, regardless of the β-blocker dosage or peak heart rate (119). However, there are limitations in using RPE alone to gauge exercise intensity. Although the subjective rating correlates well with heart rate, oxygen uptake, and workload, ischemic ST-segment depression and threatening ventricular dysrhythmias can occur without symptoms (silent ischemia) at low levels of perceived exertion (120).

DURATION

The duration of exercise required to elicit a significant training effect varies inversely with the intensity; the greater the intensity (up to about 78% $\dot{V}O_2max$), the shorter the duration of exercise necessary to achieve favorable adaptation and improvement in cardiorespiratory fitness (97). Conversely, low-intensity exercise may be compensated by a longer exercise duration. Exercise training for 10–15 minutes improves aerobic capacity, and 30-minute sessions are even more effective, but there is little additional benefit beyond this point. Moreover, longer training sessions (≥ 45 minutes) are associated with a disproportionate incidence of orthopedic injury (Fig. 3.12) (121).

FREQUENCY

Although deconditioned cardiac patients may improve cardiorespiratory fitness with only twice-weekly exercise, three or four evenly spaced workouts per week appear to represent the optimal training frequency (2). Additional benefits of five training sessions per week or more appear to be minimal, whereas the incidence of lower extremity injuries increases abruptly (Fig. 3.12) (121).

TYPES OF TRAINING ACTIVITIES

Exercise training may involve two basic types of skeletal muscle contractions or combinations thereof: a) static or isometric, when the muscle develops tension but no movement occurs; and b) dynamic or isotonic, when the tension on the muscle causes movement through a range of motion.

Isometric Exercise

Although isometric or combined static-dynamic efforts have traditionally been proscribed for patients with CAD, it appears that static exercise may be less hazardous than was once presumed, particularly in patients with minimal functional aerobic impairment and good left ventricular function (122). Recent studies (29, 123, 124) indicate that isometric exertion, regardless of the percentage of maximal voluntary contraction (MVC) used, generally fails to elicit angina, ST-segment depression, or significant ventricular dysrhythmias among selected cardiac patients. The rate-pressure product is lower during maximal isometric than during maximal isotonic exercise, primarily due to a lower peak heart rate response (123). Increased subendocardial perfusion, secondary to elevated diastolic blood pressure, may also contribute to the lower incidence of ischemic responses reported during isometric or combined isometric-dynamic effort. Furthermore, the myocardial oxygen supply/demand relationship appears to be favorably altered by superimposing static on dynamic effort, so that the rate-pressure product at ischemia is actually increased (124). These findings are changing the cautious attitude toward isometric exertion (and strength training) for coronary patients, particularly in regard to vocational counseling and exercise prescription.

Rationale for Strength Training in Cardiac Patients

Blomqvist (125) recently summarized the exercise training literature, with specific reference to strength training and training of the upper extremities. He concluded that:

> . . . in a general sense the physiologic data support the concept that therapeutic exercise programs should not be limited to dynamic leg exercise but should include upper body activi-

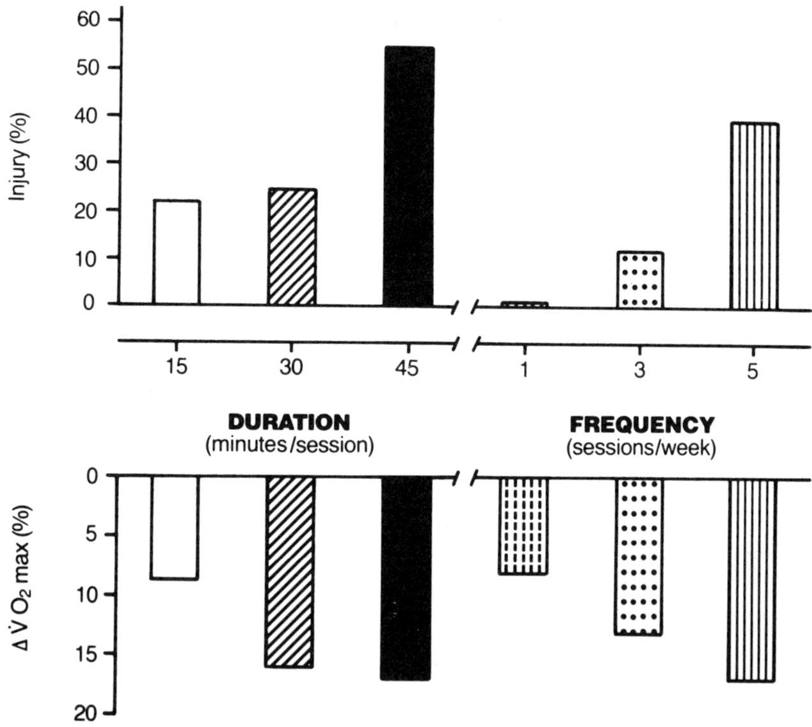

Figure 3.12. Relationships among exercise frequency and duration, improvement in maximal oxygen consumption (Δ $\dot{V}O_2max$), and the incidence of orthopedic injury. Above an exercise duration of 30 minutes/session or a frequency of 3 sessions/week, additional improvement in $\dot{V}O_2max$ is small, and the injury rate increases disproportionately. (Adapted from Pollock ML, Gettman LR, Milesis CA, et al.: Effects of frequency and duration of training on attrition and incidence of injury. *Med Sci Sports* 9:31–36, 1977.)

ties. Exercise specifically designed to improve muscle strength may be beneficial, and the exclusion of all activities requiring predominately static efforts is not warranted.

Several lines of evidence seem to support weight training as an adjunct to an aerobic exercise program in cardiac patients whose occupational or leisure-time activities require muscular strength or endurance (Fig. 3.13). Many leisure and occupational tasks require lifting, moving, or carrying a constant load (123). Since the magnitude of the pressor response to static exertion is proportionate to the percentage of MVC (126), as well as the muscle mass involved (127), any increase in strength should result in a lower rate-pressure product at any given load because the load now represents a lower percentage of MVC.

Several previous studies have reported that weight-training programs do not benefit cardiovascular function. The results from these regimens showed large increases in muscular strength but little (3–5%) if any improvement in aerobic capacity ($\dot{V}O_2max$) (128). However, these studies generally evaluated training effectiveness with dynamic lower extremity treadmill or cycle ergometer testing. When comparing heart rate and blood pressure responses to a standardized lifting or isometric test before and after isometric strength training, improvement *has* been noted (129). Such findings strongly support the specificity of measurement and specificity of fitness concept (130).

There are also intriguing data to suggest that strength training can increase muscular endurance capacity without an accompanying increase in $\dot{V}O_2max$. Hickson and associates (131) examined the effects

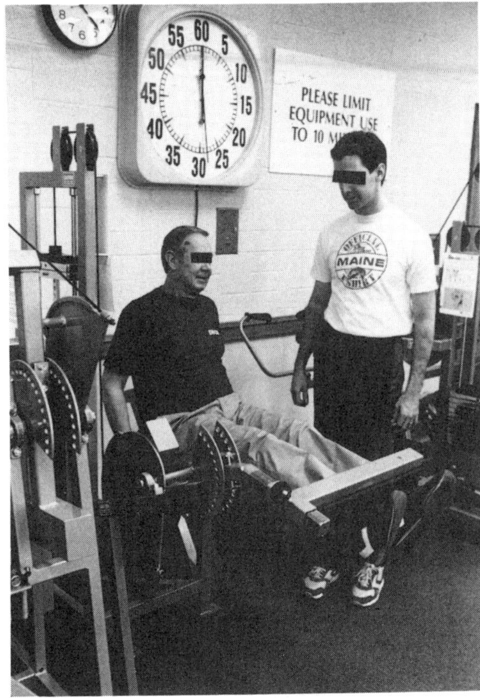

Figure 3.13. Exercise training facility at William Beaumont Hospital, Barnum Health Center, Birmingham, Michigan. Weight training (Eagle Lite-Cybex) is used to complement the physical conditioning program for selected cardiac patients.

of a lower extremity weight-training program (5 days a week for 10 weeks) on $\dot{V}O_2$max and endurance time during cycle ergometer and treadmill exercise. Although $\dot{V}O_2$max during treadmill and cycle ergometry remained essentially unchanged, endurance time to exhaustion during cycling and treadmill exercise increased 47% and 12%, respectively. These findings indicate that endurance is not a function of aerobic exercise alone, but can be significantly enhanced by weight training. This provides a further argument for the complementary use of progressive resistance training coupled with aerobic exercise.

Finally, regular progressive resistance exercise training may have a profound effect on lipid and lipoprotein levels. Using weight lifting as a model of burst-activity resistance exercise, Goldberg and associates (132) examined lipid and lipoprotein levels before and after 16 weeks of weight training in previously sedentary, healthy men. Low-density lipoprotein (LDL) cholesterol was reduced 16.2%, while the ratios of total cholesterol to high-density lipoprotein (HDL) cholesterol and LDL cholesterol to HDL cholesterol were lowered 21.6% and 28.9%, respectively. The investigators suggested that the increased HDL cholesterol concentration may have been due to a significant decrease in per cent body fat, a moderate increase in lean body mass, or both. Similar findings in cardiac patients would have important implications for secondary prevention.

Safety of Weight Training in Cardiac Patients

Although cardiac exercise programs have traditionally emphasized lower extremity dynamic aerobic exercise (i.e., walking, stationary cycle ergometry), recent research studies suggest that weight-training programs involving a substantial isometric component are safe for selected patients with CAD. Saldivar and coworkers (133) found that a low-weight, low-repetition training program was not associated with symptomatology, ST-segment abnormalities, or dysrhythmias in patients with heart disease. Similarly, Kelemen et al. (134) found no significant dysrhythmias or cardiovascular problems as a result of a 10-week circuit weight-training program in cardiac patients. More recently, Butler and associates (135), using exercise echocardiography, reported that three of 13 patients developed worsening of wall-motion scores in five left ventricular segments during aerobic exercise. In contrast, only one left ventricular segment in one patient showed a worsening in wall-motion score during circuit weight training at loads corresponding to 40–60% of one-repetition maximum.

Vander and associates (136) studied the acute hemodynamic and electrocardiographic responses to Nautilus exercise in cardiac patients and compared these responses with those obtained during symptom-limited treadmill exercise testing.

Weight loads (Fig. 3.14) during Nautilus exercise were estimated at 40–60% of MVC. Mean cardiovascular responses for all subjects (n = 21) at rest and during peak Nautilus exercise were, for the most part, unremarkable (Fig. 3.15). Peak heart rate and double product during Nautilus exercise were only 56–64% and 44–62% of treadmill values, respectively. Diastolic blood pressure during Nautilus exercise corresponded to 100–136% of values obtained during dynamic exercise testing. In contrast to dynamic exercise testing, no significant dysrhythmias, abnormal hemodynamics, ST-segment depression, or symptoms occurred during variable resistance training.

Dynamic Exercise

The most effective exercises for the endurance phase employ large muscle groups, are maintained continuously, and are rhythmic and aerobic in nature; examples include walking and jogging (even "in place"), swimming, and mobile or stationary cycle ergometry. Because of the relative consistency of energy expenditure in walking, jogging, and cycling (see chapter 1), these activities lend themselves particularly well to exercise prescription for cardiac patients. Moreover, when the exercise frequency, intensity, and duration are comparable, these activities appear to be equally effective modes of training (137).

Walking and Jogging

Walking and jogging are the most facile and easily regulated exercises for cardiorespiratory conditioning. In addition, the inherent neuromuscular limitations to the speed of walking (and, therefore, the rate of energy expenditure) establish it as the most appropriate activity for early unsupervised exercise for coronary patients (2). Even at the slowest speeds (e.g., < 2 $mi \cdot h^{-1}$), walking involves an aerobic requirement of 2 METs or more (Fig. 3.16) (138).

Advantages of a conventional walking program include a low dropout rate, an easily tolerable work intensity, and fewer musculoskeletal and orthopedic problems of the legs, knees, and feet. Moreover, brisk walk training has been shown to result in a substantial increase in aerobic capacity and a decrease in body weight and fat stores (139). Other favorable adaptations include increases in the ventilatory or anaerobic

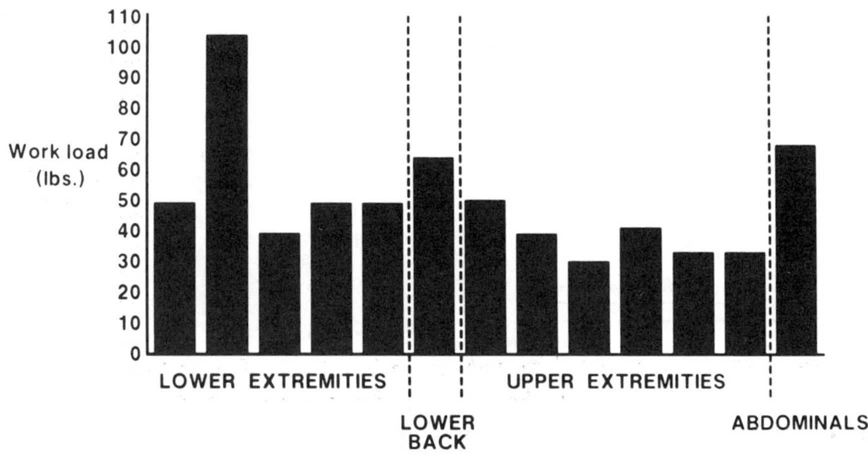

Figure 3.14. Workload (lbs) during Nautilus exercise. Lower extremity stations included (left to right) leg extension, duo-squat, leg curl, abduction, and adduction. Upper extremity stations included (left to right) pullover, lateral raise, overhead press, decline press, multicurl, and multitricep machines.(From Vander LB, Franklin BA, Wrisley D, et al.: Acute cardiovascular responses to Nautilus exercise in cardiac patients: Implications for exercise training. *Annals Sports Med* 2:165–169, 1986. Reproduced by permission.)

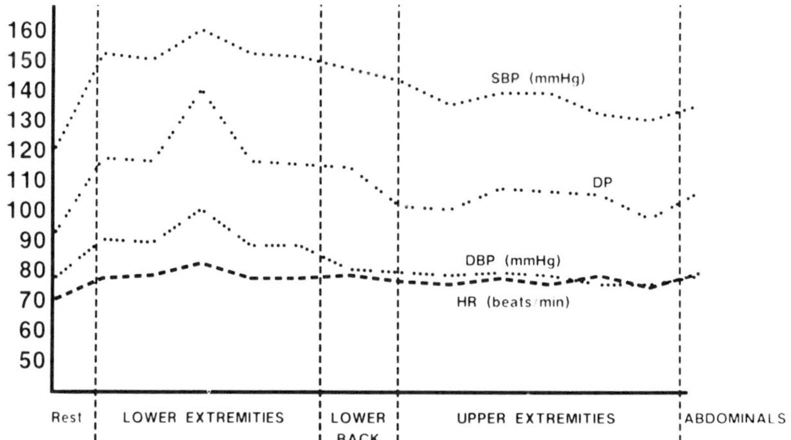

Figure 3.15. Cardiovascular response at rest and during peak Nautilus exercise. SBP, systolic blood pressure; DP, double product (HR x SBP/100); DBP, diastolic blood pressure; HR, heart rate. (From Vander LB, Franklin BA, Wrisley D, et al.: Acute cardiovascular responses to Nautilus exercise in cardiac patients: Implications for exercise training. *Annals Sports Med* 2:165–169, 1986. Reproduced by permission.)

threshold, and reductions in heart rate and somatic oxygen uptake at submaximal workloads, suggesting improved physical-work efficiency (140, 141).

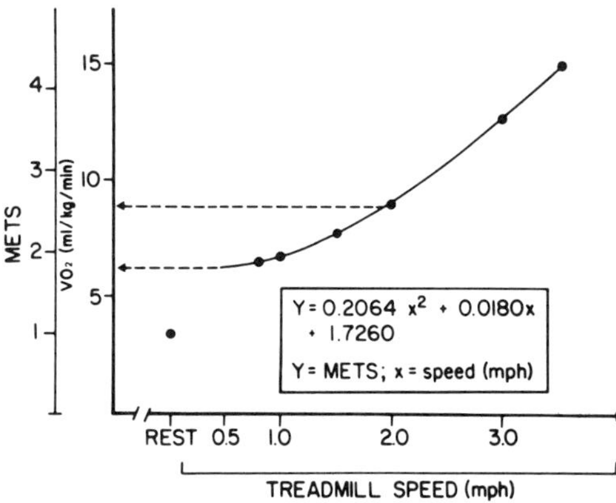

Figure 3.16. Relationship between $\dot{V}O_2$ and treadmill walking speed. The energy cost of walking at ≤ 2.0 mph, indicated by broken lines, approximates 2 METs. (From Franklin BA, Pamatmat A, Johnson S, et al.: Metabolic cost of extremely slow walking in cardiac patients: Implications for exercise testing and training. *Arch Phys Med Rehabil* 64:564–565, 1983. Reproduced with permission.)

Swimming

Although swimming is an excellent exercise for aerobic conditioning, incorporating both the upper and lower extremities, it is difficult to prescribe for two reasons: (a) energy expenditure is extremely variable and is highly dependent on skill and mechanical efficiency; and (b) training heart rates extrapolated from treadmill test data may be too high, typically by 5–10 beats·min^{-1} (142). Additional drawbacks to swim training for cardiac patients include a relatively high aerobic cost (i.e., 6.5–8.6 METs) (143), camouflaged anginal symptoms (144), and significant heart rate and blood pressure fluctuations with exposure to cold water.

Bicycling

Bicycling programs offer the flexibility of outdoor or indoor training, using a mobile bicycle or stationary-cycle ergometer. In addition, the latter can be easily adapted for arm cranking. However, with stationary-cycle ergometry, care should be taken to insure that the seat height is compatible with a slight bend in the knee at maximal leg extension, and sustained tight gripping of the handlebars should be avoided.

When compared with walking or running, the energy cost per mile (1.6 km) for outdoor cycling is relatively low: 0.60 $kcal \cdot kg^{-1} \cdot 1.6\ km^{-1}$ (Fig. 3.17) (145). For a given distance, bicycling uses approximately one-half and one-third the kilocalories of walking and running, respectively. Expressed another way, the energy cost of bicycling 4.8 km (3 miles) is the approximate energy equivalent of walking 2.4 km (1.5 miles) or running 1.6 km (1 mile).

TRAINING SPECIFICITY

Cardiorespiratory and metabolic adaptations to exercise training appear to be largely specific to the muscle groups that have been trained. For example, Clausen and coworkers (146) demonstrated that leg training caused a substantial decrease in the heart rate response to leg exercise, but not to arm exercise. Conversely, arm training resulted in an attenuated heart rate response to arm exercise, but not to leg exercise (Fig. 3.18). Similar "muscle specific" adaptations have been shown for blood lactate (147) and pulmonary ventilation (148). These findings suggest that a substantial portion of the conditioning response derives from peripheral rather than central changes, including cellular and enzymatic adaptations that increase the oxidative capacity of chronically exercised skeletal muscle (149).

Rationale for Arm Exercise Training

The lack of interchangeability of training benefits from one set of limbs to another appears to discredit the general practice of limiting exercise training to the legs alone. Many "real-life" activities require arm work to a greater extent than leg work. Consequently, cardiac patients who rely on their upper extremities for occupational or recreational activities should be advised to train the arms as well as the legs, with the expectation of improved cardiorespiratory and hemodynamic responses to both forms of effort (2).

Although upper extremity exercise training for cardiac patients has been traditionally proscribed, at a given heart rate,

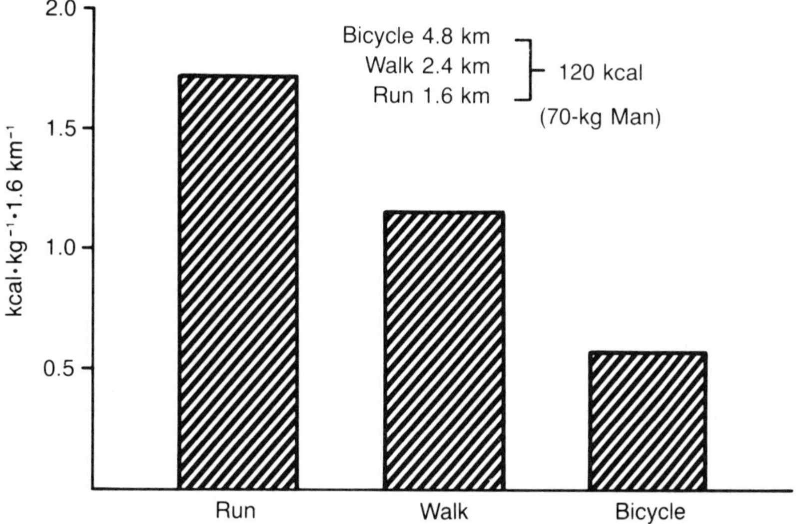

Figure 3.17. Comparison of the gross energy requirements for running, walking, or outdoor bicycling a given distance (1.6 km). (Adapted from Franklin BA, Rubenfire M: Losing weight through exercise. *JAMA* 244:377–379, 1980.)

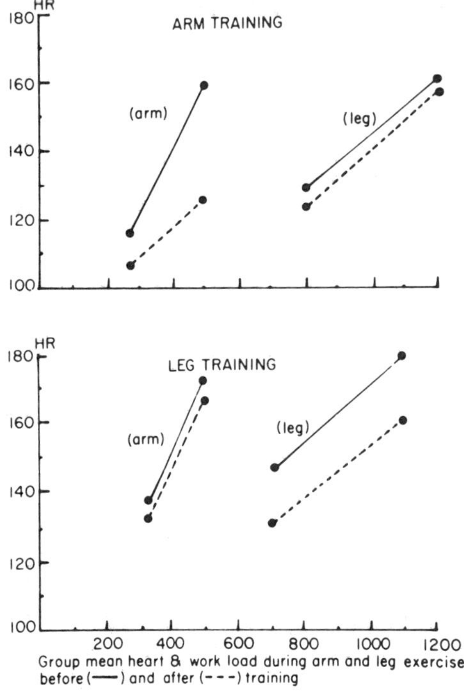

Figure 3.18. Arm training using a cycle ergometer markedly decreased the heart rate response during arm work, whereas the heart rate reduction during leg work was small. Similarly, leg training markedly decreased the heart rate during leg work, whereas the heart rate reduction during arm work was minimal. (Adapted from Clausen JP, Trap-Jensen J, Lassen NA: The effects of training on the heart rate during arm and leg exercise. *Scand J Clin Lab Invest* 26:295–301, 1970.)

arm exercise elicits no greater incidence of dysrhythmias, ischemic ST-segment depression, or angina pectoris than does leg exercise (150). Moreover, it appears that the arms respond to physical conditioning in a similar quantitative and qualitative manner as the legs (151).

ARM EXERCISE PRESCRIPTION

Guidelines for arm exercise prescription should include recommendations regarding three variables: (a) the appropriate exercise heart rate; (b) the workload (kg·m·min^{-1}) that will elicit a sufficient metabolic load for training; and (c) the proper training equipment or modalities.

Arm Exercise Training Heart Rate

Although the prescribed heart rate for arm training should ideally be derived from the results of a progressive arm ergometer test, this may not always be practical. Research indicates that a slightly lower HRmax is generally obtained during arm than during leg exercise testing (3–23 beats·min^{-1}; mean, 11 beats·min^{-1}) (18). Consequently, an arm exercise prescription based on a maximal heart rate obtained during leg ergometry may result in an inappropriately high target heart rate for arm training. As a general guideline, we have found that the prescribed heart rate for leg training should be reduced by approximately 10 beats·min^{-1} for arm training.

Since the arm and leg regressions of the percentage of relative oxygen uptake (% $\dot{V}O_2$max) on relative heart rate (% HRmax) are nearly identical (Fig. 3.19), a given percentage of HRmax during arm exercise (i.e., 70–85%) results in a percentage of arm $\dot{V}O_2$max comparable to that of leg exercise (i.e., 57–78% $\dot{V}O_2$max) (27). In addition, recent studies indicate that the heart rate-

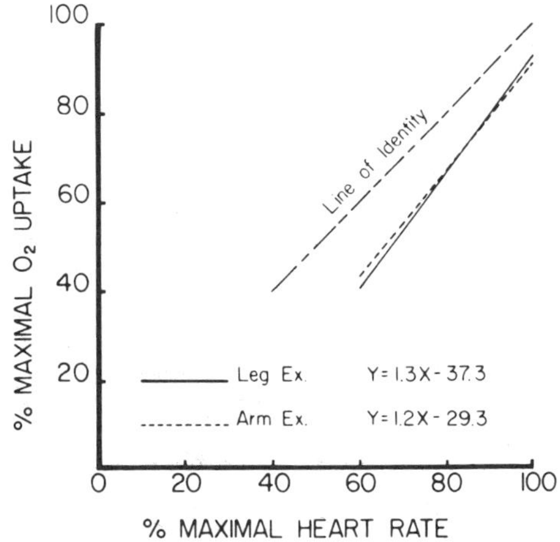

Figure 3.19 Regression lines during arm and leg exercise show a similar relationship between relative oxygen uptake, expressed as per cent $\dot{V}O_2$max, and relative heart rate, expressed as per cent HRmax. In the bivariate linear regressions, Y = per cent $\dot{V}O_2$max and X = per cent HRmax. (From Fardy PS, Webb D, Hellerstein HK: Benefits of arm exercise in cardiac rehabilitation. *Phys Sportsmed* 5:30–41, 1977. Reproduced with permission.)

oxygen uptake relation that is determined during a graded treadmill test can be generalized to *combined* arm and leg exercise when the intensity is ≅ 70% $\dot{V}O_2$max (152).

Workloads Appropriate for Arm Training

In estimating the appropriate workload for arm training, it is important to emphasize that although maximal physiologic responses are generally greater during leg exercise than arm exercise, the heart rate, blood pressure, and oxygen consumption for arm exercise are greater for any given workload. Consequently, a workload considered appropriate for leg training will generally be too high for arm training. In our experience, a workload approximately 50% of that used for leg training is appropriate for arm training (153). In other words, a patient using 300 $kg \cdot m \cdot min^{-1}$ for leg training would use 150 $kg \cdot m \cdot min^{-1}$ for arm training, demonstrating similar heart rates and perceived exertion ratings at these workloads.

Arm Exercise Training Equipment and Training Modalities

Specially designed arm or combined arm/leg ergometers (e.g., the Monarch Rehab Trainer or Schwinn Air-Dyne) are particularly good for upper extremity training. Other equipment suitable for upper body training includes rowing machines, weight training apparatus, wall pulleys, light dumbbells, vertical climbing devices (e.g., the Versa Climber), and cross-country skiing simulators (e.g., the Nordic Track). Walking or jogging while pumping handheld 1–3-lb weights can also be used to facilitate simultaneous training of the upper extremities, eliciting significantly greater increases in heart rate, oxygen consumption, and caloric expenditure over conventional walking or jogging at comparable speeds (154).

One innovative device, the Playbuoy exerciser (155), has been used as a dynamic upper-extremity conditioner in our phase III cardiac exercise program. The device includes a plastic buoy (similar to the standard swimming pool lane-divider rope buoy) on two 20-foot waxed lines attached to four plastic handles. During operation, the buoy is shuttled back and forth between two partners by alternating opening and closing of the handles.

SPECIAL CONSIDERATIONS IN EXERCISE PRESCRIPTION

Variables potentially affecting exercise trainability (that is, the qualitative and quantitative response to physical conditioning) include medications, particularly the use of β-adrenergic blockers, and left ventricular dysfunction.

β-Blockers

It has been previously suggested that β-blockade may alter or impair exercise training effects (156). Limitations may include the extent of disease, as evidenced by the need for large doses of β-blockers to relieve symptoms; the therapeutically imposed restriction of chronotropic and inotropic reserves; inhibition of skeletal muscle β-receptors, responsible for stimulating glucose metabolism (157); or the considerable fatigue reported by many of these patients. However, several recent reports have shown that cardiac patients may derive considerable physiologic benefit from an exercise training program in the presence of both cardioselective and nonselective β-blocking agents, despite therapeutic doses and a reduced training heart rate (Fig. 3.20) (158–161).

Although a sustained increase in heart rate has traditionally been acknowledged as a prerequisite to achieving an exercise training response, it should be emphasized that the chronotropic response to aerobic exercise serves merely as a hemodynamic correlate of, and monitor for, the more likely training stimulus, increased somatic oxygen uptake. Since $\dot{V}O_2$max is little affected by β-blockade, it appears that patients on such drugs can still achieve the increase in metabolic rate necessary for training by compensatory increases in stroke volume or arterial-venous oxygen difference, or both. This premise was substantiated by a

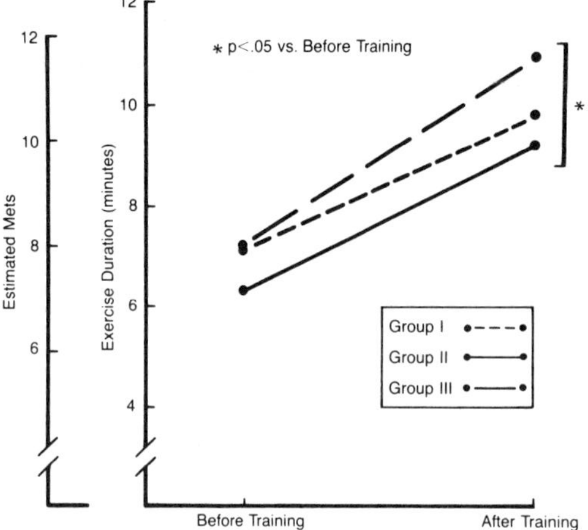

Figure 3.20 This graph shows the duration of exercise according to the Bruce protocol and estimated aerobic capacity (METs) before and after a 12-week training program in patients receiving no propranolol (Group I), patients receiving low-dose propranolol (Group II), and patients receiving high-dose propranolol (Group III). (Adapted from Pratt CM, Welton DE, Squires WG, et al.: Demonstration of training effect during chronic beta-adrenergic blockade in patients with coronary artery disease. *Circulation* 64:1125–1129, 1981.)

recent report which showed comparable cardiorespiratory and hemodynamic effects of exercise training in two groups of patients with ischemic heart disease, one with and one without β-blocker treatment (162).

The widespread clinical use of β-adrenergic blockade has prompted research on the influence of these drugs on the exercise prescription of training heart rates. It has now been shown that even β-blockade does not alter the remarkably consistent relationship between per cent $\dot{V}O_2max$ and per cent HRmax (111). Clinically, this finding is important, in that the generally accepted metabolic load for training (57–78% $\dot{V}O_2max$), associated with favorable adaptation and improvement, may be achieved by patients on β-blockade at the conventional relative heart rate recommendation for training (70–85% HRmax).

"Long-Acting" β-Blockers

Although the effect of a single morning dose (QD) of "long-acting" β-blockers may persist throughout the day, reduction of exercise heart rate is not necessarily uniform over time. Atenolol, for example, has a maximal effect between 2 and 4 hours after ingestion. Consequently, an exercise heart rate based on early morning testing for late afternoon training may be inaccurate, and vice versa. To test this hypothesis, Franklin and associates (163) subjected nine cardiac patients ($\bar{x}$ age = 54 years) on low-dose (25–50 mg) atenolol QD to morning and late afternoon testing (Bruce protocol). Mean peak exercise duration for morning and afternoon testing was similar, 11.8 versus 12.0 minutes, respectively; however, peak exercise heart rates were uniformly higher for afternoon testing (range 5–35 beats·min^{-1}, $\bar{x}$ = 19 beats·min^{-1}). Moreover, three of the nine patients demonstrated significant ST-segment depression during afternoon testing only. It was concluded that prescribed exercise heart rates for patients on QD β-blockers may be inaccurate unless the exercise testing and training time are similar.

Left Ventricular Dysfunction

Numerous studies have now demonstrated the safety and effectiveness of endurance exercise training in patients with impaired left ventricular function (ejection fraction < 45%), despite the lack of improvement in resting hemodynamics or ejection fraction (164–166).

To assess the validity of conventional methods for determining exercise training heart rates in patients with left ventricular dysfunction, Hetherington and coworkers (167) studied postmyocardial infarction patients during cycle ergometer testing in the upright position. Seventeen of the 27 patients (63%) demonstrated an abnormal stroke volume response (via impedance cardiography) at training heart rates derived by conventional methods. It was concluded that target heart rates for training based solely on the chronotropic response to exercise may subject patients with abnormal stroke volume responses to inappropriately high heart rates, excessive fatigue, or silent ischemia. The investigators suggested that the assessment of ventricular performance during exercise may provide additional useful information for prescribing training heart rates.

INCIDENCE OF CARDIOVASCULAR COMPLICATIONS DURING EXERCISE TRAINING

The incidence of cardiovascular complications during exercise is considerably greater among cardiac patients than among presumably healthy adults (168). Cobb and Weaver (169) emphasized that cardiac arrest associated with exercise testing and training in CAD patients is typically a primary arrhythmic event not due to acute myocardial infarction. Moreover, the additional risk of cardiac arrest during exercise, compared with that at other times, may be more than 100-fold during or soon after exertion.

Haskell's survey of 30 cardiac rehabilitation programs in North America revealed an average complication rate of one nonfatal and one fatal event every 34,673 and 116,402 participant-hours, respectively (92). More recently, Van Camp and Peterson (170) reported 29 cardiovascular complications (21 cardiac arrests and eight myocardial infarctions), including three fatal events, during 2,351,916 hours of outpatient cardiac exercise training. Accordingly, the incidence of complications was one cardiac arrest per 111,996 patient-hours, one myocardial infarction per 293,990 patient-hours, and one fatality per 783,972 patient-hours of exercise. It should be emphasized, however, that this seemingly low mortality rate applies only to medically supervised programs equipped with a defibrillator and appropriate emergency drugs. Recent reports indicate that up to 90% of all patients with cardiac arrests occurring under such conditions are successfully resuscitated (171).

PHYSIOLOGIC ADAPTATIONS TO ENDURANCE EXERCISE TRAINING IN CARDIAC PATIENTS

The physiologic effects of chronic exercise training are well documented and extensively reviewed elsewhere (172–174). Physical conditioning improves the patient's functional capacity and results in a reduction of the rate-pressure product at any given submaximal workload. It also promotes favorable risk factor modification, including decreases in body weight, fat stores (175), blood pressure (particularly among individuals with hypertension) (176), serum triglycerides, and low-density lipoprotein (LDL) fractions, with increases in the "protective" high-density lipoprotein (HDL) cholesterol fraction (177–179). Decreased vulnerability to dysrhythmias and increased resistance to ventricular fibrillation have also been postulated as mechanisms compatible with a specific, training-related protection against sudden cardiac death (180, 181). Accordingly, morbidity and mortality data are also encouraging (182).

A provocative study has shown that *prolonged and intense* endurance exercise training can result in a higher rate-pressure product at the onset of significant ST-segment depression (≥ 0.1 mV), implying perhaps an increase in the delivery of oxygen to the myocardium (183). Preliminary radionuclide evidence of improved myocardial perfusion and function after exercise training lends support to this hypothesis (184–186). Similar benefits have also been demonstrated with more moderate exercise-training regimens (187), although the underlying mechanisms remain unclear. Exercise training of animals with induced coronary stenosis has been shown to stimulate the development of collateral circulation (188, 189); however, a similar adaptation has yet to be demonstrated in persons with or without CAD (190, 191).

Finally, there are limitations to the benefits that exercise training offers relative to the prevention and rehabilitation of heart disease. Contrary to the speculation of a few overzealous enthusiasts (192), regular exercise training, regardless of the intensity, duration, or both, does not confer "immunity" to CAD or, for that matter, reinfarction (193). Indeed, even marathon running after myocardial infarction will not necessarily prevent progression of the disease (194).

CONCLUSION

Exercise testing and prescription appear to play an important role in the medical management and rehabilitation of patients with CAD. Multistage exercise-tolerance testing provides invaluable information in assessing the patient's functional capacity, safety of physical exertion, and effect of various interventions. Moreover, the results have long-term prognostic significance in regard to morbidity and mortality. Appropriately prescribed exercise-training programs for cardiac patients are associated with extremely low complication rates and numerous salutary effects. Although exercise guidelines should be developed as scientifically as possible, the exercise prescription should be adapted to the patient, rather than the patient to the prescription.

ACKNOWLEDGMENT

The authors thank Brenda White for typing this manuscript.

Supported in part by grants from Mr. & Mrs. Leo Demsey, Mr. & Mrs. Harry E. Figgie, Jr., Mr. & Mrs. Donald Krush, and Mr. & Mrs. Harry Mann.

REFERENCES

1. Hellerstein HK, Franklin BA: Evaluating the cardiac patient for exercise therapy: Role of exercise testing. In Franklin BA, Rubenfire M (eds): *Cardiac Rehabilitation (Clinics in Sports Medicine)*. Philadelphia, WB Saunders, 1984, p 371.
2. Hellerstein HK, Franklin BA: Exercise testing and prescription. In Wenger NK, Hellerstein HK (eds): *Rehabilitation of the Coronary Patient*, ed 2. New York, John Wiley and Sons, 1984, p 197.
3. Chaitman BR, Hanson JS: Comparative sensitivity and specificity of exercise electrocardiographic lead systems. *Am J Cardiol* 47:1335–1349, 1981.
4. Borg G: Perceived exertion as an indicator of somatic stress. *Scand J Rehabil Med* 2:92–98, 1970.
5. Fuller T, Movahed A: Current review of exercise testing: Application and interpretation. *Clin Cardiol* 10:189–200, 1987.
6. American College of Sports Medicine: *Guidelines for Graded Exercise Testing and Exercise Prescription*, ed 3. Philadelphia, Lea & Febiger, 1986, p 1.
7. Kozlowski JH, Ellestad MH: The exercise test as a guide to management and prognosis. In Franklin BA, Rubenfire M (eds): *Cardiac Rehabilitation (Clinics in Sports Medicine)*. Philadelphia, WB Saunders, 1984, p 395.
8. Ford D, Maddahi J, Berman D, et al: Differing ability of treadmill and upright bicycle exercise testing to induce clinical and electrocardiographic myocardial ischemia in patients with coronary artery disease (abst). *J Am Coll Cardiol* 1:650, 1983.
9. Wicks JR, Sutton JR, Oldridge NB, et al: Comparison of electrocardiographic changes induced by maximum exercise testing with treadmill and cycle ergometer. *Circulation* 57:1066–1070, 1978.
10. Foster C, Pollock ML, Rod JL, et al: Evaluation of functional capacity during exercise radionuclide angiography. *Cardiology* 70:85–93, 1983.
11. Bruce RA: Principles of exercise testing. In Naughton JP, Hellerstein HK, Mohler IC (eds): *Exercise Testing and Exercise Training in Coronary Heart Disease*. New York, Academic Press, 1973, p 45.
12. Handler CE, Sowton E: A comparison of the Naughton and modified Bruce treadmill exercise protocols in their ability to detect ischaemic abnormalities six weeks after myocardial infarction. *Eur Heart J* 5:752–755, 1984.
13. Zohman LR, Young JL, Kattus AA: Treadmill walking protocol for the diagnostic evaluation and exercise programming of cardiac patients. *Am J Cardiol* 51:1081–1086, 1983.
14. Franklin BA: Pitfalls in estimating aerobic capacity from exercise time or workload. *Appl Cardiol* 14:25–26, 1986.
15. Sullivan M, McKirnan MD: Errors in predicting functional capacity for postmyocardial infarction patients using a modified Bruce protocol. *Am Heart J* 107:486–492, 1984.
16. Hughson RL, Smyth GA: Slower adaptation of $\dot{V}O_2$ to steady state of submaximal exercise with Beta-adrenergic blockade. *Eur J Appl Physiol* 52:107–110, 1983.
17. Eldridge JE, Ramsey-Green CL, Hossack KF: Effects of the limiting symptom on the achievement of maximal oxygen consumption in patients with coronary artery disease. *Am J Cardiol* 57:513–517, 1986.
18. Franklin BA: Exercise testing, training and arm ergometry. *Sports Medicine* 2:100–119, 1985.
19. Asmussen E, Hemmingsen I: Determination of maximum working capacity at different ages in work with the legs or with the arms. *Scand J Clin Lab Invest* 10:67–71, 1958.
20. Schwade J, Blomqvist CG, Shapiro W: A comparison of the response to arm and leg work in patients with ischemic heart disease. *Am Heart J* 94:203–208, 1977.
21. Bar-Or O, Zwiren LD: Maximal oxygen consumption test during arm exercise–reliability and validity. *J Appl Physiol* 38:424–426, 1975.

22. Franklin BA, Vander L, Wrisley D, et al: Aerobic requirements of arm ergometry: Implications for exercise testing and training. *Phys Sportsmed* 11:81–90, 1983.
23. Shaw DJ, Crawford MH, Karliner JS, et al: Arm-crank ergometry: A new method for the evaluation of coronary artery disease. *Am J Cardiol* 33:801–805, 1974.
24. Balady GJ, Weiner DA, McCabe CH, et al: Value of arm exercise testing in detecting coronary artery disease. *Am J Cardiol* 55:37–39, 1985.
25. Glaser RM, Sawka MN, Brune MF, et al: Physiological responses to maximal effort wheelchair and arm crank ergometry. *J Appl Physiol: Respirat Environ Exercise Physiol* 48:1060–1064, 1980.
26. Wahren J, Bygdeman S: Onset of angina pectoris in relation to circulatory adaptation during arm and leg exercise. *Circulation* 44:432–441, 1971.
27. Fardy PS, Webb D, Hellerstein HK: Benefits of arm exercise in cardiac rehabilitation. *Phys Sportsmed* 5:30–41, 1977.
28. Lazarus B, Cullinane E, Thompson PD: Comparison of the results and reproducibility of arm and leg exercise tests in men with angina pectoris. *Am J Cardiol* 47:1075–1079, 1981.
29. DeBusk RF, Valdez R, Houston N, et al: Cardiovascular responses to dynamic and static effort soon after myocardial infarction: Application to occupational work assessment. *Circulation* 58:368–375, 1978.
30. Williams J, Cottrell E, Powers SK, et al: Arm ergometry: A review of published protocols and the introduction of a new weight adjusted protocol. *J Sports Med Phys Fitness* 23:107–112, 1983.
31. Fein SA, Klein NA, Frishman WH: Prognostic value and safety of exercise testing soon after uncomplicated myocardial infarction. *Cardiovasc Clin* 13:279–289, 1983.
32. Cohn PF: The role of noninvasive cardiac testing after an uncomplicated myocardial infarction. *N Engl J Med* 309:90–93, 1983.
33. Epstein SE, Palmeri ST, Patterson RE: Evaluation of patients after acute myocardial infarction: indications for cardiac catheterization and surgical intervention. *N Engl J Med* 307:1487–1492, 1982.
34. Topol EJ, Juni JE, O'Neill WW, et al: Exercise testing three days after onset of acute myocardial infarction. *Am J Cardiol* 60:958–962, 1987.
35. Topol EJ, Burek K, O'Neill WW, et al: A randomized controlled trial of hospital discharge three days after myocardial infarction in the era of reperfusion. *N Engl J Med* 318:1083–1088, 1988.
36. DeBusk RF, Haskell W: Symptom-limited versus heart rate-limited exercise testing soon after myocardial infarction. *Circulation* 61:738–743, 1980.
37. Starling MR, Crawford MH, O'Rourke RA: Superiority of selected treadmill exercise protocols predischarge and six weeks postinfarction for detecting ischemic abnormalities. *Am Heart J* 104:1054–1060, 1982.
38. Bruce RA, Hornsten TR: Exercise stress testing in evaluation of patients with ischemic heart disease. *Prog Cardiovasc Dis* 11:371–390, 1969.
39. Naughton J, Sevelius G, Balke B: Physiological responses of normal and pathological subjects to a modified work capacity test. *J Sports Med* 3:201–207, 1963.
40. Weiner DA: Predischarge exercise testing after myocardial infarction: Prognostic and therapeutic features. *Cardiovasc Clin* 15:95–104, 1985.
41. Schlant RC, Blomqvist CG, Brandenburg RO, et al: Guidelines for exercise testing. *Circulation* 74:653A–667A, 1986.
42. Cole JP, Ellestad MH: Significance of chest pain during treadmill exercise: Correlation with coronary events. *Am J Cardiol* 41:227–232, 1978.
43. Starling MR, Crawford MH, Kennedy GT, et al: Exercise testing early after myocardial infarction: Predictive value for subsequent unstable angina and death. *Am J Cardiol* 46:909–914, 1980.
44. Weld FM, Chu KL, Bigger JT Jr, et al: Risk stratification with low-level exercise testing 2 weeks after acute myocardial infarction. *Circulation* 64:306–314, 1981.
45. DeBusk RF, Blomqvist CG, Kouchoukos NT, et al: Identification and treatment of low-risk patients after acute myocardial infarction and coronary-artery bypass graft surgery. *N Engl J Med* 314:161–166, 1986.
46. McNeer JF, Margolis JR, Lee KL, et al: The role of the exercise test in the evaluation of patients for ischemic heart disease. *Circulation* 57:64–70, 1978.
47. Weiner DA, Ryan TJ, McCabe CH et al: Prognostic importance of a clinical profile and exercise test in medically treated patients with coronary artery disease. *J Am Coll Cardiol* 3:772–779, 1984.
48. Bruce RA, DeRouen TA: Exercise testing as a predictor of heart disease and sudden death. *Hosp Pract* 13(9):69–75, 1978.
49. McHenry PL, Phillips JF, Knoebel SB: Correlation of computer-quantitated treadmill exercise electrocardiogram with arteriographic location of coronary artery disease. *Am J Cardiol* 30:747–752, 1972.
50. Lester FM, Sheffield LT, Reeves TJ: Electrocardiogaphic changes in clinically normal older men following near maximal and maximal exercise. *Circulation* 36:5–14, 1967.
51. Ellestad MH, Cooke BM, Greenberg PS: Stress testing: Clinical application and predictive capacity. *Prog Cardiovasc Dis* 21:431–460, 1979.
52. Kligfield P, Okin PM, Ameisen O, et al: Evaluation of coronary artery disease by an improved method of exercise electrocardiography: The ST segment/heart rate slope. *Am Heart J* 112:589–598, 1986.

53. Ameisen O, Kligfield P, Okin PM, et al: Effects of recent and remote infarction on the predictive accuracy of the ST segment/heart rate slope. *J Am Coll Cardiol* 8:267–273, 1986.
54. Laslett LJ, Amsterdam EA: Management of the asymptomatic patient with an abnormal exercise ECG. *JAMA* 252:1744–1746, 1984.
55. Tanaka T, Friedman MJ, Okada RD, et al: Diagnostic value of exercise-induced ST segment depression in patients with right bundle branch block. *Am J Cardiol* 41:670–673, 1978.
56. Bruce RA: Editorial: Values and limitations of exercise electrocardiography. *Circulation* 50:1–3, 1974.
57. Georgopoulos AJ, Proudfit WL, Page IH: Effect of exercise on electrocardiogram of patients with low serum potassium. *Circulation* 23:567–572, 1961.
58. Sketch MH, Mooss AN, Butler ML, et al: Digoxin-induced positive exercise tests: Their clinical and prognostic significance. *Am J Cardiol* 48:655–659, 1981.
59. Jaffe MD: Effect of oestrogens on postexercise electrocardiogram. *Br Heart J* 38:1299–1303, 1977.
60. Gianelly RE, Treister BL, Harrison DC: The effect of propranolol on exercise-induced ischemic ST segment depression. *Am J Cardiol* 24:161–165, 1969.
61. Subramanian B, Bowles M, Lahiri A, et al: Long-term antianginal action of verapamil assessed with quantitated serial treadmill stress testing. *Am J Cardiol* 48:529–535, 1981.
62. Russek HI, Funk EH Jr: Comparative responses to various nitrates in the treatment of angina pectoris. *Postgrad Med* 31:150–155, 1962.
63. Chaitman BR, Waters DD, Theroux P, et al: S-T segment elevation and coronary spasm in response to exercise. *Am J Cardiol* 47:1350–1358, 1981.
64. Yasue H, Omote S, Takizawa A, et al: Comparison of coronary arteriographic findings during angina pectoris associated with S-T elevation or depression. *Am J Cardiol* 47:539–546, 1981.
65. McHenry PL, Morris SN, Kavlier M, et al: Comparative study of exercise-induced ventricular arrhythmias in normal subjects and patients with documented coronary artery disease. *Am J Cardiol* 37:609–616, 1976.
66. Califf RM, McKinnis RA, McNeer JF, et al: Prognostic value of ventricular arrhythmias associated with treadmill exercise testing in patients studied with cardiac catheterization for suspected ischemic heart disease. *J Am Coll Cardiol* 2:1060–1067, 1983.
67. McHenry PL, Fisch C: Clinical applications of the treadmill exercise test. *Mod Concepts Cardiovasc Dis* 46:21–25, 1977.
68. Naughton J, Haider R: Methods of exercise testing. In Naughton JP, Hellerstein HK, Mohler IC (eds): *Exercise Testing and Exercise Training in Coronary Heart Disease.* New York, Academic Press, 1973, p 79.
69. Chin CF, Messenger JC, Greenberg PS, et al: Chronotropic incompetence in exercise testing. *Clin Cardiol* 2:12–18, 1979.
70. Wiens RD, Lafia P, Marder CM, et al: Chronotropic incompetence in clinical exercise testing. *Am J Cardiol* 54:74–78, 1984.
71. Hinkle LE, Carver ST, Plakum A: Slow heart rates and increased risk of cardiac death in middle-aged men. *Arch Intern Med* 129:732–748, 1972.
72. Ellestad MH, Wan MKC: Predictive implications of stress testing. Follow-up of 2700 subjects after maximum treadmill stress testing. *Circulation* 51:363–369, 1975.
73. Sheps DS, Ernst JC, Briese FW, et al: Exercise-induced increase in diastolic pressure: indicator of severe coronary artery disease. *Am J Cardiol* 43:708–712, 1979.
74. Irving JB, Bruce RA, DeRouen TA: Variations in and significance of systolic pressure during maximal exercise (treadmill) testing: relation to severity of coronary artery disease and cardiac mortality. *Am J Cardiol* 39:841–848, 1977.
75. Comess KA, Fenster PE: Clinical implications of the blood pressure response to exercise. *Cardiology* 68:233–244, 1981.
76. Amon KW, Richards KL, Crawford MH: Usefulness of the postexercise response of systolic blood pressure in the diagnosis of coronary artery disease. *Circulation* 70:951–956, 1984.
77. Weiner DA, McCabe C, Hueter D, et al.: The predictive value of chest pain as an indicator of coronary disease during exercise testing (abst). *Circulation* 54[Suppl II]:10, 1976.
78. Rochmis P, Blackburn H: Exercise tests. A survey of procedures, safety and litigation experience in approximately 170,000 tests. *JAMA* 217:1061–1066, 1971.
79. Stuart RJ Jr, Ellestad MH: National survey of exercise stress testing facilities. *Chest* 77:94–97, 1980.
80. Young DZ, Lampert S, Graboys TB, et al: Safety of maximal exercise testing in patients at high risk for ventricular arrhythmia. *Circulation* 70:184–191, 1984.
81. Franklin BA, Hellerstein HK, Gordon S, et al: Exercise prescription for the myocardial infarction patient. *J Cardiopulmonary Rehabil* 6:62–79, 1986.
82. Fletcher BJ, Thiel J, Fletcher GF: Phase II intensive monitored cardiac rehabilitation for coronary artery disease and coronary risk factors—A six-session protocol. *Am J Cardiol* 57:751–756, 1986.
83. DeBusk RF, Haskell WL, Miller NH, et al: Medically directed at-home rehabilitation soon after clinically uncomplicated acute myocardial in-

farction: A new model for patient care. *Am J Cardiol* 55:251–257, 1985.
84. Wenger NK: Early ambulation after myocardial infarction: The in-patient exercise program. In Franklin BA, Rubenfire M (eds): *Cardiac Rehabilitation (Clinics in Sports Medicine).* Philadelphia, WB Saunders, 1984, p 333.
85. Barnard RJ, Gardner GW, Diaco NV, et al: Cardiovascular responses to sudden strenuous exercise: Heart rate, blood pressure, and ECG. *J Appl Physiol* 34:833–837, 1973.
86. Barnard RJ, MacAlpin R, Kattus AA, et al: Ischemic response to sudden strenuous exercise in healthy men. *Circulation* 48:936–942, 1973.
87. Foster C, Anholm JD, Hellman CK, et al: Left ventricular function during sudden strenuous exercise. *Circulation* 63:592–596, 1981.
88. Foster C, Dymond DS, Carpenter J, et al: Effect of warm-up on left ventricular response to sudden strenuous exercise. *J Appl Physiol: Respirat Environ Exercise Physiol* 53:380–383, 1982.
89. Stein RA, Berger HJ, Zaret BL: The cardiac response to sudden strenuous exercise in the post-myocardial infarction patient receiving beta blockers. *J Cardiopulmonary Rehabil* 6:336–342, 1986.
90. Belcastro AN, Bonen A: Lactic acid removal rates during controlled and uncontrolled recovery exercise. *J Appl Physiol* 39:932–936, 1975.
91. Dimsdale JE, Hartley H, Guiney T, et al: Postexercise peril: Plasma catecholamines and exercise. *JAMA* 251: 630–632, 1984.
92. Haskell WL: Cardiovascular complications during exercise training of cardiac patients. *Circulation* 57:920–924, 1978.
93. Franklin BA: Motivating and educating adults to exercise. *Journal of Physical Education and Recreation* 49:13–17, 1978.
94. Stoedefalke KG: Physical fitness programs for adults. *Am J Cardiol* 33:787–790, 1974.
95. Pollock ML, Ward A, Foster C: Exercise prescription for rehabilitation of the cardiac patient. In Pollock ML, Schmidt DH (eds): *Heart Disease and Rehabilitation.* Boston, Houghton Mifflin, Professional Medical Division, 1979, p 413.
96. Pollock ML, Pels AE: Exercise prescription for the cardiac patient: An update: In Franklin BA, Rubenfire M (eds): *Cardiac Rehabilitation (Clinics in Sports Medicine).* Philadelphia, WB Saunders, 1984, p 425.
97. Pollock ML: Quantification of endurance training programs. In Wilmore JH (ed): *Exercise and Sport Sciences Reviews.* New York, Academic Press, 1973, p 155.
98. Hagberg JM, Ehsani AA, Holloszy JO: Effect of 12 months of intense exercise training on stroke volume in patients with coronary artery disease. *Circulation* 67:1194–1199, 1983.
99. Ehsani AA, Biello DR, Schultz J, et al: Improvement of left ventricular contractile function by exercise training in patients with coronary artery disease. *Circulation* 74:350–358, 1986.
100. Rogers MA, Yamamoto C, Hagberg JM, et al: The effect of 7 years of intense exercise training on patients with coronary artery disease. *J Am Coll Cardiol* 10:321–326, 1987.
101. Kilbom A, Hartley LH, Saltin B, et al: Physical training in sedentary middle-aged older men: I. Medical evaluation. *Scand J Clin Lab Invest* 24:315–322, 1969.
102. Hossack KF, Hartwig R: Cardiac arrest associated with supervised cardiac rehabilitation. *J Cardiac Rehabil* 2:402–408, 1982.
103. Wenger NK: Is strenuous physical activity appropriate for patients with coronary heart disease? *Adv Cardiol* 31:199–204, 1982.
104. Wilmore JH: Exercise prescription: Role of the physiatrist and allied health professional. *Arch Phys Med Rehabil* 57:315–319, 1976.
105. Karvonen M, Kentala K, Mustala O: The effects of training on heart rate: A longitudinal study. *Annals Medicinae Experimentalis et Biologiae Fenniae* 35:307–315, 1957.
106. Davis JA, Convertino VA: A comparison of heart rate methods for predicting endurance training intensity. *Med Sci Sports* 7:295–298, 1975.
107. Dressendorfer RH, Smith JL: Predictive accuracy of the maximum heart rate reserve method for estimating aerobic training intensity in early cardiac rehabilitation. *J Cardiac Rehabil* 4:484–489, 1984.
108. American Heart Association Committee on Exercise: *Exercise Testing and Training of Individuals with Heart Disease or at High Risk for its Development: A Handbook for Physicians.* Dallas, American Heart Association, 1975, p 1.
109. Hellerstein HK, Hirsch EZ, Ader R, et al: Principles of exercise prescription for normals and cardiac subjects. In Naughton JP, Hellerstein HK (eds): *Exercise Testing and Exercise Training in Coronary Heart Disease.* New York, Academic Press, 1973, p 129.
110. Taylor HL, Haskell W, Fox SM III, et al: Exercise tests: A summary of procedures and concepts of stress testing for cardiovascular diagnosis and function evaluation. In Blackburn H (ed): *Measurement in Exercise Electrocardiography (The Ernst Simonson Conference).* Springfield, Illinois, Thomas, 1969, p 259.
111. Hossack KF, Bruce RA, Clark LJ: Influence of propranolol on exercise prescription of training heart rates. *Cardiology* 65:47–58, 1980.
112. Chang K, Hossack KF: Effect of diltiazem on heart rate responses and respiratory variables during exercise: Implications for exercise prescription and cardiac rehabilitation. *J Cardiac Rehabil* 2:326–332, 1982.

113. Franklin B, Hodgson J, Buskirk ER: Relationship between percent maximal O_2 uptake and percent maximal heart rate in women. *Research Quarterly for Exercise and Sport* 51:616–624, 1980.
114. Londeree BR, Ames SA: Trend analysis of the % $\dot{V}O_2$max-HR regression. *Med Sci Sports* 8:122–125, 1976.
115. Katch V, Weltman A, Sady S, et al: Validity of the relative percent concept for equating training intensity. *Eur J Applied Physiol* 39:219–227, 1978.
116. Coplan NL, Gleim GW, Nicholas JA: Using exercise respiratory measurements to compare methods of exercise prescription. *Am J Cardiol* 58:832–836, 1986.
117. Gutman MC, Squires RW, Pollock ML, et al: Perceived exertion-heart rate relationship during exercise testing and training in cardiac patients. *J Cardiac Rehabil* 1:52–59, 1981.
118. Hage P: Perceived exertion: One measure of exercise intensity. *Phys Sportsmed* 9:136–143, 1981.
119. Pollock ML, Foster C: Exercise prescription for participants on propranolol (abst). *J Am Coll Cardiol* 1:624, 1983.
120. Williams MA, Fardy PS: Limitations in prescribing exercise. *The Journal of Cardiovascular and Pulmonary Technology* 8:36–38, 1980.
121. Pollock ML, Gettman LR, Milesis CA, et al: Effects of frequency and duration of training on attrition and incidence of injury. *Med Sci Sports* 9:31–36, 1977.
122. Fardy PS: Isometric exercise and the cardiovascular system. *Phys Sportmed* 9:43–56, 1981.
123. Ferguson RJ, Cote P, Bourassa MG, et al: Coronary blood flow during isometric and dynamic exercise in angina pectoris patients. *J Cardiac Rehabil* 1:21–27, 1981.
124. DeBusk RF, Pitts W, Haskell W, et al: Comparison of cardiovascular responses to static-dynamic and dynamic effort alone in patients with ischemic heart disease. *Circulation* 59:977–984, 1979.
125. Blomqvist CG: Upper extremity exercise testing and training. In Wenger NK (ed): *Exercise and the Heart* (ed 2). Philadelphia, FA Davis, 1985, p 175.
126. Lind AR, McNichol GW: Muscular factors which determine the cardiovascular responses to sustained and rhythmic exercise. *Can Med Assoc J* 96:706–715, 1967.
127. Mitchell JH, Payne FC, Saltin B, et al: The role of muscle mass in the cardiovascular response to static contractions. *J Physiol* 309:45–54, 1980.
128. Pollock ML, Wilmore JH, Fox SM: *Health and Fitness Through Physical Activity*. New York, John Wiley and Sons, 1978, p 45.
129. Lewis S, Nygaard E, Sanchez J, et al: Static contraction of the quadriceps muscle in man: cardiovascular control and responses to one-legged strength training. *Acta Physiol Scand* 122:341–353, 1984.
130. Sharkey BJ: Specificity of testing. In Grana A (ed): *Advances in Sports Medicine and Physical Fitness*. Chicago, Year Book Medical Publishers, 1988, p 25.
131. Hickson RC, Rosenkoetter MA, Brown MM: Strength training effects on aerobic power and short-term endurance. *Med Sci Sports Exerc* 12:336–339, 1980.
132. Goldberg L, Elliot DL, Schutz RW, et al: Changes in lipid and lipoprotein levels after weight training. *JAMA* 252:504–506, 1984.
133. Saldivar M, Frye WM, Pratt CM, et al: Safety of a low weight, low repetition strength training program in patients with heart disease (abst). *Med Sci Sports Exerc* 15:119, 1983.
134. Kelemen MH, Stewart KJ, Gillilan RE, et al: Circuit weight training in cardiac patients. *J Am Coll Cardiol* 7:38–42, 1986.
135. Butler RM, Beierwaltes WH, Rogers FJ: The cardiovascular response to circuit weight training in patients with cardiac disease. *J Cardiopulmonary Rehabil* 7:402–409, 1987.
136. Vander LB, Franklin BA, Wrisley D, et al: Acute cardiovascular responses to Nautilus exercise in cardiac patients: Implications for exercise training. *Ann Sports Med* 2:165–169, 1986.
137. Pollock ML, Dimmick J, Miller HS, et al: Effects of mode of training on cardiovascular function and body composition of adult men. *Med Sci Sports* 7:139–145, 1975.
138. Franklin BA, Pamatmat A, Johnson S, et al: Metabolic cost of extremely slow walking in cardiac patients: Implications for exercise testing and training. *Arch Phys Med Rehabil* 64:564–565, 1983.
139. Pollock ML, Miller HS, Janeway R, et al: Effects of walking on body composition and cardiovascular function of middle-aged men. *J Appl Physiol* 30:126–130, 1971.
140. Ciske PE, Dressendorfer RH, Gordon S, et al: Attenuation of exercise training effects in patients taking beta blockers during early cardiac rehabilitation. *Am Heart J* 112:1016–1025, 1986.
141. Dressendorfer RH, Smith JL, Amsterdam EA, et al: Reduction of submaximal exercise myocardial oxygen demand post-walk training program in coronary patients due to improved physical work efficiency. *Am Heart J* 103:358–362, 1982.
142. Thompson DL, Boone TW, Miller HS: Comparison of treadmill exercise and tethered swimming to determine validity of exercise prescription. *J Cardiac Rehabil* 2:363–370, 1982.
143. Fletcher GF, Cantwell JD, Watt EW: Oxygen consumption and hemodynamic response of exercises used in training of patients with recent myocardial infarction. *Circulation* 60:140–144, 1979.
144. Magder S, Linnarsson D, Gullstrand L: The effect of swimming on patients with ischemic heart disease. *Circulation* 63:979–986, 1981.

145. Franklin BA, Rubenfire M: Losing weight through exercise. *JAMA* 244:377–379, 1980.
146. Clausen JP, Trap-Jensen J, Lassen NA: The effects of training on the heart rate during arm and leg exercise. *Scand J Clin Lab Invest* 26:295–301, 1970.
147. Klausen K, Rasmussen B, Clausen JP, et al: Blood lactate from exercising extremities before and after arm or leg training. *Am J Physiol* 227:67–72, 1974.
148. Rasmussen B, Klausen K, Clausen JP, et al: Pulmonary ventilation, blood gases and blood pH after training of the arms or the legs. *J Appl Physiol* 38:250–256, 1975.
149. Henriksson J, Reitman JS: Time course of changes in human skeletal muscle succinate dehydrogenase and cytochrome oxidase activities and maximal oxygen uptake with physical activity and inactivity. *Acta Physiol Scand* 99:91–97, 1977.
150. Fardy PS, Doll NE, Reitz NL, et al: Prevalence of dysrhythmias during upper, lower and combined upper and lower extremity exercise in cardiac patients (abst). *Med Sci Sports* 13:137, 1981.
151. Wrisley D, Franklin BA, Vander L, et al: Effects of exercise training on arm and leg aerobic capacity in cardiac patients (abst). *Med Sci Sports* 15:92, 1983.
152. Goss FL, Robertson RJ, Auble TE, et al: Are treadmill-based exercise prescriptions generalizable to combined arm and leg exercise? *J Cardiopulmonary Rehabil* 7:551–555, 1987.
153. Franklin BA, Scherf J, Pamatmat A, et al: Arm-exercise testing and training. *Practical Cardiology* 8:43–70, 1982.
154. Makalous SL, Araujo J, Thomas TR: Energy expenditure during walking with hand weights. *Phys Sportsmed* 16:139–148, 1988.
155. Frost G: The Playbuoy exerciser. *American Corrective Therapy Journal* 31:156, 1977.
156. Zohman LR: Exercise stress test interpretation for cardiac diagnosis and functional evaluation. *Arch Phys Med Rehabil* 58:235–240, 1977.
157. Hossack KF, Bruce RA, Kusumi F: Altered exercise ventilatory responses by apparent propranolol-diminished glucose metabolism: Implications concerning impaired physical training benefit in coronary patients. *Am Heart J* 102:378–382, 1981.
158. Pratt CM, Welton DE, Squires WG, et al: Demonstration of training effect during chronic beta-adrenergic blockage in patients with coronary artery disease. *Circulation* 64:1125–1129, 1981.
159. Stuart RJ, Koyal SN, Lundstrom R, et al: Does exercise training alter maximal oxygen uptake in coronary artery disease during long-term beta-adrenergic blockade? *J Cardiopulmonary Rehabil* 5:410–414, 1985.
160. Froelicher V, Sullivan M, Myers J, et al: Can patients with coronary artery disease receiving beta blockers obtain a training effect? *Am J Cardiol* 55: 155D–161D, 1985.
161. Fletcher GF: Exercise training during chronic beta blockade in cardiovascular disease. *Am J Cardiol* 55:110D–113D, 1985.
162. Vanhees L, Fagard R, Amery A: Influence of beta-adrenergic blockade on the hemodynamic effects of physical training in patients with ischemic heart disease. *Am Heart J* 108:270–275, 1984.
163. Franklin BA, Borysyk L, Kornegger G, et al: Variable responses to exercise testing in patients on "long-acting" beta-blockade: Implications for exercise prescription (abst). *Med Sci Sports* 18(2)Suppl:S68, 1986.
164. Conn E, Williams RS, Wallace AG: Exercise responses before and after physical conditioning in patients with severely depressed left ventricular function. *Am J Cardiol* 49:296–300, 1982.
165. Le Tac B, Cribier A, Desplaches JF: A study of left ventricular function in coronary patients before and after physical training. *Circulation* 56:375–378, 1977.
166. Lee A, Ice R, Blessey R, et al: Long-term effects of physical training on coronary patients with impaired ventricular function. *Circulation* 60:1519–1526, 1979.
167. Hetherington M, Haennel R, Teo KK, et al: Importance of considering ventricular function when prescribing exercise after acute myocardial infarction. *Am J Cardiol* 58:891–895, 1986.
168. Franklin BA: Safety of outpatient cardiac exercise therapy: Reducing the incidence of complications. *Phys Sportsmed* 14:235–248, 1986.
169. Cobb LA, Weaver WD: Exercise: A risk for sudden death in patients with coronary heart disease. *J Am Coll Cardiol* 7:215–219, 1986.
170. Van Camp SP, Peterson RA: Cardiovascular complications of outpatient cardiac rehabilitation programs. *JAMA* 256:1160–1163, 1986.
171. Haskell WL: Safety of outpatient cardiac exercise programs: Issues regarding medical supervision. In Franklin BA, Rubenfire M (eds): *Cardiac Rehabilitation (Clinics in Sports Medicine)*. Philadelphia, WB Saunders, 1984, p 445.
172. Franklin BA, Wrisley D, Johnson S, et al: Chronic adaptations to physical conditioning in cardiac patients: Implications regarding exercise trainability. In Franklin BA, Rubenfire M (eds): *Cardiac Rehabilitation (Clinics in Sports Medicine)*. Philadelphia, WB Saunders, 1984, p 471.
173. Franklin BA, Gordon S, Timmis GC: Adaptations to chronic exercise training in cardiac patients: An update. In Oldridge NB, Foster C, Schmidt DH (eds): *Cardiac Rehabilitation and Clinical Exercise Programs: Theory and Practice*. Ithaca, New York, Mouvement Publications, 1988, p 111.

174. Franklin BA, Dressendorfer RH, Holloszy JO, et al: Physiological adaptations to chronic endurance exercise training in patients with coronary artery disease (A round table). *Phys Sportsmed* 15:129–154, 1987.
175. Franklin B, Buskirk E, Hodgson J, et al: Effects of physical conditioning on cardiorespiratory function, body composition and serum lipids in relatively normal weight and obese middle-aged women. *Int J Obes* 3:97–109, 1979.
176. Boyer JL, Kasch FW: Exercise therapy in hypertensive men. *JAMA* 211:1668–1671, 1970.
177. Streja D, Mymin D: Moderate exercise and high-density lipoprotein cholesterol: Observations during a cardiac rehabilitation program. *JAMA* 242:2190–2192, 1979.
178. Heath GW, Ehsani AA, Hagberg JM, et al: Exercise training improves lipoprotein lipid profiles in patients with coronary artery disease. *Am Heart J* 105:889–894, 1983.
179. Cowan GO: Influence of exercise on high-density lipoproteins. *Am J Cardiol* 52:13B–16B, 1983.
180. Blackburn H, Taylor HL, Hamrell B, et al: Premature ventricular complexes induced by stress testing: Their frequency and response to physical conditioning. *Am J Cardiol* 31:441–449, 1973.
181. Noakes TD, Higginson L, Opie LH: Physical training increases ventricular fibrillation thresholds of isolated rat hearts during normoxia, hypoxia and regional ischemia. *Circulation* 67:24–30, 1983.
182. Hammond HK: Exercise for coronary heart disease patients: Is it worth the effort? *J Cardiopulmonary Rehabil* 5:531–539, 1985.
183. Ehsani AA, Heath GW, Hagberg JM, et al: Effects of 12 months of intense exercise training on ischemic ST-segment depression in patients with coronary artery disease. *Circulation* 64:1116–1124, 1981.
184. Froelicher V, Jensen D, Atwood JE, et al: Cardiac rehabilitation: Evidence for improvement in myocardial perfusion and function. *Arch Phys Med Rehabil* 61:517–522, 1980.
185. Froelicher V, Jensen D, Genter F, et al: A randomized trial of exercise training in patients with coronary heart disease. *JAMA* 252:1291–1297, 1984.
186. Froelicher V, Jensen D, Sullivan M: A randomized trial of the effects of exercise training after coronary artery bypass surgery. *Arch Intern Med* 145:689–692, 1985.
187. Laslett LJ, Paumer L, Amsterdam EA: Increase in myocardial oxygen consumption indexes by exercise training at onset of ischemia in patients with coronary artery disease. *Circulation* 71:958–962, 1985.
188. Bloor CM, White FC, Sanders TM: Effects of exercise on collateral development in myocardial ischemia in pigs. *J Appl Physiol: Respirat Environ Exercise Physiol* 56:656–665, 1984.
189. Eckstein RW: Effect of exercise and coronary artery narrowing on coronary collateral circulation. *Circ Res* 5:230–235, 1957.
190. Conner JF, LaCamera F, Swanick EJ, et al: Effects of exercise on coronary collateralization—angiographic studies of six patients in a supervised exercise program. *Med Sci Sports* 8:145–151, 1976.
191. Ferguson RJ, Petitclerc R, Choquette G, et al: Effect of physical training on treadmill exercise capacity, collateral circulation and progression of coronary disease. *Am J Cardiol* 34:764–769, 1974.
192. Bassler TJ: Marathon running and immunity to heart disease. *Phys Sportsmed* 3:77–80, 1975.
193. Gamble P, Froelicher VF: Can an exercise program worsen heart disease? *Phys Sportsmed* 10:69–77, 1982.
194. Noakes TD, Opie LH, Rose AG: Marathon running and immunity to coronary heart disease: Fact versus fiction. In Franklin BA, Rubenfire M (eds): *Cardiac Rehabilitation (Clinics in Sports Medicine)*. Philadelphia, WB Saunders, 1984, p 527.

CHAPTER 4

Nonischemic Cardiovascular Disease

T. William Moir, M.D.

Exercise testing and exercise training programs are now standard procedures in the diagnosis and treatment of ischemic heart disease. The established value of these applications has prompted a growing interest in their use in nonischemic cardiovascular disease. The purpose of this chapter is to evaluate the diagnostic efficacy of exercise testing and to assess the value of exercise training programs in nonischemic cardiovascular conditions. The conditions of interest are essential hypertension, valvular heart disease, mitral valve prolapse, congenital heart disease, cardiomyopathy, cardiac arrhythmias and conduction defects, and electronic pacemakers. The role of exercise testing and training for cardiac transplant patients is also considered.

ESSENTIAL HYPERTENSION

Hypertension is a major public health problem for the United States with at least 35 million people affected (1). This number includes patients with mild hypertension (defined as diastolic blood pressures between 90 and 104 mm Hg) for whom drug therapy has been ineffective in reducing overall mortality risk or preventing the development of clinical complications such as ischemic heart disease. Detection is usually achieved incidentally through casual blood pressure measurements by physicians or other health care personnel. Nonetheless, it is important to identify such patients so that hygienic measures, such as dietary sodium restriction, weight control, discontinuance of cigarette smoking, and, perhaps, exercise conditioning, might be recommended as efforts to reduce cardiovascular risk. If these measures are beneficial, then such interventions prior to the development of established hypertension would be of value. Recent experience with exercise testing in certain populations indicates that selected individuals predisposed to established hypertension can be identified. There is also growing interest in the use of exercise testing to predict future blood pressure trends in patients with established hypertension. Moreover, there is evidence that exercise training can reduce blood pressure in mild hypertension and, extrapolating from that, may prevent the development of established hypertension in patients identified by exercise testing as predisposed.

The objectives of this section are to review the data that support the efficacy of exercise testing for identifying and categorizing hypertensive and hypertension-prone individuals, and to assess the value of exercise training as a hygienic measure in the prevention and treatment of borderline or mild hypertension, here defined as systolic pressure greater than 140 mm Hg and diastolic pressure of 90 to 100 mm Hg.

Exercise Testing

Abnormal blood pressure responses to dynamic exercise in subjects who are normotensive at rest may be predictive of future established hypertension. As summarized in Table 4.1, population studies suggest a small but definite power to predict subsequent resting hypertension in patients who have exaggerated blood pressure responses to dynamic exercise. This is true for both an exaggerated systolic pressure rise (greater than 200 to 230 mm Hg) and/or abnormal diastolic pressure (in-

Table 4.1
Hypertensive Response to Dynamic Exercise in Normotensive Populations and Prediction of Subsequent Resting Hypertension

Study (Type)	Normotensive at Rest (No.)	Hypertensive with Exercise (No.)	Prevalence of Hypertensive Response (%)	Follow-up (months)	Subsequent Hypertension (%)	
					Exercise Normotensive	Exercise Hypertensive
Wilson and Meyer (2) (prospective)	2746	341	12.4	32	9	21.0
Dlin et al. (3) (case control)	5098	102	2.0	70	0	10.6
Jackson et al. (4) (case control)	4856	53	1.1	48	15	51.0

crease more than 10 mm Hg or greater than 90 mm Hg). In the prospective study of Wilson and Meyer (2), 21% of the exercise hypertensive responders subsequently developed resting hypertension, corresponding to a relative risk of 2.28 when compared with those who had normal resting and exercise blood pressure. In one of the two case control studies summarized in Table 4.1 (3, 4) the predictive accuracy is as high as 51%. However, the predictive value of a positive test is generally low, that is, most subjects found to have an exaggerated blood pressure response to exercise do not develop resting hypertension on follow-up evaluation. On the other hand, these studies show a high degree of specificity, that is, in the absence of an abnormal blood pressure response to exercise there is a low probability of subsequent development of resting hypertension.

The mechanism underlying the exaggerated blood pressure response to exercise prior to development of resting hypertension is unknown. However, an obvious area of interest in this regard is the sympathetic nervous system. Plasma catecholamines have been found to be higher in patients with essential hypertension (5, 6), and it is postulated that exercise testing provokes an exaggerated sympathetic response that may serve as a marker for the subsequent development of established hypertension (7). Consequently, exercise testing may be an effective tool for screening selected populations, particularly those with a familial predilection to hypertension and those with other known coronary risk factors for whom predictive knowledge of the future development of hypertension would be of clinical value.

A practical impediment to large-scale application of such prehypertensive screening is the availability and cost of exercise testing. For wide application, guidelines and methodologies will have to be developed that are simpler than those currently recommended by the American Heart Association and the American College of Cardiology (8). The development of a field test, as suggested by the American College of Sports Medicine, may provide a practical means of exercise testing in large populations (9). Personal characteristics can serve as predictors of an exaggerated systolic pressure response to exertion and identify those who might benefit from exercise testing (10). For example, among both men and women, age, obesity, and cigarette smoking, and, in women, alcohol consumption (10) are positively associated with a disproportionate systolic blood pressure response to exercise and are themselves risk factors for hypertension.

Exercise testing is widely used in hypertensive patients as a method for detecting occult or suspected coronary artery disease. More recently, however, dynamic exercise testing has been used as a noninvasive method for studying hypertensive responses and hemodynamics in hypertensive patients, especially to predict future blood pressure trends in hypertensive adolescents.

Fixler et al. (11) followed 131 adolescents who were found to be hypertensive during a blood pressure screening of 10,641 eighth grade students. Hypertensive students had repeat blood pressure measurements and an exercise test 1 year later, and follow-up resting blood pressure measurements at 2 years. Regression analysis was used to examine the association between earlier resting pressures and exercise pressures with the final outcome resting pressures. Blood pressure during dynamic exercise did not significantly contribute to prediction of future systolic or diastolic pressures; rather, the average resting systolic pressure on the earlier screening was the best predictor of systolic pressure 2 years later.

In a study of 63 young women (average age 21 years) who were hypertensive during an adolescent pregnancy and then studied 3 to 6 years later, both resting blood pressure and systolic blood pressure responses to exercise were higher than those observed in a control group of women who had had normotensive pregnancies (12). Although it is clear that hypertension during an adolescent pregnancy denotes an increased risk of future established hypertension, an exaggerated postpartum exercise blood pressure response does not add to detection since the resting blood pressure usually remains elevated above normal in these subjects (12). Similarly, the study of Nudel et al. (13), in which adolescents with sustained essential hypertension were shown to have exaggerated exercise blood pressures as compared with normal children or those with labile blood pressures, indicates that exercise testing adds little to that which is already known except, perhaps, the identification of the occasional young hypertensive who may develop a "dangerously high blood pressure during exercise."

In patients with established hypertensive cardiovascular disease, exercise testing may help in categorizing cardiac performance during exercise. Wong et al. (14) showed that with isolated blood pressure elevation there is no impairment of exercise performance or evidence of subendocardial ischemia. With left ventricular hypertrophy, however, maximal exercise duration is decreased and there frequently is evidence for myocardial ischemia. Wu et al's (15) study of 40 subjects with varying degrees of hypertension showed a higher prevalence of exercise-induced ST-segment abnormalities in patients with evidence for more advanced hypertension as reflected in left ventricular hypertrophy. Moreover, antihypertensive therapy was associated with regression of left ventricular hypertrophy in the resting electrocardiogram of some patients and an impressive reduction in the prevalence of exercise-related ST-segment abnormalities. However, as shown by other investigators, regression of ventricular repolarization abnormalities is also evident on the resting electrocardiograms of patients who demonstrate reductions in blood pressure with antihypertensive therapy (16–18). Therefore, although exercise testing of patients with hypertensive cardiovascular disease is of physiologic interest, it cannot be recommended as an integral component of an antihypertensive program unless an exercise training program is planned. However, some clinicians believe that exercise testing has a role in assessing the response to antihypertensive therapy, although it is admittedly impractical on a routine basis (19).

Isometric tests such as handgrip cause elevations of blood pressure and are estimates of sympathetic adjustments. However, they have no proven utility in prediction of hypertension or evaluation of the sympathetic nervous system status in patients with established hypertension. The handgrip test has been studied in hypertensive patients and found to be a relatively poor index of autonomic function as compared with autonomic sympathetic adjustments to upright tilt or the Valsalva maneuver (20).

Exercise Prescription

Recent epidemiologic studies show that high levels of physical fitness are associated with lower blood pressures, predominantly systolic, as compared with subjects with lower levels of fitness. This is true for selected population prevalence data (21), as well as for subjects studied prospectively

(22, 23). Although a natural selection bias—"them that has, does"—cannot be entirely excluded, the inverse relationship between physical fitness obtained by vigorous exercise and hypertension risk has focused attention on exercise training as possibly therapeutic for borderline and mild hypertension. Considering that there is as yet no unanimity of opinion with respect to drug therapy at these blood pressure levels (diastolic 90 to 100 mm Hg), the use of exercise training as a component of a hygienic approach that also emphasizes salt restriction and weight control is entirely appropriate (24). An intensification of efforts to further document the efficacy of nonpharmacologic measures in the management of hypertension, including exercise training, is timely considering a recent study that shows more than 25% of patients normotensive on medication remain so for at least a year after discontinuance of drug therapy (25).

Table 4.2 is a modified summary of recent studies of the effect of relatively low-level intensity exercise training on blood pressure (26). These data show modest but statistically significant blood pressure decreases following aerobic exercise training programs in hypertensive patients (27–34). Because of the small numbers of patients and slight reductions in blood pressure (13 and 9 mm Hg average declines in systolic and diastolic pressure, respectively), it is difficult to attribute clinical significance to these changes. A Gertrude Stein aphorism is pertinent here—"a difference to be significantly different must make a difference"—and it remains to be shown whether decreases in blood pressure of this magnitude reduce the cardiovascular risks of hypertension. Additionally, there are similarly conducted studies that show no significant reduction in blood pressure as a result of exercise training (35–38). Nonetheless, these data support further study of exercise training as a potential alternative to drug treatment in mild hypertension.

Patients with diastolic blood pressure of 100 mm Hg or more should be treated pharmacologically as a primary intervention. However, concomitant hygienic measures, such as salt restriction and weight reduction, must be stressed. If this combination antihypertensive management program is successful in reducing blood pressure, an exercise training program is then appropriate. Under these circumstances an exercise test is recommended to ascertain that exaggerated blood pressure responses are not provoked by exercise.

Successful antihypertensive drug ther-

Table 4.2
Effect of Aerobic Exercise Training on Resting Blood Pressure[a]

Study	No. of Patients	Blood Pressure (mm Hg)					P
		Pretraining		Posttraining		Change (%) Systolic/Diastolic	
		Systolic	Diastolic	Systolic	Diastolic		
Boyer and Kasch (27)	23	159	105	146	93	−13(8%)/−12(11%)	<0.01
Choquette and Ferguson (28)	37	136 ± 13	90 ± 7	122 ± 14	82 ± 10	−14(10%)/−9(9%)	<0.01
Bonanno and Lies (29)	12	148	97	135	83	−13(9%)/−14(14%)	<0.01
Krotkiewski et al. (30)	27	134 ± 20	87 ± 8	125 ± 20	80 ± 9	−9(7%)/−7(8%)	<0.01
Roman et al. (31)	27	182 ± 16	113 ± 9	154 ± 7	97 ± 5	−28(15%)/−16(4%)	<0.01
Kukkonen et al. (32)	12	145 ± 14	99 ± 3	136 ± 10	88 ± 10	−9(6%)/−11(11%)	<0.01
Hagberg et al. (33)	25	137 ± 5	80 ± 10	129 ± 5	75 ± 10	−8(6%)/−5(6%)	<0.01
Duncan et al. (34)	44	146 ± 1	94 ± 1	134 ± 1	87 ± 1	−12(8%)/−7(7%)	<0.01

[a] **Modified from Seals D, Hagberg J: The effect of exercise training on human hypertension: a review. *Med Sci Sports Exerc* 16:207–215, 1984.**

apy is associated with reduction of mean arterial blood pressure both at rest and during exercise, but the mechanisms of benefit of medications differ. Although total peripheral resistance is decreased with diuretics and vasodilators (both direct and centrally acting), β-blockers' antihypertensive effect is associated with reduction in both resting and exercise cardiac output and heart rate. As is well recognized, these latter effects may be significant impediments to exercise performance, and the limitation of heart rate response by β-blockade requires exercise intensity end points for training programs other than attainment of selected percentages of age-predicted heart rates. In these circumstances, attainment of an optimal level of exercise as judged by perceived exertion during exercise testing (the Borg Rating of Perceived Exertion) can be effectively used (39). Finally, because of the ventricular arrhythmia risk associated with prolongation of the electrocardiographic Q-T interval, hypokalemia must be avoided by potassium supplementation or by the use of potassium-sparing diuretics among treated patients in exercise training programs.

Isometric exercises cause significant increases in blood pressure in both untreated and treated hypertensive subjects. Recent studies of the isometric handgrip test during use of various combinations of antihypertensive agents (β-blockers plus diuretics, β-blockers plus diuretics plus vasodilators, α-methyldopa alone, and labetalol) show no significant attenuation of the isometric hypertensive reflex (40). These findings, together with evidence that prolonged isometric exercise is associated with excessive renal retention of sodium and potassium (41), support the generally held view that isometric types of training programs should be avoided by hypertensive patients.

VALVULAR HEART DISEASE

Nowadays a major clinical problem in the management of patients with valvular heart disease is the need for accurate assessment of the optimal time for valve surgery. Generally, the functional status of the patient, as judged by the symptomatic classification of the New York Heart Association, and the graphic information obtained from chest x-rays, electrocardiograms, and echocardiograms remain the most important predictors. Recently, the noninvasive measurement of left ventricular function during exercise by exercise radionuclide angiography has proven to be of value in the preoperative assessment of patients with valvular heart disease. The purpose of this section is to review the efficacy of exercise testing as part of the selection process in the timing of valvular heart surgery and the appropriateness of its use in postoperative evaluation. Additionally, the role of exercise training of patients with prosthetic heart valves will be examined.

Exercise Testing

Aortic Valve Disease

Hochreiter and Borer (42) state that the goal of exercise testing in valvular heart disease is to obtain information with regard to exercise tolerance, exercise-related arrhythmias, chronotropic capacity, ventricular function, and, in some cases, adequacy of myocardial perfusion during exercise. In the case of aortic stenosis, the benefits of acquiring these data through exercise testing must be balanced against the inherent risk of exercise stress. At the present time, in adults, the additional information obtained by exercise testing does not outweigh the risk, and candidates for aortic valve replacement should continue to be evaluated on the basis of functional status and the results of other noninvasive clinical assessments (43). However, as will subsequently be discussed, this is not the case with congenital aortic stenosis in children.

With aortic valvular regurgitation, valve replacement may or may not be recommended for patients who are asymptomatic or minimally symptomatic (functional classes I and II). Thus, noninvasive methods, including exercise testing, should be considered to evaluate the major determinant of benefit and survivorship after valve replacement, namely, left ventricular function. Although the duration of graded exercise, particularly when used in conjunction with echocardiographic assessment of left ventricular function, is a good predictor of postoperative survival (44), the determination of left ventricular ejection fraction by exercise radionuclide angiography is more effective in assessing early signs of left ventricular dysfunction. This is particularly true for asymptomatic patients whose left ventricular function is normal at rest but shows unchanged or decreased ejection fraction during exercise (45). However, this is an impractical recommendation for all patients with aortic regurgitation. Rather, it is more appropriately used in those patients who, although asymptomatic, show echocardiographic signs of increasing left ventricular end-systolic dimension (greater than 55 mm). If the radionuclide exercise ejection fraction is abnormal, a recommendation for valve replacement might be considered. Finally, for aortic regurgitation patients who fail to thrive hemodynamically after aortic valve replacement, radionuclide exercise angiography serves as a noninvasive evaluation of left ventricular function that can establish the need for invasive study to evaluate candidacy for possible reoperation.

Mitral Valve Disease

There is a limited role for exercise testing in mitral stenosis. Generally, functional classification based on symptoms remains the major criterion for recommending surgical therapy (mitral valvuloplasty or mitral valve replacement). The validity of symptoms as a guideline for surgical intervention is supported by the studies of Bishop and Wade (46) that show a good correlation between functional classification and the mean pulmonary artery pressure, both at rest and during exercise, which is an accepted index of severity of mitral stenosis. Although treadmill testing has been used in the evaluation of patients with mitral stenosis, there is a poor correlation between the degree of mitral stenosis and the duration of symptom-limited treadmill exercise. Therefore, present data support the continued use of functional classification as the major guideline to surgical intervention in mitral stenosis (47), together with graphic information acquired noninvasively by x-ray, electrocardiography, and echocardiography.

As in mitral stenosis, the need for valve replacement in patients with mitral regurgitation is generally determined by symptomatic status. However, in contrast to valve surgery in mitral stenosis, surgical results with mitral regurgitation are often disappointing because of residual left ventricular dysfunction. This is a result of volume overload of the left ventricle and irreversible structural change that may occur prior to the appearance of symptoms that would ordinarily prompt mitral valve surgery. Therefore, there is a growing acceptance of the use of exercise radionuclide angiography to evaluate left ventricular function by measurement of exercise ejection fraction; the resting ejection fraction is not sufficient since a normal value may merely reflect a large amount of mitral regurgitation rather than a decreased forward flow (48, 49). While such monitoring of left ventricular function in patients with mitral regurgitation is of value for recommending valvular surgery at an opportune time, there are technical limitations with respect to availability of equipment, complexity, and cost. Although the use of this radionuclide procedure may become more prevalent in the future, a technical breakthrough with the development of exercise echocardiography may simplify the acquisition of these important data in patients (50).

Table 4.3 summarizes the author's opinion regarding the clinical value of dynamic exercise testing and exercise radionuclide angiography for the pre- and postoperative evaluation of patients with valvular heart disease.

Exercise Prescription

There is now considerable information regarding the effect of cardiac valve surgery on exercise capacity (51–53). Generally, these studies show that functional capacity is substantially increased following aortic valve replacement; in contrast, patients undergoing mitral and mitral/aortic valve surgery show little or no improvement (51). An improvement in oxygen uptake in response to cycle ergometer exercise follow-

Table 4.3
Clinical Value of Noninvasive Dynamic Exercise Testing in Valvular Heart Disease

Valve Disease	Preoperative		Postoperative	
	Treadmill/Bike	Bike Radionuclide Angiography	Treadmill/Bike	Bike Radionuclide Angiography
Aortic stenosis	No	No	No	No
Aortic regurgitation	No	Yes	No	Yes
Mitral stenosis	No	No	No	No
Mitral regurgitation	No	Yes	No	Yes

ing aortic valve replacement as compared with preoperative testing appears to be due to an altered oxygen uptake kinetics associated with favorable changes in exercise heart rate and arterial venous oxygen difference (52). Additionally, analysis of the effect of aortic valve replacement on exercise capacity assessed by anaerobic threshold measurements shows that about one-third of the patients have an improvement in this variable, especially those who are at lower preoperative thresholds (53).

Postoperative exercise training studies are limited in number and scope, and the results are not sufficiently favorable with respect to improvement of aerobic capacity to suggest that patients enter such programs. In large part this may be due to associated irreversible myocardial damage, particularly as might be the case with rheumatic heart disease. A single study of physical training after heart valve replacement, consisting of a 24-week period of daily, low-intensity aerobic exercise (Royal Canadian Air Force program), showed improvement beyond the immediate postoperative recovery phase in patients who were in the long-term exercise program as compared with patients who carried on usual activity (54). However, the improvement in aerobic capacity in these patients was of insufficient magnitude to recommend postoperative aerobic fitness programs in valvular surgery patients. Because many patients are on anticoagulants, have prosthetic valves that may cause mechanical hemolysis during exercise-induced tachycardia, and have limited valve orifice sizes, caution is suggested in recommending moderate- to high-intensity exercise training programs.

MITRAL VALVE PROLAPSE

It is generally accepted that the myxomatous "floppy mitral valve" associated with mitral prolapse is now the commonest cause of mitral regurgitation, at least in populations from which rheumatic heart disease has virtually disappeared. However, this end point, although eventually reached by an unknown number of patients, is a relatively infrequent clinical consequence of mitral valve prolapse. More prevalent are problems related to ventricular ectopy, both at rest and with exercise, and electrocardiographic abnormalities under these same circumstances (55). However, recent and more rigorous epidemiologic study shows that although there is a mitral valve prolapse "syndrome," it is seen in small numbers of patients who are referred to tertiary care centers for evaluation of symptoms, electrocardiographic abnormalities, and arrhythmias.

In most mitral valve prolapse patients, the frequency of symptoms and electrocardiographic findings is not significantly different from that in an unselected population (56). However, there are an unknown number of patients with what has been termed the "primary mitral valve prolapse syndrome" characterized by atypical chest pain, palpitations, auscultatory systolic clicks, and echocardiographic evidence of prolapse without any other cardiac abnormality (57). This symptom complex frequently leads to exercise testing for evaluation of the atypical chest pain and the cardiac dysrhythmia, usually ventricular premature beats.

Exercise Testing

In contrast to asymptomatic patients with mitral valve prolapse who generally show no significant abnormalities or functional aerobic impairment on exercise testing (58), symptomatic patients have a relatively high prevalence of exercise-induced electrocardiographic ST-segment abnormalities and ventricular ectopy. However, simultaneous myocardial perfusion scintigraphy with thallium demonstrates that these are false-positive electrocardiographic changes with respect to coronary artery disease, although, of course, the two may coexist (59). These data show a significant lowering of the specificity and predictive values of abnormal exercise tests in patients with mitral valve prolapse, and suggest that testing should not be done without a simultaneous thallium myocardial perfusion study if the indication is solely to evaluate chest pain. Although ventricular ectopy is frequently found in patients with mitral valve prolapse, life-threatening arrhythmias are rare (60, 61). Therefore, routine attempts to detect arrhythmias by exercise provocation serve no useful purpose unless patients have symptoms during exercise and the nature of the arrhythmia needs to be known for consideration of appropriate therapy. Finally, exercise radionuclide angiography for evaluation of left ventricular function is not warranted in these patients unless coexisting coronary artery disease is suspected; wall motion abnormalities in mitral valve prolapse patients are usually associated with arteriographic evidence of coronary artery disease (62).

Exercise Prescription

Generally, in asymptomatic patients with mitral valve prolapse, there is no need for exercise testing prior to beginning a physical training program. In contrast, exercise testing appears to be warranted among patients with a history of exercise-induced symptoms, particularly palpitations. It has been suggested that aerobic exercise training may be beneficial for mitral valve prolapse patients without functionally significant mitral regurgitation. Limited data demonstrate that such patients completing a 12-week jogging program achieve a cardiovascular training effect and a decrease in both the prevalence and complexity of preexercise ventricular ectopy (63). If, as suggested by Wooley (64), some of the components of the mitral valve prolapse syndrome are due to a hyperadrenergic state, then an enhanced parasympathetic (vagal) state after training with regular aerobic exercise should be of therapeutic value. Clearly, this possibility needs further investigation.

CONGENITAL HEART DISEASE

There are increasing numbers of patients with congenital heart disease reaching adult life as a result of the remarkable achievements of cardiovascular surgery. Indeed, total physiologic correction has been attained in a variety of congenital heart defects. The purpose of this section is to review the need and utility of exercise testing to document the efficacy of these repairs. The defects of most clinical interest and importance include transposition of the great vessels, tetralogy of Fallot, congenital aortic stenosis, coarctation of the aorta, pulmonary valvular stenosis, and both atrial and ventricular septal defects. The role of exercise training after successful surgery in these patients will also be briefly reviewed.

Exercise Testing

Tetralogy of Fallot

Definitive repair of tetralogy of Fallot has been successfully achieved for more than 20 years. Advances in surgical techniques have allowed closure of the ventricular septal defect, reconstruction of the ventricular outflow tract, and avoidance of damage to the cardiac conduction system. Long-term evaluation of the outcome of this surgery documents excellent late clinical results in almost 90% of hospital survivors after surgery (65); late mortality is predominantly due to cardiac causes with a significant frequency of sudden death. Garson et al. (66) studied 104 patients who underwent treadmill testing at an average of 7 years after repair of tetralogy of Fallot. In 14% of the patients, ventricular arrhythmias were evident at rest but increased to 30% with treadmill exercise. Uniform ventricular premature beats were the most prevalent, but multiform beats were also seen and ventricular tachycardia occurred in one patient. Hemodynamic evaluation by cardiac catheterization shortly after treadmill testing revealed a significant correlation between the prevalence of ventricular ectopy and the levels of both systolic and diastolic pressures in the right ventricle. More recently, a study of exercise testing performed 1 to 16 years after correction of tetralogy confirms a relatively high prevalence (25%) of ventricular ectopy in postoperative tetralogy patients; the arrhythmia was variously seen just prior to, during, or after exercise (67). Additional hemodynamic information obtained in selected patients confirmed the probability of abnormal ventricular function as the etiology of the arrhythmia. Thus, it appears that exercise testing is an effective screening method for ventricular arrhythmias in these patients and that complex forms of ectopy are associated with the risk of sudden cardiac death. Therefore, it is clear that exercise testing has an important role in the postoperative management of tetralogy patients (68), and is a valuable testing method in efforts to suppress this arrhythmia with pharmacologic therapy. Limited data suggest that phenytoin appears to have the most beneficial antiarrhythmic effect (69), although the newer classes of suppressive agents may be found to be even more useful after appropriate evaluation.

Congenital Aortic Valvular Stenosis

Electrocardiographic responses to exercise testing in children with aortic stenosis are of value in estimating the severity of aortic obstruction. With dynamic exercise this is manifested by electrocardiographic evidence of subendocardial ischemia at a time when resting hemodynamic evaluation of the left ventricular aortic gradient may show only a mild degree of obstruction. In some patients, the abnormal electrocardiographic response to exercise returns toward normal during postoperative follow-up (70). The presumed mechanism for the electrocardiographic change is subendocardial ischemia due to an imbalance between myocardial oxygen demand and supply in the inner layers of the left ventricle during the increased pressure conditions (both systolic and diastolic) in that chamber during exercise (71).

In addition to electrocardiographic abnormalities as predictors of hemodynamically significant aortic stenosis, these patients also show a lower than normal blood pressure response to dynamic exercise that has potential use for the noninvasive evaluation of children with this defect. The postexercise systolic blood pressure minus the preexercise systolic pressure (the "delta" pressure), when used in conjunction with electrocardiographic changes during exercise, increases the clinician's ability to select for catheterization assessment those patients who are likely to require aortic valve surgery (72). Clearly, these data confirm an important role for noninvasive exercise testing in patients with congenital valvular aortic stenosis. It is useful both as a component of preoperative procedures to select proper timing for aortic valve surgery as well as serving a monitoring function during long-term follow-up postoperatively.

Coarctation of the Aorta

Exercise-induced hypertension occurs frequently after surgical repair of coarctation of the aorta and may be accompanied by electrocardiographic ST-segment depression (73, 74). In exercise studies with normal controls, blood pressure increases significantly in both groups but is significantly higher in the coarctectomy patients (75). Additionally, blood pressure in the leg increases significantly from resting in the normal control subject but is unchanged in the coarctectomy patients. These findings suggest that a residual obstruction across the site of the coarctectomy causes the observed postexercise systolic hypertension in the arm as compared to controls. Therefore, exercise testing with blood pressure measurements should be performed in all children after coarctectomy, and repeat catheterization advised for consideration of reoperation if the postexercise systolic pressure rise is excessive, that is, greater than 200 mm Hg (75). Alternatively, some restriction of physical activities and/or use of antihypertensive drugs might be advised.

Atrial and Ventricular Septal Defects

Upright exercise studies in patients with defects of cardiac septation are limited. Existing hemodynamic data have been obtained with dynamic, upright exercise in patients following operative correction of secundum atrial septal defects. These studies show that in spite of normal hemodynamic findings at rest, patients may have impairment of cardiac output during exercise in the absence of residual shunts, cardiac arrhythmias, or pulmonary hypertension (76). However, many of these patients were symptomatic before surgery, some in functional class II of the New York Heart Association, although they became asymptomatic and in functional class I postoperatively. Nonetheless, irreversible changes in function concomitant with their preoperative symptomatic state may have already been established, and these data should not be used to limit physical activity in patients with asymptomatic atrial septal defects. Dynamic exercise testing is, however, probably a prudent recommendation for such patients who wish to begin a training program.

Ventricular septal defects are the sole abnormality in 20 to 25% of children with congenital heart disease (77). Recent catheterization studies of adolescents with small-to-moderate ventricular defects (left to right shunt smaller than 50% of left ventricular output and normal pulmonary vascular resistance) indicate that the pulmonary and systemic blood flows both increase but the left to right shunt remains unchanged, implying that the shunt volume per beat decreases during exercise (78). Because the systemic blood flow rises normally without a corresponding increase in left to right shunt flow, it is concluded that the hemodynamic effects of dynamic exercise are favorable, and patients with such defects should not be restricted in aerobic exercise activities. This is particularly true because in a significant percentage of patients, shunt flow decreases with advancing age and the septal defect may close spontaneously (79, 80).

Pulmonary Stenosis

Isolated pulmonary valvular stenosis is less prevalent than some of the aforementioned defects and accounts for about 8% of congenital heart disease. However, its natural history is not well known, and patients may exhibit varying degrees of abnormalities from minimal signs of pulmonary stenosis to rapid appearance of right-sided heart failure due to fibrosis or hypertrophy. Supine exercise studies have been obtained during cardiac catheterization of both children and adults in an attempt to categorize the hemodynamic consequences of pulmonary stenosis over time (81). These studies reveal significant hemodynamic differences at rest and during exercise between adults and children with severe pulmonary stenosis (valve area less than 0.5 cm^2/m^2). Exercise heart rates and cardiac index were lower in adults than in children as was the maximum elevation of right ventricular systolic pressure during exercise. These data suggest that long-standing severe pulmonary stenosis causes hemodynamic abnormalities probably due to right ventricular myocardial dysfunction; therefore, early relief of severe pulmonary stenosis in childhood should be recommended (81). Noninvasive dynamic exercise does not have a clear role in evaluating the functional status of patients with isolated pulmonic stenosis other than to document reductions in aerobic capacity.

The author's opinion of the clinical value of exercise testing in the aforementioned congenital defects is summarized in Table 4.4. Dynamic exercise is of general value in ascertaining aerobic capacity irrespective of etiology; moreover, it may reveal specific

Table 4.4
Clinical Value of Noninvasive Dynamic Exercise Testing for Provocation of Abnormalities in Common Congenital Heart Diseases

Cardiac Defect	O_2 Capacity	Stenotic Gradients	Arrhythmias	ECG Abnormalities
Aortic stenosis	Yes	Yes	Yes	Yes
Coarctation of aorta	Yes	Yes	No	Yes
Tetralogy of Fallot	Yes	No	Yes	Yes
Ventricular septal defect	Yes	No	No	No
Atrial septal defect	Yes	No	No	No
Pulmonary stenosis	Yes	No	No	No

cardiovascular abnormalities that have significant diagnostic value, including stenotic gradients, arrhythmias, and ECG abnormalities.

Exercise Prescription

Regular dynamic exercise is generally considered a component of programs recommended for the primary prevention of cardiovascular diseases, particularly coronary artery disease. These preventive measures should be initiated in childhood to attain the earliest possible cardiovascular benefit and establish a lifelong pattern of hygienic habits, including regular exercise. For those reasons it is inappropriate arbitrarily to exclude all children with congenital heart defects from regular physical training programs. Rather, clinical situations should be individualized for patients with mild defects who do not require surgical intervention as well as for those who have had successful operative repairs.

In a remarkable study of 830 children with congenital heart defects, Cumming (82) has shown that a significant number of patients have reasonably normal exercise capacity as measured by the Bruce exercise protocol. This is true for the most prevalent congenital heart defects, including atrial septal defect, ventricular septal defect, congenital aortic stenosis, and pulmonary stenosis; however, treadmill endurance did not separate mild from significant disease as judged by prior catheterization studies in these patients. Only children with defects associated with persistent cyanosis or other more obviously severe disease had consistent reductions in exercise capacity. In contrast, in the majority of children with congenital defects Goldberg et al. (83) found a significant limitation of maximal exercise capacity that was remarkably improved after surgical repair.

Considering the significant advances in pediatric cardiac surgery, it is evident that most children with congenital defects should have total correction at a young age with the expectation of an improvement in exercise capacity. After successful surgical repair, children with congenital heart disease have shown increases in physical work capacity following dynamic exercise programs with improvement in cardiopulmonary efficiency, lipid profiles, and psychosocial adjustment (84–86). Considering these advances, it is timely for the American Heart Association to update its 1971 report that recommends recreational and occupational activity guidelines for physician use when counseling young patients with heart disease (87).

CARDIOMYOPATHY

Ischemic heart disease is the major cause of cardiomyopathy manifested by congestive heart failure. However, similar degrees of heart failure are seen with the syndrome of idiopathic dilated cardiomyopathy in sufficient numbers to be of clinical importance. By definition, the cause of the left ventricular disease is unknown, but it occurs without evidence of coronary artery disease. An additional but uncommon form of cardiomyopathy, the hypertrophic variety, is also of undetermined cause and is characterized by advanced left ventricular hypertrophy with and without outflow tract obstruction. The purpose of this section is to describe the role of exercise testing in these two forms of nonischemic cardiomyopathy. Additionally, the role that physical training might play as part of a management program for patients with left ventricular dysfunction will be discussed.

Exercise Testing

Idiopathic Dilated Cardiomyopathy

Consideration of the efficacy of exercise testing in this form of cardiomyopathy requires an examination of the experience with the more common cause of congestive heart failure, namely, ischemic heart disease. There is now an extensive experience with exercise testing of ischemic heart disease patients with either marked left ventricular dysfunction manifested by abnormally low ejection fractions or clinically apparent heart failure. Generally, these studies have been performed to correlate symptomatic functional classification with various indices of left ventricular dysfunction in order to establish hemodynamic data that can be compared after entering such patients in exercise training programs (88). For that purpose, exercise testing in ischemic heart disease has proved effective, but its role in functional evaluation in idiopathic dilated cardiomyopathy has had limited investigation.

In patients with class II or III heart failure associated with idiopathic dilated cardiomyopathy on therapy, radionuclide exercise ventriculography and hemodynamic monitoring show that the left ventricular ejection fraction remains essentially unchanged during exercise, and that high resting systemic and pulmonary vascular resistance persist (89). Moreover, functional capacity as measured by exercise duration is well preserved in one-half of the patients (10 of 20 subjects); these patients have significantly lower resting heart rates and, during exercise, higher cardiac outputs and lower systemic vascular resistance. This finding suggests a blunted sympathetic response in some of these subjects, but this is not unique to this etiology of heart disease (90–92). That being the case, exercise testing to assess functional capacity should be used for these patients, as is the case with ischemic heart disease, only when needed to assess response to change in therapy or any other intervention.

Hypertrophic Cardiomyopathy

Although an uncommon type of cardiomyopathy as compared with the idiopathic dilated variety, the hypertrophic form is associated with a high mortality rate. Many of these patients die suddenly, especially during vigorous exercise (about 4% per year), and the disease is the leading cause of unexpected death during competition among young athletes (93, 94). There is extensive experience with both invasive and noninvasive exercise testing in patients with hypertrophic cardiomyopathy. Such studies have been done to establish prognostic indicators, particularly as related to recommendations for exercise activity, and to evaluate both medical and surgical therapeutic interventions.

Hypertrophic cardiomyopathy patients can be classified into three groups: (*a*) those with generalized left ventricular hypertrophy without outflow tract obstruction; (*b*) those without obstruction at rest but with the development of a significant systolic gradient provoked by exercise; and (*c*) those with signs of obstruction both at rest and during exercise (95). As compared with patients with nonobstructive hypertrophic cardiomyopathy, those with resting left ventricular outflow tract gradients or with signs of obstruction provoked by exercise have evidence of left ventricular systolic dysfunction and shortened exercise duration. However, this distinction is not always clear-cut with respect to the correlation of hemodynamic evidence of outflow tract obstruction and symptomatic functional classification (96). Therefore, neither invasive nor noninvasive exercise evaluation can discriminate with sufficient accuracy so that exercise recommendations can be confidently made for hypertrophic cardiomyopathy patients with variable hemodynamic compromise during effort. However, exercise testing has proven value in assessing the efficacy of treatment modes in these patients.

Treadmill exercise capacity and symptomatic status have been evaluated in hypertrophic cardiomyopathy patients treated with β-blockade (propranolol) or a calcium channel blocker (verapamil). Verapamil treatment produces a significant decrease in the left ventricular outflow tract obstruction, and this is accompanied by an improved exercise capacity (97–99). Although propranolol similarly enhances exercise capacity, it is associated with deterioration of functional capacity in some patients (98).

Exercise capacity determined by treadmill testing shows a consistent improvement after septal myotomy and myectomy in patients with obstructive hypertrophic cardiomyopathy (100). Simultaneously measured cardiac output during testing suggests improved left ventricular function as the most significant contributor to the increased exercise capacity. Postoperative noninvasive study with radionuclide angiography during maximal exercise shows a normal ejection fraction response and demonstrates that global left ventricular function is not compromised by the surgical procedure (101).

Exercise Prescription

Williams (88) has summarized the rationale for considering exercise training of patients with left ventricular dysfunction and clinical heart failure. This approach is based on myocardial ischemia animal model data that suggest improvement in function and reduction of cardiac arrhythmias after training (102, 103). Whether an exercise training program is of benefit to patients with ischemia-related left ventricular dysfunction is not particularly relevant with respect to the idiopathic form of cardiomyopathy. One obvious difference is the segmental nature of the myocardial lesions in ischemic heart disease due to specific coronary artery lesions, compared with dilated cardiomyopathy where there generally is a global abnormality of left ventricular contractility.

The natural history of dilated cardiomyopathy reveals that patients who present with significant heart failure (functional classes III and IV) will have an accelerated course with almost two-thirds dying within 2 years (104, 105). Therefore, rest and avoidance of strenuous exertion are obvious parts of their management. However, these natural history data also show that almost one-fourth of patients show clinical improvement and reduction in heart size. This is particularly true for patients whose cardiomyopathy may be alcohol-related and in whom abstinence is maintained during treatment. Therefore, a small percentage of patients with idiopathic dilated cardiomyopathy may be potential candidates for an exercise training program, but it is unlikely that this would be of specific benefit as compared with abstinence from tobacco and alcohol, antiarrhythmics for control of ventricular ectopy, and reduction of left ventricular preload and afterload by vasodilators. Although it is attractive to consider that the benefits of aerobic training (slower heart rates at rest and with effort, reduction of peripheral vascular resistance, etc.) may be of benefit in the management of ischemic cardiomyopathy (106), it should not at this time be extended to patients with the idiopathic variety.

At present there are no clinical variables that are reliable for identifying those patients with hypertrophic cardiomyopathy who are at risk of sudden death (107). Additionally, no hemodynamic variable, such as magnitude of the left ventricular outflow tract obstruction or left ventricular end-diastolic pressure, characterizes patients with this disease who die suddenly. The majority of the patients who die suddenly are young (under 30 years) and without significant functional limitations. Finally, even in patients who have obtained symptomatic benefit from medical therapy (propranolol) or by surgical reduction of the left ventricular outflow tract obstruction, there is no demonstrated protection against sudden death (107, 108). Therefore, exercise training programs should not be recommended for patients with hypertrophic cardiomyopathy irrespective of their clinical status.

ARRHYTHMIAS AND CONDUCTION ABNORMALITIES

Cardiac arrhythmias, particularly ventricular ectopy, are the most common isolated abnormalities of cardiac function among persons without apparent heart disease. Although arrhythmias are clearly an important clinical feature in the natural history of the nonischemic cardiovascular conditions already considered, their significance as an isolated abnormality remains a perplexing clinical problem. This section evaluates the role of exercise testing as a method of detecting and categorizing these arrhythmias, and reviews the usefulness of exercise training as a primary intervention in their treatment. Although exercise testing has a limited role in evaluating primary cardiac conduction defects in otherwise presumably normal subjects, its utility in that regard will also be examined. Exercise training for patients with conduction defects managed by permanent transvenous pacemakers will also be considered.

Exercise Testing

Ventricular Ectopy

Premature ventricular beats occur in approximately 40 to 75% of normal persons as detected by continuous ambulatory electrocardiography (109–114). Although most of this ectopy is simple, that is, infrequent and without repetitive forms, a significant number of subjects have complex ectopy including frequent premature beats, multiforms, and brief runs of tachycardia (115). In long-term follow-up, the prognosis for such asymptomatic individuals is similar to that of a population without this arrhythmia (116). Dynamic exercise testing has also been used to expose the complexity of ventricular ectopy and to evaluate associated clinical features and prognosis in apparently healthy subjects. Additionally, exercise testing is being increasingly used to evaluate the risk of exertional-induced ventricular tachycardia. The prevalence of ventricular tachycardia associated with maximal treadmill exercise testing has been studied in a cohort of subjects without apparent heart disease from the Baltimore Longitudinal Study on Aging (117). Only 1.1% of subjects had exercise-induced ventricular tachycardia and this was not associated with increased cardiovascular morbidity or mortality over a 2-year period as compared with a group of age- and sex-matched control subjects. These data are similar to other studies of patients with ventricular arrhythmias exposed by treadmill testing, all of whom subsequently had cardiac catheterization; in those without significant coronary artery disease, no relation was found between exercise-induced ventricular arrhythmias and survival (118).

The traditional view that subjects with ventricular arrhythmias aggravated by exercise are more likely to have underlying heart disease than those in whom the arrhythmias are suppressed has been reevaluated since the work of Mann and Burchell in 1952 (119). It appears that an increase in preexisting ventricular arrhythmias is associated with a higher frequency of underlying cardiovascular disease than is suppression of ventricular ectopy during exercise (119–121). Nonetheless, the prognosis for future cardiac events did not differ between the two groups of patients, and suppression of ventricular arrhythmias by exercise does not guarantee freedom from occult cardiovascular disease (121). Therefore, for exercise testing of apparently normal subjects with complex ventricular arrhythmias, the addition of a radioactive thallium myocardial perfusion study should be considered, particularly if the person has coronary risk factors.

Of particular importance is the role of exercise testing in evaluating ventricular tachycardia in a young population without apparent heart disease. This arrhythmia is exercise related in a significant number of young patients with a history of tachycardia and can be reproduced by treadmill testing (122). Additionally, in some patients without ventricular tachycardia, it may appear during the recovery period. In contrast with adults, exercise-related cardiac dysrhythmias are rare in children without apparent heart disease (123) and should be evaluated by treadmill testing as well as by electrophysiologic studies, if indicated. Although a primary cardiomyopathy is the most common cause of ventricular ectopy in children, arrhythmogenic right ventricular dysplasia is increasingly recognized as an occult cardiac etiology of ventricular tachycardia, particularly that associated with exercise (124–127). Exercise testing is also an important procedure in the evaluation of patients with ventricular arrhythmias associated with prolonged Q-T or QT-U intervals (128). This is particularly true for the uncommon but clinically important congenital etiologies such as the Jervell and Lange-Nielsen (129) and the Romano and Ward syndromes (130) in which exercise may provoke reentrant ventricular arrhythmias because of an exaggeration of a preexisting cardiac sympathetic nerve imbalance. This may occur either during or immediately after exercise (128).

Podrid and Graboys (131) recommend the incorporation of exercise testing as an important tool in the selection of an antiarrhythmic program for patients with arrhythmias during exercise or recovery in spite of apparent control of ectopy at rest. Other individuals requiring therapy are those who have symptomatic ventricular tachycardia either at rest or with exertion, and those with heart disease who exhibit a high prevalence of asymptomatic ventricular premature beats, particularly salvos of nonsustained ventricular tachycardia that are not suppressed during exercise. Ambulatory electrocardiographic monitoring is also recommended as part of a systematic testing of drug efficacy, but the elimination or decreased frequency of ventricular arrhythmias during exercise is the major goal. Although sustained ventricular tachyarrhythmias requiring immediate medical treatment occurred in 9% of patients during exercise testing, there was no mortality or significant morbidity (131).

Of special interest with regard to exercise-related ventricular arrhythmias is their high prevalence among well-trained and apparently healthy endurance athletes. Ambulatory electrocardiography among apparently healthy runners during exercise reveals frequencies of 50 to 60% for isolated and simple ventricular premature beats with a lower frequency (5 to 10%) of more complex ectopy, including couplets and, uncommonly, short runs of ventricular tachycardia (132–135). Exercise testing is significantly less sensitive in exposing these ventricular arrhythmias than is ambulatory electrocardiography during a distance run (132). Therefore, exercise testing appears to have a limited utility for ventricular arrhythmia detection in trained subjects, although it has proven value for documenting the efficacy of suppressive drug therapy of these arrhythmias in symptomatic patients (131).

Figure 4.1 is a suggested algorithm for the noninvasive evaluation and management of apparently healthy subjects (without heart disease) with ventricular arrhythmias that are detected either incidentally or during the investigation of symptoms. An age criterion is suggested as a guideline for the extent of evaluation of simple ventricular premature beats because of epidemiologic evidence that it may be a risk factor associated with coronary artery disease in men age 40 or over (136, 137). Although this recommendation is controversial (138), an age criterion seems reasonable, especially for persons who are or wish to be involved in vigorous athletic activities.

Supraventricular Arrhythmias

Atrial and junctional premature beats occur in up to 27% of normal individuals during exercise testing (139, 140). Sustained episodes of exertion-induced supraventricular tachycardia or atrial fibrillation are relatively rare and occur in less than 2% of normal individuals during exercise testing (139). Moreover, there is no evidence that these arrhythmias are specific markers for occult heart disease, and insurance studies report no adverse effect of these evoked arrhythmias on mortality rates (141). As with ventricular premature beats, exercise testing to expose supraventricular arrhythmias is not as effective as 24-hour ambulatory electrocardiography (132). Therefore, exercise testing for su-

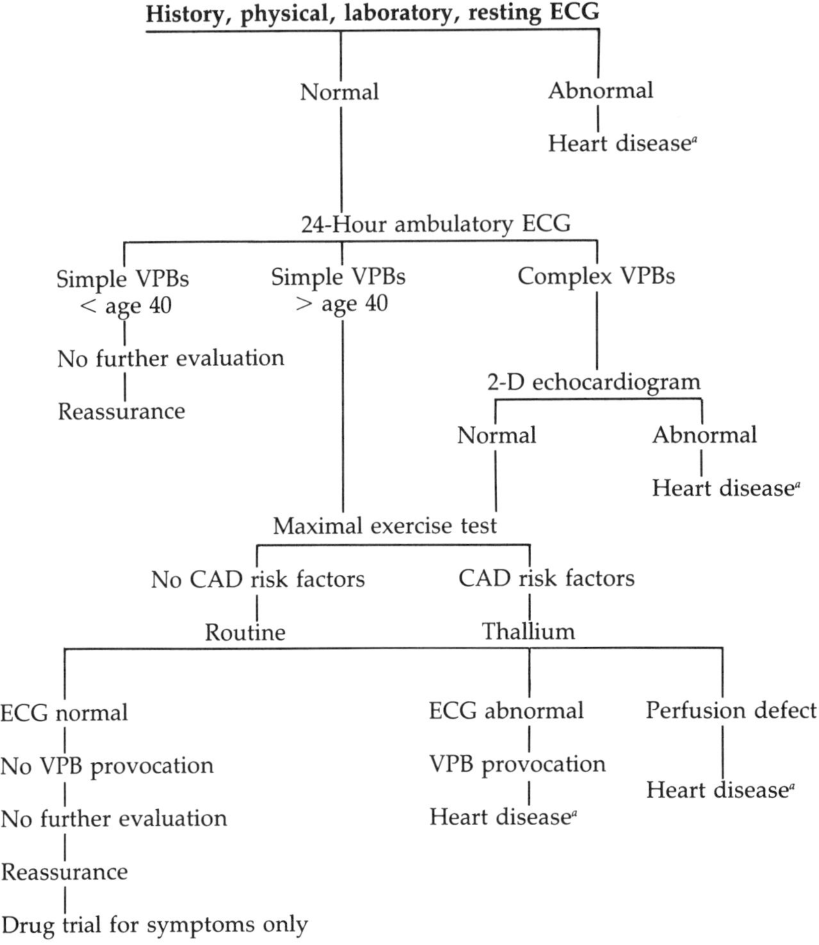

[a] **Further evaluation, including cardiac catheterization and electrophysiologic study, if indicated.**

Figure 4.1. Role of exercise testing in the evaluation of patients with ventricular premature beats (VPBs) without apparent heart disease. *Simple* indicates infrequent, uniform beats without repetitive forms. *Complex* indicates frequent, multiform beats, repetitive forms, and ventricular tachycardia. *CAD*, coronary artery disease.

praventricular arrhythmias should be used only as a detection method in patients who have exercise-related symptoms and in whom it may be important to distinguish supraventricular from ventricular arrhythmias. This would be the case for patients with Wolff-Parkinson-White syndrome who have a very high prevalence of supraventricular arrhythmias, particularly atrial fibrillation. Because exercise testing in these patients generally does not provoke supraventricular arrhythmias (142), its use should be limited to those patients who have palpitations during physical activity. In contrast, exercise testing may provoke supraventricular arrhythmias such as atrial fibrillation in patients with sinus node dysfunction, so screening for this anomaly might be considered (143). Additionally, exercise testing may provoke supraventricular arrhythmias in patients with either cardiac or cerebral symptoms during activity.

Conduction Defects

In sedentary but normal individuals atrioventricular (AV) block is rare. When present it is most frequently a manifestation of ischemic heart disease, although it may be due to primary degenerative diseases of the His-Purkinje system as is seen in etiologies such as Lev's and Lenegre's diseases (144, 145). However, in presumably normal populations the most frequent type of AV block other than prolonged P-R interval is second-degree Wenckebach with 2 to 1 conduction; it is usually due to an enhanced vagal effect on the AV node and is seen predominantly among well-trained endurance athletes (146, 147). Characteristically, this conduction phenomenon, which is usually found on both resting and ambulatory electrocardiograms, is abolished by the lessened vagal and increased sympathetic effect during exercise testing. Advanced AV block (Mobitz II type) may rarely occur during exercise testing and is due to disease of the His-Purkinje system; it is not a manifestation of excess vagal effect at the AV junction (148). Therefore, rate-related AV block may be detected by exercise testing, which should be considered in the evaluation of exercise-related cerebral symptoms.

Preexisting bundle branch block usually persists during exercise, and conventional exercise testing adds little to the determination of its etiology. However, exercise radionuclide angiography during cycle ergometer exercise may reveal an abnormality of left ventricular wall motion from which underlying heart disease can be diagnosed; this may be due to coronary disease, but occasionally it is a manifestation of nonischemic cardiomyopathy of undetermined etiology (149). Exercise-related right bundle branch block also occurs and is generally considered less likely to represent occult heart disease than is the left bundle variety. However, among children and young adults, exercise-related right bundle branch block is more prevalent than left, and is usually associated with a congenital heart defect or cardiomyopathy (150).

Complete heart block without associated cardiac disease is uncommon and usually congenital in origin. Generally the site of the block is proximal to the His bundle and is due to a discontinuity between the atrial musculature and the atrial conduction system or to fibrous tissue separating the AV node from the bundle of His (144, 151). Patients without any other associated heart defects lead normal lives and are generally able to participate in strenuous physical activities without apparent limitations. However, exercise testing is advisable in such cases not only to ascertain functional capacity but to detect the presence of ventricular ectopy that occurs in a significant number of these patients (152). An increase in ventricular rate is obviously limited in these patients, but cardiac output is augmented by virtue of an enhanced stroke volume, and syncope due to cerebral underperfusion is uncommon (153).

Cardiac Pacemakers

Exercise testing is required for cardiac pacemaker patients who wish to participate in exercise programs. The purposes of testing are to acquire information with regard to the "spontaneous" heart rate and blood pressure responses and to provoke symptoms. However, prior to exercise testing it is essential to know the conduction abnormality for which the pacemaker was placed, that is, whether it was for chronotropic incompetence because of sinus node disease or ventricular bradycardia due to high degree AV block. Additionally, knowledge of possible underlying heart disease and left ventricular function and an understanding of the pacemaker type and programming are critical.

With the commonly used fixed rate asynchronous ventricular pacemaker, the heart rate response to exercise is limited by the programmed ventricular rate. Consequently, the heart rate cannot be used as a guide to exercise intensity, and other variables, such as blood pressure, symptoms, or ratings of perceived exertion, must be utilized. However, the use of an atrioventricular synchronous pacemaker with a normally functioning sinus node provides appropriate increases in ventricular rate during exercise. Recommended exercise test end points for patients with asynchronous fixed rate or synchronous variable rate pacemakers are listed in Table 4.5.

Recent studies of exercise performance in patients with atrial synchronized ventricular pacemakers show that the main-

Table 4.5
Exercise Testing of Patients with Asynchronous Fixed Rate or Synchronous Variable Rate Pacemakers

Dynamic Exercise Testing End Points	
Asynchronous Ventricular	Synchronous Atrioventricular
Peripheral underperfusion symptoms (cerebral, muscular)	Cardiopulmonary symptoms (dyspnea, chest pain)
Maximal systolic BP	% Age predicted maximal HR
Cardiopulmonary symptoms (dyspnea, chest pain)	Arrhythmias
Arrhythmias	Rating of perceived exertion
Rating of perceived exertion	

BP, blood pressure; HR, heart rate.

tenance of a normal chronotropic response to exercise produces a significant improvement in patients as compared with asynchronous ventricular pacing (153). Therefore, exercise testing of patients with the former type of pacemaker allows a more appropriate assessment of physical capacity with respect to recommendations for exercise training. Additionally, exercise testing is also useful for patients with these atrial synchronous physiologic pacemakers for evaluating the dependability of atrial sensing at increased heart rates (154).

Exercise Prescription

As previously discussed, both simple and complex ventricular premature beats are highly prevalent in both normal sedentary adults and trained athletes. Although these arrhythmias may be provoked by exercise, they seldom lead to sustained repetitive forms that cause serious hemodynamic consequences in subjects with normal ventricular function. Therefore, after appropriate evaluation (Fig. 4.1), patients without evident heart disease should be permitted to participate in regular aerobic activity, including various types of endurance events. For a minority of individuals in this category, symptoms both at rest and with exercise may require suppressive drug therapy that reduces exercise capacity, as may occur with β-blocking agents. However, specific antiarrhythmic agents, such as quinidine, procainamide, and disopyramide, and the newer classes of agents, may be effective in controlling symptomatic ventricular premature beats without reducing chronotropic capacity during exercise. Although the efficacy of suppressive drug treatment may be evident by cessation of symptoms during physical effort, exercise testing should be used to document this benefit and to monitor the possibility of proarrhythmic effects that can occur with the use of these agents (155). This being the case, it is important to emphasize that for patients (and athletes), drug therapy generally should be used only for symptoms related to ventricular ectopy.

Exercise training has been suggested as a component of nondrug, hygienic interventions for normal patients with ventricular premature beats. However, as shown during a 6-week multifactor, hygienic intervention program, including supervised aerobic physical conditioning, there is no significant reduction in the frequency or type of ventricular ectopy in these patients as compared with a control group (156). This failure to modify ventricular ectopy favorably in normal men is similar to that found after a 6-month exercise training program in coronary artery disease patients with similar ventricular arrhythmias (157).

As with ventricular arrhythmias, for supraventricular rhythms and conduction defects that are identified by exercise testing as the cause of exercise-related symptoms without apparent heart disease, physical training programs need only be restricted or modified to the extent that associated symptoms are relieved. Similarly, the indications for drug therapy pertain in this situation as well, although a β-blocker may be needed to control the ventricular rate during exercise for patients with atrial fibrillation. As with ventricular arrhythmias, the efficacy of drug therapy in supraventricular rhythms should be monitored by serial exercise testing during long-term exercise training.

For patients with permanent transvenous pacemakers, aerobic exercise programs can be devised that will improve aerobic capacity. Because of the inherent differences in the physiologic effect of asynchronous fixed rate pacemakers as contrasted with atrioventricular synchronized pacemakers, training programs must be appropriately tailored and require careful pretraining exercise testing. However, preliminary studies indicate that for both types of permanent pacemakers, a training effect can be achieved and body composition improved (158).

The purpose of exercise training programs for pacemaker patients is to improve the quality of life by increasing exercise tolerance for activities of everyday living as well as for participation in selected low-intensity recreational sports programs. Exercise guidelines for pacemaker patients are becoming available (158–160), and recommendations for exercise training are outlined in Table 4.6. Noteworthy is the need for careful monitoring of systolic blood pressure rather than heart rate, using a modified Karvonen equation (161), as an intensity guideline for patients with asynchronous single chamber ventricular pacemakers, as well as close observation for symptomatic evidence of cerebral underperfusion. Because frequent blood pressure measurement during training is not practical, patients with fixed-rate pacemakers must use the appropriate rating of perceived exertion (e.g., "fairly light" to "somewhat hard") or other subjective end points as determined by pretraining exercise testing. Testing also provides direct measurement or estimation of oxygen uptake from which recommendations for occupational and recreational activities can be made using published tables of metabolic costs (162).

Table 4.6
Exercise Training of Patients with Asynchronous Fixed Rate or Synchronous Variable Rate Pacemakers

Dynamic Exercise Training Guidelines[a]	
Asynchronous Ventricular	Synchronous Atrioventricular
Intensity	Intensity
Target rating of perceived exertion	60–80% target maximal HR[b]
60–80% target maximal systolic BP[b]	Target rating of perceived exertion
Training duration: 30–40 min	
Training frequency: 3–4 times/week	

[a] **Karvonen equation for calculation of target HR or systolic BP for training based on pretraining exercise testing:**
Target HR = $(HR_{max} - HR_{rest})(0.6 \text{ to } 0.8) + HR\ rest$
Target systolic BP = $(BP_{max} - BP_{rest})(0.6 \text{ to } 0.8) + BP\ rest$
[b] **BP, blood pressure; HR, heart rate.**

CARDIAC TRANSPLANTATION

Exercise is an important component in the postoperative management of cardiac transplantation patients. Dynamic exercise testing has been used as the primary method for studying the cardiopulmonary physiology of transplantation in human subjects, and more recently for the prescription of postoperative exercise training programs for transplantation patients. In this section the cardiovascular physiology of dynamic exercise in transplant patients will be briefly reviewed along with an examination of the role of exercise training as a component of posttransplantation rehabilitation.

Exercise Testing

The physiologic responses to dynamic supine exercise in patients with orthotopic transplanted hearts are well documented. More recent upright exercise studies have verified and extended these observations (163, 164).

Denervation of the myocardium as a consequence of orthotopic transplantation is marked by the loss of the modulating effects of the parasympathetic and sympathetic nervous system. Consequently, there is a high resting heart rate and a diminished chronotropic reserve. Early in exercise an increase in cardiac output is due to an enhanced stroke volume through the Frank-Starling mechanism to increased venous return. With continued exercise an increase in circulating catecholamines gradually increases heart rate, which causes a further elevation of cardiac output. However, when compared with the mechanisms in normal control subjects, these fail to yield the same maximal exercise response seen with an intact native circulatory system (163). In transplant patients there is some elevation of serum lactate, which may contribute to earlier fatigue and decreased duration of exercise as compared with normal subjects. Although there is no increase in the prevalence of significant cardiac arrhythmias or electrocardiographic signs of ischemia in these patients as compared with normal subjects, they demonstrate a significantly decreased maximal systolic blood pressure during exercise. There is conjecture that this limitation and early fatigue of peripheral muscle function may be the consequence of some element of graft rejection or the immunosuppressive drugs, particularly steroids. The availability of cyclosporine has significantly reduced the need for the latter drug therapy and may allow a more normal muscular performance during exercise.

Although there are some limitations, it appears that selected cardiac transplantation patients can participate in aerobic exercise training programs as part of a comprehensive postoperative cardiac rehabilitation effort.

Exercise Prescription

The rationale for aerobic exercise training for transplant patients is identical to that for postmyocardial infarction, angioplasty, and cardiac bypass surgery patients. The goals are an improvement in exercise tolerance, an increased sense of well-being, motivation to return to normal activities, and the possible achievement of secondary prevention, particularly as relates to risk factors for coronary artery disease involving the donor heart.

Although limited, there are studies that show benefits for cardiac transplant patients entered into treadmill walking and cycle ergometry programs (165, 166). Exercise tolerance, as evaluated mainly by systolic blood pressure responses and perceived exertion ratings, is consistently improved for any given exercise intensity after training. Moreover, the feasibility of exercise rehabilitation for these patients appears established, with good patient compliance and a reasonably high rate of return to work (167). Although systematic data are not yet available, it appears that exercise as part of the rehabilitation of these patients may be helpful for secondary prevention through changes in life-style (167). However, this important justification for exercise rehabilitation of transplant patients remains to be determined by appropriate controlled studies.

Finally, under close supervision, selected cardiac transplant patients appear capable of participating safely in rigorous endurance aerobic events, such as marathon running (168). However, as is the case with similar exercise feats by postmyocardial infarction patients, such an effort is more of a demonstration than a recommended goal for rehabilitation.

SUMMARY

Abnormal blood pressure responses to dynamic exercise testing in patients who are normotensive at rest are predictive of future hypertension in a small number of subjects. Although of low sensitivity in identifying prehypertensive individuals, a normal blood pressure response to exercise is associated with a lessened likelihood of future hypertension. Although dynamic exercise training is associated with only modest reductions in blood pressure, it appears to be an appropriate component of nonpharmacologic treatment programs for hypertensive patients.

The routine use of exercise testing in valvular heart disease generally is not clinically warranted except when used in conjunction with radionuclide angiography in patients with aortic and mitral regurgitation. Exercise training studies in valvular heart disease patients, including those with heart valve replacements, are limited and do not suggest significant benefits. In the mitral valve prolapse syndrome, there is a high prevalence of nonspecific exercise-induced electrocardiographic changes and cardiac arrhythmias, although the latter are rarely life threatening. Unless such patients are symptomatic during activity, routine exercise testing probably adds little to clinical management, although exercise testing and training programs may be beneficial.

Exercise testing is clinically useful in both preoperative assessment and postoperative management of a variety of congenital heart defects, including tetralogy of Fallot, aortic stenosis, coarctation of the aorta, pulmonary stenosis, and atrial and ventricular septal defect. With complete surgical correction of many of these defects, exercise training programs are possible and appropriate.

For patients with idiopathic dilated cardiomyopathy, exercise testing is of limited value and should be used only to assess changes in therapy or other interventions. Similarly, testing is not effective in assessing the risk of sudden cardiac death among patients with hypertrophic cardiomyopathy, and exercise training programs should not be recommended.

For patients with cardiac arrhythmias, particularly ventricular ectopy, exercise testing is of value in diagnosis, risk assessment, and evaluation of treatment efficacy. However, exercise training does not reduce the prevalence of cardiac arrhythmias in otherwise normal subjects. Exercise testing and training are of benefit for carefully selected individuals with cardiac pacemakers, and can be used effectively as components of a postoperative rehabilitation program for cardiac transplant patients.

REFERENCES

1. Chobanian A: Antihypertensive therapy in evolution. *N Engl J Med* 314:1701–1702, 1986.
2. Wilson N, Meyer E: Early prediction of hypertension using exercise blood pressure. *Prev Med* 10:62–68, 1981.
3. Dlin R, Hanne N, Silverberg, et al.: Follow-up of normotensive men with exaggerated blood pressure response to exercise. *Am Heart J* 106:316–320, 1983.
4. Jackson A, Squires W, Grimes G, et al.: Prediction of future resting hypertension from exercise blood pressure. *J Cardiac Rehabil* 3:263–268, 1983.
5. Franco-Marselli R, Elghazi E, Joly S, et al.: Increased plasma adrenaline concentrations in benign essential hypertension. *Br Med J* 2:1251–1254, 1977.
6. DeChamplain J, Couseneau M, van Ameringen M, et al.: The role of the sympathetic nervous system in experimental and human hypertension *Postgrad Med J* 53(Suppl):15–30, 1977.
7. Davidoff R, Schamroth C, Goldman T, et al.: Postexercise blood pressure as a predictor of hypertension. *Aviat Space Environ Med* 53:591–594, 1982.
8. Special Report, Subcommittee on Exercise Testing and Prescription. *Circulation* 74:653A–667A, 1986.
9. American College of Sports Medicine: *Guidelines for Exercise Testing and Prescription*, ed 3. Philadelphia, Lea & Febiger, 1986, p 9.
10. Criqui M, Haskell W, Heiss G, et al.: Predictors of systolic blood pressure response to treadmill exercise: the Lipid Research Clinics Program Prevalence Study. *Circulation* 68:225–233, 1983.
11. Fixler D, Laird W, Dana K: Usefulness of exercise stress testing for prediction of blood pressure trends. *Pediatrics* 75:1071–1075, 1985.
12. Cottrill C, Kotchen J, Guthrie G: Cardiovascular response to exercise following adolescent hypertensive pregnancy. *J Adolesc Health Care* 1:91–95, 1980.
13. Nudel D, Gootman N, Brunson C, et al.: Exercise performance of hypertensive adolescents. *Pediatrics* 65:1073–1078, 1980.
14. Wong H, Kasser I, Bruce R: Impaired maximal exercise performance with hypertensive cardiovascular disease. *Circulation* 39:633–638, 1969.
15. Wu S, Secchi M, Mancarella S, et al.: Usefulness of stress testing for the evaluation of hypertensive heart disease in young hypertensive subjects. *Cardiology* 71:277–283, 1984.
16. Guazzi M, Palese A, Magrini F, et al.: Correlation of electrocardiographic changes and hemodynamic functions in the treatment of primary arterial hypertension. *Am J Med Sci* 267:299–309, 1974.
17. Ibrahim M, Tarazi R, Dustan H, et al.: Electrocardiograms in evaluation of resistance to antihypertensive therapy. *Arch Intern Med* 137:1125–1129, 1977.
18. Yamada T, Kubota T, Endo T, et al.: Effects of antihypertensive treatment on left ventricular hypertrophy in patients with essential hypertension. *J Am Geriatr Soc* 27:500–506, 1979.
19. Miller A, Kaplan B, Upton M, et al.: Treadmill exercise testing in hypertensive patients treated with hydrochlorothiazide and β-blocking drugs. *JAMA* 250:67–70, 1983.
20. Chrysant S: The value of grip test as an index of autonomic function in hypertension. *Clin Cardiol* 5:139–143, 1982.
21. Fraser G, Phillips R, Harris R: Physical fitness and blood pressure in school children. *Circulation* 67:405–412, 1983.
22. Paffenbarger R, Wing A, Hyde R, et al.: Physical activity and incidence of hypertension in college alumni. *Am J Epidemiol* 117:245–256, 1983.
23. Blair S, Goodyear N, Gibbons L, et al.: Physical fitness and incidence of hypertension in healthy normotensive men and women. *JAMA* 252:487–490, 1984.
24. Kaplan N: Nondrug treatment of hypertension. *Ann Intern Med* 102:359–373, 1985.
25. Alderman M, Davis T, Gerber L, et al.: Antihypertensive drug therapy withdrawal in a general population. *Arch Intern Med* 146:1309–1311, 1986.

26. Seals D, Hagberg J: The effect of exercise training on human hypertension: a review. *Med Sci Sports Exerc* 16:207–215, 1984.
27. Boyer J, Kasch F: Exercise therapy in hypertensive men. *JAMA* 211:1668–1671, 1970.
28. Choquette G, Ferguson R: Blood pressure reduction in borderline hypertensives following physical training. *Can Med Assoc J* 108:699–703, 1973.
29. Bonanno J, Lies J: Effects of physical training on coronary risk factors. *Am J Cardiol* 33:760–763, 1974.
30. Krotkiewski M, Mandroukas L, Sjostrome L, et al.: Effects of long-term physical training on body fat, metabolism, and blood pressure in obesity. *Metabolism* 28:650–658, 1979.
31. Roman O, Comuzzi E, Villalon E, et al.: Physical training program in arterial hypertension. A long-term prospective follow-up. *Angiology* 67:230–243, 1981.
32. Kukkonen K, Rauramaa E, Voutilainen E, et al.: Physical training of middle-aged men with borderline hypertension. *Ann Clin Res* 14(Suppl):139–145, 1982.
33. Hagberg J, Goldring A, Ehsani A, et al.: Effect of exercise training on the blood pressures and hemodynamics of adolescent hypertensives. *Am J Cardiol* 52:763–768, 1983.
34. Duncan J, Farr J, Upton J, et al.: The effects of aerobic exercise on plasma catecholamines and blood pressure in patients with mild hypertension. *JAMA* 254:2609–2613, 1985.
35. Hanson J, Nedde W: Preliminary observations on physical training for hypertensive males. *Circ Res* 27(Suppl):49–53, 1970.
36. Sonnerstadt R, Wasir H, Henning R, et al.: Systemic haemodynamics in mild arterial hypertension before and after physical training. *Clin Sci Mol Med* 45:145–149, 1973.
37. Ressl J, Chrostek J, Jandova R: Hemodynamic effects of physical training in essential hypertension. *Cardiologica* 32:121–133, 1977.
38. DePlaen J, Detry JM: Hemodynamic effects of training in established hypertension. *Acta Cardiol (Brux)* 35:179–188, 1980.
39. Hartzell A. Freund B, Jilka S, et al.: The effect of beta-adrenergic blockade on ratings of perceived exertion during submaximal exercise before and following endurance training. *J Cardiopul Rehabil* 6:444–456, 1986.
40. O'Hare J, Murnaghan D: Failure of antihypertensive drugs to control blood pressure rises with isometric exercise in hypertension. *Postgrad Med J* 57:522–555, 1981.
41. Parfrey P, Wright P, Ledingham J: Prolonged isometric exercise. Part 1: Effect on circulation and on renal excretion of sodium and potassium in mild essential hypertension. *Hypertension* 3:182–187, 1981.
42. Hochreiter C, Borer J: Exercise testing in patients with aortic and mitral valve disease: current applications. *Cardiovasc Clin* 13:291–300, 1983.
43. Areskog N: Exercise testing in the evaluation of patients with valvular heart disease. *Clin Physiol* 4:201–208, 1984.
44. Borer J, Bachrach S, Green M, et al.: Exercise-induced left ventricular dysfunction in symptomatic and asymptomatic patients with aortic regurgitation: assessment by radionuclide cineangiography. *Am J Cardiol* 42:351–357, 1978.
45. Bonow R, Borer J, Rosing D, et al.: Preoperative exercise capacity in symptomatic patients with aortic regurgitation as a predictor of postoperative left ventricular function and long term prognosis. *Circulation* 62:1280–1290, 1980.
46. Bishop J, Wade O: Relationships between cardiac output and rhythm, pulmonary vascular pressures and disability in mitral stenosis. *Clin Sci* 24:391–404, 1963.
47. Almendral J, Garcia-Andoin J, Sanchez-Cascos A, et al.: Treadmill stress testing in the evaluation of patients with valvular heart disease. *Cardiology* 69:42–51, 1982.
48. Kennedy J, Doces J, Stewart D, et al.: Left ventricular function before and following surgical treatment of mitral valve disease. *Am Heart J* 97:592–598, 1979.
49. Borer J, Gottdiener J, Rosing D, et al.: Left ventricular function in mitral regurgitation: determination during exercise (abst). *Circulation* 60:II–38, 1979.
50. Nishida K, Kitamura H, Higami M, et al.: Exercise echocardiography to evaluate left ventricular function in mitral and aortic regurgitation. *J Cardiogr* 15:123–133, 1985.
51. Carstens V, Behrenbeck D, Helger H: Exercise capacity before and after cardiac valve surgery. *Cardiology* 70:41–49, 1983.
52. Niemela K, Ikakeimo M, Linnaluoto M, et al.: Response to progressive bicycle exercise before and following aortic valve replacement. *Cardiology* 70:110–118, 1983.
53. Niemela K, Ikakeimo M, Takkunen J: Determination of the anaerobic threshold in the evaluation of functional status before and following valve replacement. *Cardiology* 72:165–173, 1985.
54. Newell J, Kappagoda C, Stoker J, et al.: Physical training after heart valve replacement. *Br Heart J* 44:638–649, 1980.
55. Wei J, Bulkley B, Schaeffer A, et al.: Mitral valve prolapse syndrome and recurrent ventricular tachyarrhythmia. *Ann Intern Med* 89:6–9, 1978.
56. Savage D, Devereux R, Garrison R, et al.: Mitral valve prolapse in the general population. II. Clinical features: The Framingham Study. *Am Heart J* 106:577–581, 1983.
57. Barlow J, Pocock W: The mitral valve prolapse

enigma—two decades later. *Mod Concepts Cardiovasc Dis* 53:13–17, 1984.

58. Barzilay J, Froone P, Gross M, et al.: Exercise testing and physical fitness in mitral valve prolapse. *J Cardiopul Rehabil* 6:465–468, 1986.
59. Massie B, Botvinick E, Shomes D, et al.: Myocardial perfusion scintigraphy in patients with mitral valve prolapse. *Circulation* 57:19–26, 1978.
60. Beton D, Brear S, Edwards J, et al.: Mitral valve prolapse: an assessment of clinical features, associated conditions, and prognosis. *Q J Med* 52:150–164, 1983.
61. Jeresaty R: Mitral valve prolapse. An update. *JAMA* 254:793–795, 1985.
62. Newman G, Gibbons R, Jones R: Cardiac function during rest and exercise in patients with mitral valve prolapse. *Am J Cardiol* 47:14–19, 1981.
63. Alexander L, Schaal S: Effects of exercise on mitral valve prolapse syndrome patients (abst). *Med Sci Sports Exerc* 14:164, 1982.
64. Wooley C: Where are the diseases of yesteryear? Da Costa's syndrome, soldier's heart, the effort syndrome, neurocirculatory asthenia and the mitral valve prolapse syndrome. *Circulation* 53:749–751, 1976.
65. Fuster V, McGoon D, Kennedy M, et al.: Long-term evaluation (12–22 years) of open heart surgery for tetralogy of Fallot. *Am J Cardiol* 46:635–642, 1980.
66. Garson A, Gillette P, Gutgesell H, et al.: Stress-induced ventricular arrhythmia after repair of tetralogy of Fallot. *Am J Cardiol* 46:1006–1012, 1980.
67. Hannon J, Danielson G, Puga F, et al.: Cardiorespiratory response to exercise after repair of tetralogy of Fallot. *Tex Heart Inst J* 12:393–400, 1985.
68. Kavey R, Blackman M, Sondheimer H: Incidence and severity of chronic ventricular dysrhythmias after repair of tetralogy of Fallot. *Am Heart J* 103:342–350, 1982.
69. Garson A, Gillette P, McNamara D: Control of late postoperative ventricular arrhythmias with phenytoin in young patients. *Am J Cardiol* 46:290–294, 1980.
70. Whitmer J, James F, Kaplan S, et al.: Exercise testing in children before and after surgical treatment of aortic stenosis. *Circulation* 63:254–263, 1981.
71. Kveselis D, Rocchinei A, Rosenthal A, et al.: Hemodynamic determinants of exercise-induced ST-segment depression in children with valvular aortic stenosis. *Am J Cardiol* 55:1133–1139, 1985.
72. Alpert B, Kartodihardjo W, Harp R, et al.: Exercise blood pressure response—a predictor of severity of aortic stenosis in children. *J Pediatr* 98:763–765, 1981.
73. Connor T: Evaluation of persistent coarctation of aorta after surgery with blood pressure measurement and exercise testing. *Am J Cardiol* 43:74–78, 1979.
74. James F, Kaplan S: Systolic hypertension during submaximal exercise after correction of coarctation of the aorta (abst). *Circulation* 50 (Suppl II):34, 1974.
75. Freed M, Rocchini A, Rosenthal A, et al.: Exercise-induced hypertension after surgical repair of coarctation of the aorta. *Am J Cardiol* 43:253–258, 1979.
76. Epstein S, Besier G, Goldstein R, et al.: Hemodynamic abnormalities in response to mild and intense upright exercise following operative correction of an atrial septal defect or tetralogy of Fallot. *Circulation* 47:1065–1075, 1973.
77. Nadas A, Fyler D: *Pediatric Cardiology*, ed 3. Philadelphia, WB Saunders, 1972, p 348.
78. Bendien C, Bossina K, Buurma A, et al.: Hemodynamic effects of dynamic exercise in children and adolescents with moderate-to-small ventricular septal defects. *Circulation* 70:929–934, 1984.
79. Bloomfield D: The natural history of ventricular septal defect in patients surviving infancy. *Circulation* 29:914–955, 1964.
80. Weidman W, Blunt S, DuShane J, et al.: Clinical course in ventricular septal defects. *Circulation* 56 (Suppl):I–56–69, 1977.
81. Krabill K, Wang Y, Enzig S, et al.: Rest and exercise hemodynamics in pulmonary stenosis: comparison of children and adults. *Am J Cardiol* 56:360–365, 1985.
82. Cumming G: Maximal exercise capacity of children with heart defects. *Am J Cardiol* 42:613–619, 1978.
83. Goldberg B, Fripp R, Lister G, et al.: Effect of physical training on exercise performance of children following surgical repair of congenital heart disease. *Pediatrics* 68:691–699, 1981.
84. Ruttenberg H, Adams T, Orsmond G, et al.: Effects of exercise training on aerobic fitness in children after open-heart surgery. *Pediatr Cardiol* 4:19–24, 1983.
85. Mathews R, Nixon P, Stephenson R, et al.: An exercise program for pediatric patients with congenital heart disease: organizational and physiological aspects. *J Cardiac Rehabil* 3:467–475, 1983.
86. Donovan E, Mathews R, Nixon P, et al.: An exercise program for pediatric patients with congential heart disease: psychosocial aspects. *J Cardiac Rehabil* 3:476–480, 1983.
87. Committee Report of the American Heart Association Ad Hoc Committee on Rehabilitation of the Young Cardiac: Recreational and occupational recommedations for use by physicians counseling young patients with heart disease. *Circulation* 43:459–464, 1971.

88. Williams RS: Exercise training of patients with ventricular dysfunction and heart failure. In Wenger NK (ed): *Exercise and the Heart,* ed 2. Philadelphia, FA Davis, 1985, p 219.
89. Kirlin P, Das S, Zijnen P, et al.: The exercise response to idiopathic dilated cardiomyopathy. *Clin Cardiol* 7:205–210, 1984.
90. Benge W, Litchfield R, Marcus M: Exercise capacity in patients with severe left ventricular dysfunction. *Circulation* 61:955–959, 1980.
91. Higginbotham M, Morris K, Conn E, et al.: Determinants of variable exercise performance among patients with severe left ventricular dysfunction. *Am J Cardiol* 51:52–60, 1983.
92. Litchfield R, Kerber R, Benge J, et al.: Normal exercise capacity in patients with severe left ventricular dysfunction. Compensatory mechanisms. *Circulation* 66:129–134, 1982.
93. Orinius E: Prognosis in hypertrophic cardiomyopathy. *Acta Med Scand* 206:289–292, 1979.
94. Maron B, Roberts W, McAllister H, et al.: Sudden death in young athletes. *Circulation* 62:218–229, 1980.
95. Manyari D, Paulsen W, Boughner D, et al.: Resting and exercise left ventricular function in patients with hypertrophic cardiomyopathy. *Am Heart J* 105:980–987, 1983.
96. Losse B, Kuhn H, Loogan F, et al.: Exercise performance in hypertrophic cardiomyopathies. *Eur Heart J* 4: 197–208, 1983.
97. Rosing D, Kent K, Borer J, et al.: Verapamil therapy: a new approach to the pharmacologic treatment of hypertrophic cardiomyopathy. I. Hemodynamic effects. *Circulation* 60:1201–1207, 1979.
98. Rosing D, Kent K, Maron B, et al.: Verapamil therapy: a new approach to the pharmacologic treatment of hypertrophic cardiomyopathy. II. Effects on exercise capacity and symptomatic status. *Circulation 60:1208–1213, 1979.*
99. Hanroth P, Schluter M, Sonntag F, et al.: Influence of verapamil therapy on left ventricular performance at rest and during exercise in hypertrophic cardiomyopathy. *Am J Cardiol* 52:544–548, 1983.
100. Redwood D, Goldstein R, Hirshfeld J, et al.: Exercise performance after septal myotomy and myectomy in patients with obstructive hypertrophic cardiomyopathy. *Am J Cardiol* 44:215–220, 1979.
101. Borer J, Bacharach S, Green M, et al.: Effect of septal myotomy and myectomy on left ventricular systolic function at rest and during exercise in patients with IHSS. *Circulation* 60 (Suppl):82–87, 1979.
102. Noakes T, Higginson L, Opie L: Physical training increases ventricular fibrillation thresholds of isolated rat hearts during normoxia, hypoxia, and regional ischemia. *Circulation* 67:24–30, 1983.
103. Bersohn M, Scheuer J: Effects of ischemia on the performance of hearts from physically trained rats (abst). *Am J Physiol* 234:H215, 1970.
104. Fuster V, Gersh B, Giuliani E, et al.: The natural history of idiopathic dilated cardiomyopathy. *Am J Cardiol* 47:525–531, 1981.
105. Unverferth D, Magorien R, Moeschberger M, et al.: Factors influencing the one-year mortality of dilated cardiomyopathy. *Am J Cardiol* 54:147–152, 1984.
106. Likoff M: Can patients with chronic congestive heart failure benefit from physical conditioning? A review of the potential adaptations to training. *Heart Failure* 1:125–130, 1985.
107. Maron B, Roberts W, Epstein S: Sudden death in hypertrophic cardiomyopathy: a profile of 78 patients. *Circulation* 65:1388–1394, 1982.
108. Maron B, Merrill W, Freier P, et al.: Long-term clinical course and symptomatic status of patients after operation for hypertrophic subaortic stenosis. *Circulation* 57:1205–1213, 1978.
109. Brodsky M, Wu D, Denes P, et al.: Arrhythmias documented by 24 hour continuous electrocardiographic monitoring in 50 male medical students without apparent heart disease. *Am J Cardiol* 39:390–395, 1977.
110. Sobotka P, Mayer J, Bauernfeind R, et al.: Arrhythmia documented by 24 hour continuous ambulatory electrocardiographic monitoring in young women without apparent heart disease. *Am Heart J* 101:753–759, 1981.
111. Raftery E, Cashman P: Long term recording of the electrocardiogram in a normal population. *Postgrad Med J* 52 (Suppl):32–37, 1976.
112. Kostis J, McCrone K, Moreyra A, et al.: Premature ventricular complexes in the absence of identifiable heart disease. *Circulation* 63:1351–1356, 1981.
113. Bjerragaard P: Premature beats in healthy subjects 40–79 years of age. *Eur Heart J* 3:493–503, 1982.
114. Fleg J, Kennedy H: Cardiac arrhythmias in a healthy elderly population: detection by 24 hour ambulatory electrocardiography. *Chest* 81:302–307, 1982.
115. Kennedy H, Underhill S: Frequent and complex ventricular ectopy in apparently healthy subjects: a clinical study of 25 cases. *Am J Cardiol* 38:141–148,1976.
116. Kennedy H, Whitlock J, Sprague M, et al.: Long-term follow-up of asymptomatic healthy subjects with frequent and complex ventricular ectopy. *N Engl J Med* 312:193–197, 1985.
117. Fleg J, Lakatta E: Prevalence and prognosis of exercise-induced non-sustained ventricular tachycardia in apparently healthy volunteers. *Am J Cardiol* 54:762–764, 1984.
118. Califf R, McKinnis R, McNeer F, et al.: Prognostic value of ventricular arrhythmias associated with treadmill exercise testing in patients studied with

cardiac catheterization for suspected ischemic heart disease. *J Am Coll Cardiol* 2:1060–1067, 1983.

119. Mann R, Burchell H: Premature ventricular contractions and exercise. *Proc Mayo Clinic* 27:383–389, 1952.
120. Udall J, Ellestad M: Predictive implications of ventricular premature contractions associated with treadmill stress testing. *Circulation* 56:985–989, 1977.
121. Sonnkeg C, Nylander E: Significance and reproducibility of exercise related idiopathic ventricular arrhythmias. *Eur Heart J* 1:183–193, 1980.
122. Deal B, Miller S, Scagliotti D, et al.: Ventricular tachycardia in a young population without overt heart disease. *Circulation* 73:1111–1118, 1986.
123. Monarrez C, Strong W, Roes A: Exercise electrocardiography in the evaluation of cardiac dysrhythmias in children. *Paediatrician* 7:116–125, 1978.
124. Marcus F, Fontaine G, Guiraudon G, et al.: Right ventricular dysplasia: a report of 24 adult cases. *Circulation* 65:384–398, 1982.
125. Rossi P, Massumi A, Gillette P, et al.: Arrhythmogenic right ventricular dysplasias: clinical features, diagnostic techniques and current management. *Am Heart J* 103:415–420, 1982.
126. Rosenfeld L, Botsford W: Intraventricular Wenckebach conduction and localized reentry in a case of right ventricular dysplasia with recurrent ventricular tachycardia. *J Am Coll Cardiol* 2:585–591, 1983.
127. Rakovec P, Rossi L, Fontaine C, et al.: Familial arrhythmogenic right ventricular disease. *Am J Cardiol* 58:377–378, 1986.
128. Moss A, Schwartz P: Delayed repolarization (QT or QTU prolongation) and malignant ventricular arrhythmias. *Mod Concepts Cardiovasc Dis* 51:85–90, 1982.
129. Jervell A, Lange-Nielsen F: Congenital deaf mutism, functional heart disease with prolongation of the QT interval, and sudden death. *Am Heart J* 57:59–68, 1937.
130. Ward O: New familial cardiac syndrome in children. *J Irish Med Assoc* 54:103–106, 1974.
131. Podrid P, Graboys T: Exercise stress testing in the management of cardiac rhythm disorders. *Med Clin North Am* 68:1139–1151, 1984.
132. Pantano J, Oriel R: Prevalence and nature of cardiac arrhythmias in apparently normal well trained runners. *Am Heart J* 104:762–768, 1982.
133. Pilcher G, Cook J, Johnston B, et al.: Twenty-four hour continuous electrocardiography during exercise and free activity in 80 apparently healthy runners. *Am J Cardiol* 51:859–861, 1983.
134. Talan D, Bauernfiend R, Ashley W, et al.: Twenty-four hour continuous ECG recordings in long distance runners. *Chest* 82:19–24, 1982.
135. Ekblom B, Hartley L, Day W: Occurrence and reproducibility of exercise induced ventricular ectopy in normal subjects. *Am J Cardiol* 43:35–40, 1979.
136. Hinkle L, Carver S, Stevens M: The frequency of asymptomatic disturbances of cardiac rhythm and conduction in middle aged men. *Am J Cardiol* 24:629–650, 1969.
137. Rabkin S, Mathewson F, Tate R: Relationship of ventricular ectopy in men without apparent heart disease to occurrence of ischemic heart disease and sudden death. *Am Heart J* 101:135–142, 1981.
138. Crow R, Prineas R, Blackburn H: The pragmatic significance of ventricular ectopic beats among the apparently healthy. *Am Heart J* 101:244–248, 1981.
139. McHenry P, Fisch C, Jordan J, et al.: Cardiac arrhythmias observed during maximal exercise testing in clinically normal men. *Am J Cardiol* 29:331–336, 1978.
140. Whinnery J: Dysrhythmia comparison in apparently healthy males during and after treadmill and accelerated stress test. *Am Heart J* 105:732–737, 1983.
141. Rodstein M, Wollach L, Gubner R: Mortality study of the significance of extrasystoles in an insured population. *Circulation* 44:617–625, 1971.
142. Strasberg B, Ashley W, Wyndham C, et al.: Treadmill testing in the Wolff-Parkinson-White syndrome. *Am J Cardiol* 45:742–748, 1980.
143. Abbott J, Hirschfeld D, Kunkel F: Graded exercise testing in patients with sinus node dysfunction. *Am J Med* 62:330–338, 1977.
144. Lev M: The pathology of complete atrioventricular block. *Prog Cardiovasc Dis* 6:317–326, 1964.
145. Lenegre J: Bilateral bundle branch block. *Cardiologia* 48:134–147, 1966.
146. Zeppilli P, Fenici R, Sassara M, et al.: Wenckebach second degree A-V block in top ranking athletes: an old problem revisited. *Am Heart J* 100:281–293, 1980.
147. Viitasalo M, Kala R, Eisalo A: Ambulatory electrocardiographic recording in endurance athletes. *Br Heart J* 47:213–220, 1982.
148. Woelfel A, Simpson R, Gettes L: Exercise induced distal atrioventricular block. *J Am Coll Cardiol* 2:578–581, 1983.
149. Rowe D, DePuey E, Sonnemaker R, et al.: Left ventricular performance during exercise in patients with left bundle branch block: evaluation by gated radionuclide ventriculography. *Am Heart J* 105:66–71, 1983.
150. Bricker J, Traweek M, Danford D, et al.: Exercise-related bundle branch block in children. *Am J Cardiol* 56:796–797, 1985.
151. Rosen K, Mehta S, Rahimtoola S, et al.: Sites of congenital and surgical heart block as defined by His bundle electrocardiography. *Circulation* 44:833–841, 1971.
152. Hanne-Paparo N, Kellerman J: Complete heart block and physical performance. *Int J Sports Med* 3:9–13, 1983.

153. Fananapazer L, Bennett D, Monks P: Atrial synchronized ventricular pacing: contribution of the chronotropic response to improved exercise performance. *PACE* 6:601–608, 1983.

154. Bricker J, Garson A, Traweek M, et al.: The use of exercise testing in children to evaluate abnormalities of pacemaker function not apparent at rest. *PACE* 6:601–608, 1983.

155. Velebit V, Podrid P, Lown B, et al.: Aggravation and provocation of ventricular arrhythmias by antiarrhythmic drugs. *Circulation* 65:886–894, 1982.

156. DeBacker G, Jacobs D, Prineas R, et al.: Ventricular premature contractions: a randomized nondrug intervention trial in normal men. *Circulation* 59:762–769, 1979.

157. Laslett L, Bauer P, Paumer L, et al.: Ventricular ectopy frequency and complexity not altered by exercise training in coronary disease patients. *Cardiology* 70:284–290, 1983.

158. Superko H: Effects of cardiac rehabilitation in permanently paced patients with third degree heart block. *J Cardiac Rehabil* 3:561–568, 1983.

159. Obma R, Keritzinsky G, Anderson R: Exercise for pacemaker patients. *Phys Sportsmed* 12:127–130, 1984.

160. American College of Sports Medicine: *Guidelines for Exercise Testing and Prescription*, ed 3. Philadelphia, Lea & Febiger, 1986, p 65.

161. Karvonen M, Kentala E, Mustala O: The effects of training on heart rate. *Ann Med Exp Biol Fenn* 35:307–315, 1957.

162. The Committee on Exercise: *Exercise Testing and Training of Individuals with Heart Disease or High Risk for its Development*. Dallas, American Heart Association, 1975, p 42.

163. Savin W, Haskell W, Schroeder J, et al.: Cardiorespiratory responses of cardiac transplant patients to graded symptom-limited exercise. *Circulation* 62:55–60, 1980.

164. Bexton R, Milne J, Cory-Pearce R, et al.: Effect of beta blockade on exercise response after cardiac transplantation. *Br Heart J* 49:584–588, 1983.

165. Squires R, Arthur P, Gau G, et al.: Exercise after cardiac transplanation: a report of two cases. *J Cardiac Rehabil* 3:570–574, 1983.

166. Roos R: Exercise training for heart transplant patients. *Phys Sportsmed* 14:165–174, 1986.

167. Kavanagh T, Yacoub M, Tuck J: Receptiveness and compliance of cardiac transplant patients to an exercise rehabilitation program (abst). *Circulation* 74 (Suppl):II–10, 1986.

168. Kavanagh T, Yacoub M, Campbell R, et al.: Marathon running after cardiac transplantation: a case history. *J Cardiopul Rehabil* 6:16–20, 1986.

CHAPTER 5

Patients with Peripheral Vascular Disease

R. James Barnard, Ph.D.
John A. Hall, M.S.

INTRODUCTION

Atherosclerotic peripheral vascular disease (PVD) of the lower extremities is a major clinical problem. Boyd (1) found that the life expectancy of 1476 PVD patients followed for 10 years was about 10 years less than that of the general population. In the Framingham study, the incidence of intermittent claudication was found to be 2.6/1000 for men, and 1.1/1000 for women (2). However, according to Friedman (3), PVD is often overlooked in routine screening of patients, and many patients with absent peripheral pulses are asymptomatic. Thus, the true incidence of this disease is not precisely known. Approximately 25% of all patients with coronary atherosclerosis have PVD manifested by intermittent claudication (2, 4).

Since PVD is a form of atherosclerosis, it is not surprising that risk factors such as hyperlipidemia, smoking, hypertension, and diabetes, which are commonly associated with coronary atherosclerosis, are also associated with PVD. Diabetes mellitus is the most prominent of the associated findings in patients with PVD. Peripheral atherosclerosis was found to be 11 times more frequent in diabetic than nondiabetic individuals (5), and gangrene 40 times more common in diabetic patients (6).

The clinical diagnosis of PVD has generally been based on subjective complaints of discomfort, pain, or fatigue in the legs with walking, diminished or nonpalpable pulses, and/or the presence of systolic bruits at rest. Intermittent claudication is the only specific symptom of PVD. Like angina, claudication pain is the result of an inadequate delivery of oxygen to muscle. The term claudication comes from the Latin *claudicare*, which means to limp. This is really not an accurate description of the symptoms of PVD patients since limping is rarely observed. According to Friedman (3) the nature of claudication is variable. Some patients feel only a sense of aching or weakness in the legs with walking. In others a tightening or pressing pain develops in the calves or buttocks, while others complain of sharp, cramping calf pain, which may be excruciating. The pain disappears quickly with the cessation of walking.

The palpatation of peripheral pulses has been a standard technique used to detect PVD during routine screening of patients. The posterior tibial pulse was found always to be present in normal individuals, while dorsalis pedis pulses were absent in up to 20% of normal individuals (7). Several reasons may account for the lack of dorsalis pedis pulses, including peripheral vasoconstriction, inability of the examiner to locate the pulse, and/or the population studied. Even in young individuals the dorsalis pedis pulse may be absent in 5 to 12% of the population (3, 7). Thus, the posterior tibial pulse is the one most commonly examined in clinical practice. However, this takes skill and practice. In 1961 Franklin et al. (8) described an ultrasonic flowmeter based on the Doppler effect, and in 1963

Watson and Rushmer (9) demonstrated that blood flow could be detected through human skin by pulsed ultrasound. Since then the transcutaneous Doppler flowmeter has been found to be far superior to simply palpating pulses (10) and is now used extensively to evaluate patients with PVD. Taking measurements at various levels of the limb gives a better indication of the site of arterial obstruction. Colt (11) recommended measurements at the femoral, popliteal, and both anterior and posterior tibial arteries in patients with lower limb PVD. According to Strandness (12) the transcutaneous Doppler flowmeter may be used in the clinical evaluation of patients with arterial disease at all levels of the upper and lower extremities.

The Doppler flowmeter provides an output signal, which can be recorded to give a flow velocity wave form. The recorded velocity depends on many factors and thus is really not a highly accurate measure of blood flow velocity. It is, however, useful to record because changes in wave form are obvious in patients with arterial obstruction (10). However, analysis of the wave form has not provided precise information about the extent of vascular obstruction, only whether or not obstruction is present. A recent attempt at evaluating the Doppler wave form by Laplace transformation has also been found to have major limitations (13).

The best use of the Doppler flowmeter in PVD patients is for the accurate measurement of blood pressure in the legs. According to Strandness, "the measurement of blood pressure at several levels of the limb is one of the simplest, most reliable and useful methods for the evaluation of arterial narrowing and occlusion." These standard clinical techniques for the diagnosis of PVD at rest, however, do not provide precise information as to the degree of hemodynamic impairment, and underestimate the prevalence of PVD since they provide information only in cases of severe or complete occlusion (14, 15).

EXERCISE TESTING

In 1960 it became apparent to Strandness (12) that better testing methods were needed for the detection and evaluation of PVD patients. He undertook a series of studies in normal individuals and in claudication patients that led to the development of the Strandness test. Subjects walked on a treadmill at 2 mi·h^{-1}, 12% grade until the development of claudication or for 5 min. Immediately after the test, the subjects were asked to lie down and blood pressure was measured at the ankle. Pre- and postexercise measurements were compared. Strandness and his associates confirmed earlier observations by Leary and Allen in 1941 (16), Ejrup in 1948 (17), and Winsor in 1950 (18), who reported that following exercise in claudication patients, pedal pulses either diminished or transiently disappeared. In normal individuals, ankle pressures increased at low workloads but fell at higher, more exhaustive workloads. Strandness and his associates then used the test to evaluate the response of claudication patients to exercise training and reconstructive surgery.

In 1950, Winsor (18) introduced the concept of the *blood pressure index.* He found that in normal healthy individuals the ratio of systolic pressure in the lower extremity to the systolic pressure in the upper extremity was always greater than 1.0. Blood pressure gradients less than 1.0 were found in 24% of patients with PVD in the lower limbs. In 1968, a more comprehensive study by Carter (19) found the resting ankle systolic pressure always to be ≥97% of the brachial systolic pressure in individuals without PVD. In claudication patients with angiographically documented complete arterial occlusion, the ankle pressure was always less than 85% of the brachial pressure. In patients with mild to severe arterial stenosis, the ankle pressure ranged from 45 to 120% of the brachial pressure. Similar results were reported by Yao et al. (20) in 1969 and again by Carter (21), also in 1969. Thus, under resting conditions the ankle pressure may remain normal in patients with mild to severe atherosclerosis. Similar results have been obtained with actual blood flow measurements (12). May et al. (22) have suggested that in order to observe any consistent reduction in resting pressure or flow, a major artery must be stenosed by at least 80%. Thus, when PVD is detected by the resting Doppler, the disease has already reached an advanced stage.

The value of exercise testing for the early detection of PVD was documented by Carter in 1972 (23). In 10 limbs with arterial stenosis of ≥25% of the lumen diameter, the resting pressure index was normal in 6 and abnormal in 4. With exercise, abnormal indices were found in all 10 limbs. The exercise used by Carter consisted of up to 2.5 min of foot flexion and extension at a rate of one per second. Resistance was created during the first 30 sec by the hand of the examiner. Thus, this test may be used for screening, but due to variations in the exact amount of work performed, would not be good for serial tests.

We (24) have used the approach outlined initially by Strandness with some modification. Our patients are first given a symptom-limited progressive treadmill test using a modified Bruce protocol starting at 1.0 $mi \cdot h^{-1}$, 0% grade. This test is given for two purposes. The first is to evaluate the cardiac status of the patient and to assign a maximum training heart rate. This is important since many patients with PVD also have coronary disease. The second reason for the symptom-limited test is to determine the workload to be used for the Doppler test. If the results of the symptom-limited test indicate that the patient can complete the Strandness 2 $mi \cdot h^{-1}$, 12% grade test, this test is used. If the patient cannot tolerate this workload, a lower workload is used which the patient can tolerate. Since it is sometimes difficult to pick a workload for the Doppler test that the patient can maintain for 5 min and still develop claudication, we have developed a two-stage test as outlined in Table 5.1. This two-stage test enables the technician to increase the workload after 2.5 min if the patient has not started to develop signs of claudication. This approach also reduces the risk of ECG or blood pressure abnormalities that might require termination of the test.

Doppler testing should be done in a quiet room with the temperature at approximately 75° F. On the day of testing, the patients are instructed not to exercise for at least 6 hrs prior to the test to preclude a warm-up effect (25). The patients are also instructed not to eat for at least 2 hrs prior to the test.

Table 5.1.
Doppler Stress Test Protocol

Max Stress Test MET Level	Doppler Test[a]			
	Stage 1		Stage 2	
	$mi \cdot h^{-1}$	(%) Grade	$mi \cdot h^{-1}$	(%) Grade
≤3.5	1.0	0	1.5	2
3.6–5.5	1.5	2	2.0	6
5.6–7.5	1.5	4	2.0	8
7.6–9.5	1.5	6	2.0	12
<9.5	2.0	12	2.0	12

[a] Each stage of the Doppler Test is 2.5 min. At the end of Stage 1 the work load is increased to Stage 2 unless the patient has developed grade 2 claudication pain or there is a contraindication from the ECG or blood pressure recordings.

When the patient arrives at the testing room, ECG electrodes are attached to monitor the resting and exercise ECG. The patient is then rested for 5-min in the supine position while blood pressure cuffs are placed around the left arm and both ankles. If the room temperature is cool, a blanket should be placed over the patient. At the end of the 5-min rest, brachial artery pressure is obtained by standard auscultatory techniques. Ankle pressures are obtained by using a Parks, Model 909, Ultrasonic Velocity Detector (Beverton, Oregon) to detect flow in the posterior tibial arteries.

Following the resting measurements, the patient is instructed to inform the technician about any symptoms that may develop during the Doppler exercise test. Symptoms, both cardiac and leg, are graded on a scale of 1-4, 1 being the onset of pain and 4 being the most severe. Patients are never taken beyond grade 2 angina pain but may be taken to grade 4 leg pain. The patient then performs the 5-min Doppler exercise test with continuous ECG monitoring. At the end of the test the patient is instructed to quickly lie down. Left brachial and right and left posterior tibial artery pressures are immediately taken and repeated each minute thereafter until ankle pressures return to resting levels. With practice, a skilled technician can record all 3 pressures in less than 45 sec. Two technicians are preferable, one recording ankle pressures and one brachial. Using this format, both ankle and brachial pressures may be recorded almost simultaneously.

At the end of the test an ankle/arm index (AAI) is generated for each limb by dividing the tibial systolic pressure by the brachial systolic pressure. Figure 5.1 shows the brachial and tibial systolic blood pressure responses obtained from 8 normal, healthy adults (16 limbs) performing the Strandness 2 mi·h^{-1}, 12% grade test. The tibial systolic pressure was always higher than the brachial systolic pressure, resulting in an AAI of 1.15 ± 0.01 at rest and 1.16 ± 0.02 immediately after exercise. At this low workload, tibial pressure increased in proportion to the brachial pressure. However, at higher workloads tibial pressure will fall even in normal individuals as shown by Strandness. An AAI > 1.0 has been consistently reported by other investigators.

Figure 5.2 shows the response from patients with PVD. Arterial obstruction was severe enough in every patient (11 limbs) to reduce resting tibial pressure (AAI = 0.78 ± 0.04). Upon exercise, brachial pressure increased but tibial pressure fell, resulting in an AAI of 0.57 ± 0.07. In cases of complete arterial occlusion or more severe exercise, the tibial pulse may disappear immediately following exercise if the activity creates severe enough ischemia (12).

Figure 5.3 shows the response of 25 limbs suspected of having only arterial occlusion based on symptoms or the presence of PVD in the contralateral leg. Resting AAI was normal (1.05 ± 0.01); however, with exercise, tibial pressure fell, resulting in an abnormal AAI of 0.76 ± 0.03 and suggesting the presence of mild atherosclerosis.

We try to pick a workload for our tests that will result in a decrease in tibial pressure but not a complete disappearance of the pulse. This gives us a measurable value which can then be compared following either exercise or surgical intervention when the patient is retested at the same work load.

Treadmill walking is the exercise of choice for Doppler testing of PVD patients for several reasons. First, it is an activity that most patients can do easily if the speed and grade are adjusted appropriately for the work capacity of the patient. Secondly, walking uses primarily the calf muscles, which results in the shunting of blood from the foot and other leg muscles to the gastrocnemius-plantaris when ischemia produces vasodilation. This reduces the tibial artery pressure. Third, the workload (speed and grade) can be precisely controlled and used for retest purposes following intervention.

Bicycle ergometry is not recommended because it uses primarily the thigh muscle. With ischemia, blood may be shunted from muscles in the upper leg, and the tibial pulse may not change appreciably. Alpert et al. (26) have also emphasized the im-

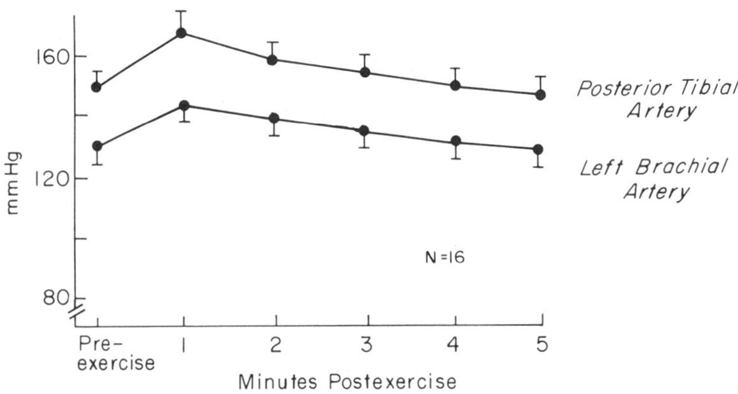

Fig. 5.1. Normal systolic pressure responses at rest and following completion of the 5-min Strandness 2 mi·h^{-1}, 12% grade test in 8 healthy adults. The ankle/arm index was 1.15 ± 0.01 at rest and 1.16 ± 0.02 immediately following exercise.

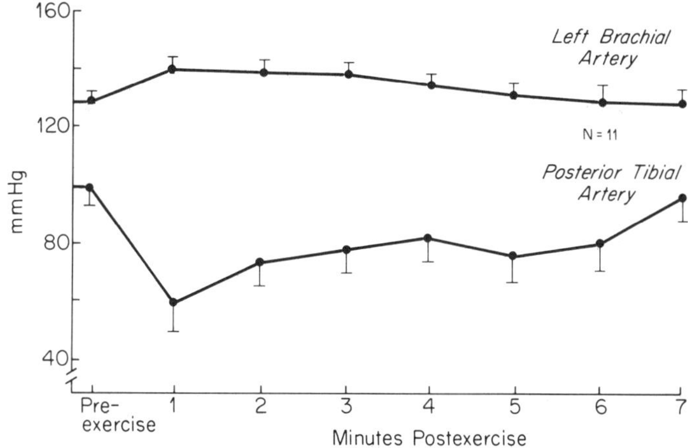

Fig. 5.2. Systolic pressure responses at rest and following the Doppler test in 11 limbs with PVD. The resting ankle/arm index (0.78 ± 0.04) was abnormal at rest and became grossly abnormal (0.57 ± 0.07) immediately following exercise.

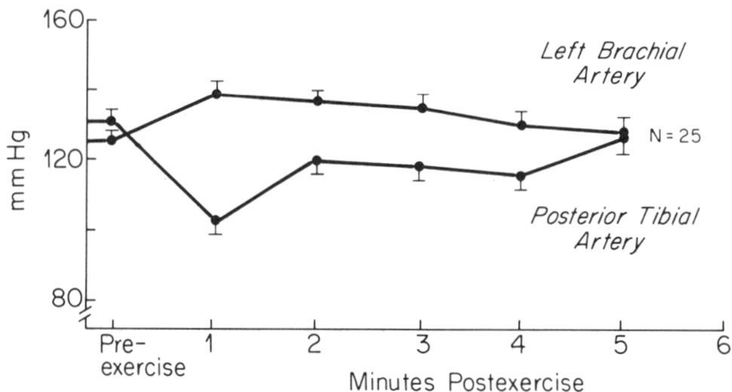

Fig. 5.3. Systolic pressure responses in 25 limbs suspected of having PVD. The resting ankle/arm index (1.05 ± 0.01) was normal. However, immediately following the Doppler test the ankle/arm index was abnormal (0.76 ± 0.03).

portance of upright exercise. In one patient with claudication symptoms and aortic occlusion, lower limb blood flow was normal during supine flexion-extension foot exercise but was clearly abnormal during walking.

While treadmill walking is the preferable mode of exercise for testing PVD patients, the lack of a treadmill should not discourage physicians from exercise testing patients with symptoms of PVD. Either foot flexion-extension as described by Carter (23) and earlier by Lassen et al. (27) or a simple exercise in which patients raise up on their toes every few seconds can be used for screening. The main objective is to use the calf muscles. According to Strandness, exercise testing can be very valuable for the early detection of patients with PVD. However, he points out that even an exercise test may not detect patients with PVD when the occlusive disease is localized below the level of the popliteal artery.

EXERCISE PRESCRIPTION

The fact that regular exercise can increase the performance capacity of patients with intermittent claudication is well documented in the literature. The amount of improvement has been variable, ranging from a few minutes increase in walking to the ability to complete a marathon as we reported in one case study (28). The exercise prescription given the patient is probably the major factor determining the amount of improvement achieved.

Walking is the exercise of choice as it

uses the calf muscles and results in the development of lower leg ischemia. According to Scheel (29), ischemia is the primary factor that stimulates the development of collateral vessels. *Thus, it is important for PVD patients to walk to the point of severe pain to create as much ischemia as can be tolerated.* Unfortunately, many training studies have not emphasized this point.

We tell our patients to walk as long as they can at the point of severe pain, sit down and rest until the pain subsides, and then walk again to the point of severe pain. This process is repeated until the patient has completed 20-30 min of exercise. Two daily sessions are recommended initially. After 1 week the sessions are lengthened to 30-40 min depending on the work capacity of the individual. By 4 weeks major improvements are usually seen in performance capacity and the prescription is reduced to one 40-60-min bout of daily walking. We emphasize to the patients that unless they consistently walk into their leg pain, they will not achieve a significant improvement in performance capacity and a reduction in leg pain.

The patients are of course reminded to check their heart rate to be sure they remain in their training zone. For those who are asymptomatic and suffer only from leg fatigue, the prescription for walking rate is assigned according to the heart rate response observed on the initial stress and Doppler exercise tests.

Schoop (30) theorized that the velocity of blood flow and the pressure gradient across a stenosis were important factors in the development of collateral circulation. He recommended interval training with its work-rest pauses as a means of increasing collateral circulation and improving performance capacity. While this method of training would produce the greatest rise in blood pressure and blood velocity, it would also create an ischemic response in the legs in a shorter period of time. However, this approach to training could be hazardous for patients with coronary atherosclerosis if they exceed the appropriate heart rate for their cardiac condition. Interval training could possibly be the most effective program for asymptomatic PVD patients with no restrictions due to coronary disease.

While cycle ergometry has been used in some training studies with PVD patients and has resulted in increases in performance capacity, we recommend walking either on a treadmill or, preferably, outside as the primary modality for training. Cycle ergometry may be used as an adjunct in selected patients who are severely limited by claudication. Many times these individuals can do more work on an ergometer, which may result in a better training effect on the heart. In such cases 2-3 days of ergometer work combined with daily walking would provide an optimal overall training response.

CHRONIC ADAPTATIONS TO TRAINING

Numerous studies on humans (31–42) and animals (43-45) with peripheral arterial obstruction in the legs have demonstrated that regular exercise can produce significant increases in performance capacity. In many patients claudication symptoms disappear. The mechanisms responsible for the increase in performance capacity are still incompletely understood. In their early work Strandness and Bell (46) demonstrated an improvement in both resting and postexercise ankle pressures immediately following reconstructive bypass surgery. Thus, when Skinner and Strandness (32) observed the same type of improvement in ankle pressures following exercise training, they ascribed the improved hemodynamic response to the development of collateral vessels and the resultant increase in oxygen delivery to the muscles.

Unfortunately, there is little information available to document the formation of collateral vessels in humans as a result of regular exercise. In a case report (28) we described a 46-year-old male who had complete occlusion of both femoral arteries just below the branch of the deep femoral. Collateral vessels had formed from small vertebral arteries branching from the lower abdominal aorta and had joined the popliteal to perfuse the lower limb. On first examination at the Pritikin Longevity Center in January 1977, this individual had no palpable pulses in the ankles, experienced severe claudication pain, and was limited to less than 100 yards of walking. After completing two 45-60-min daily walks and walking to the point of severe pain for 3 weeks, he was able to walk 3 miles in one hour with minimal leg pain. After leaving the Center he continued with his walking program and soon started jogging. In 1978, he ran in several 20-km road races and completed the Chicago marathon. In 1986, we tested this individual and found his resting pulses to be diminished but clearly palpable in both legs at rest. With exercise there was a slight drop in the pressure in the right posterior tibial artery but no drop in pressure on the left side. A digital angiogram showed a more massive collateral network and dilation of the major collateral vessels, which obviously accounted for the increase in distal pulses at rest and the improvement in exercise capacity.

In an additional study of 16 patients with abnormal ankle/arm indices both at rest and immediately postexercise, we found significant improvements in both indices following the 26-day intensive Pritikin Longevity Center Program (24). Figure 5.4 shows the blood pressure responses before and after the program. We attributed the improvement to collateral formation resulting from daily walking to the point of severe pain. Unfortunately, we were unable to document collateral formation by angiograms; however, the improvement in resting and postexercise ankle/arm indices would suggest that this was the case.

Studies on animals with acute arterial occlusion have shown that exercise training enhances collateral development (43,44). In one animal study of acute stenosis, Mathien and Terjung (45) demonstrated increased blood flow (microsphere technique) following training that was presumably the result of collateral formation. Unfortunately, there was no significant difference in blood flow during tetanic contraction between the trained and control animals. The lack of difference between the two groups may have been due to the nature of the tetanic muscle test used and its effect on blood flow. The trained animals clearly had a significant increase in performance as measured by treadmill running. One interesting observation was a redistribution of blood flow in the trained muscles. Blood flow was increased to the white portion of the gastrocnemius and decreased to the red portion during tetanic muscle stimulation.

Blood flow measurements have been made in humans with PVD following exercise training. Using a Xenon-131 washout

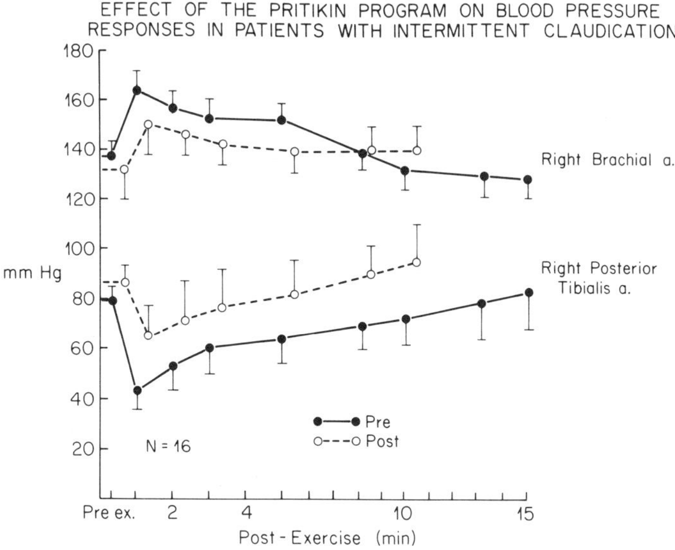

Fig. 5.4. Effect of 26 days of exercise and diet intervention, Pritikin Program (24), on patients with bilateral PVD. In the right limb resting AAI increased from 0.59 ± 0.04 to 0.64 ± 0.04 while the immediate postexercise AAI increased from 0.25 ± 0.04 to 0.40 ± 0.08. (From Hall JA, Barnard RJ: The effects of an intensive 26-day program of diet and exercise on patients with peripheral vascular disease. *J Cardiac Rehabil* 2:571, 1982.)

technique to estimate blood flow, Larsen and Lassen (31) found slightly higher maximum flow to the anterior tibial muscle in trained compared with control PVD patients, but the difference was not statistically significant. Using the same technique in a second study, they were able to show a significant effect from training when blood flow to the calf was measured. Ericsson et al. (34) reported a significant increase in blood flow to the lower limb following training in PVD patients who were studied by venous occlusion plethysmography. Others, however, have not been able to document an increase in blood flow even though a significant increase in performance capacity was observed.

Despite no change in maximum flow, Zetterquist (35) found an increase in peripheral oxygen utilization and suggested a redistribution of blood flow to the active muscles. This agrees with the recent animal data from Mathien and Terjung (45). Sorlie and Myhre (39) found a lower popliteal venous O_2-saturation and lower lactate in their patients. Dahllof et al. (36) found an increase in gastrocnemius succinic dehydrogenase activity with training despite no change in lower limb blood flow. In a follow-up study, Holm et al. (47) found that reconstructive surgery to increase blood supply to the legs resulted in a regression of succinate dehydrogenase activity back to control levels as the patients stopped their walking program. Those patients who complied with their walking program continued to have elevated levels of succinate dehydrogenase activity.

Thus, there is no doubt that regular exercise increases performance capacity and decreases symptoms of claudication; however, the mechanism(s) responsible are still incompletely defined. In addition to increasing performance capacity, Foley (48) suggested that gangrenous feet healed faster when patients were put on an exercise program. Twenty-two patients were placed on a walking program in the hospital and then were encouraged to walk on a daily basis after discharge. One patient was considered to be a failure as he discontinued walking and had to have his leg amputated. Since blood flow to the feet is decreased in PVD patients during exercise, any improvement in gangrene would likely be due to increased blood flow at rest. This, of course, would only occur if collateral development is enhanced by walking. A majority of lower limb amputations are done on diabetic patients with gangrene. Thus, regular walking exercise may prevent the need for amputation as reported by Foley.

SPECIAL PRECAUTIONS, LIMITATIONS, AND PROBLEMS

There is no evidence to suggest that severe ischemia during exercise results in any tissue damage in the legs. This obviously is different from the situation that exists in the heart where prolonged ischemia may result in myocardial infarction. Since many patients with PVD also have coronary atherosclerosis, attention must focus on limitations to exercise dictated by the presence of coronary disease. We have seen a few cases in which PVD was the limiting factor for performance capacity on initial testing. After a few weeks of intensive walking therapy, a significant increase in performance capacity enabled the patients to work to a much higher heart rate during a standard treadmill test and to exhibit an ischemic response in the electrocardiogram. Thus, the importance of regular treadmill testing is obvious.

The exact length of time that regular exercise will result in an increase in performance capacity is not known. Most training studies reported have lasted from a few weeks to six months. The long-term effects are not known. Based on the known progressive nature of atherosclerosis, one would speculate that the improvement seen with regular exercise might diminish as atherosclerosis produces more and more closure of the vessels. Thus, exercise should only be one aspect of a rehabilitative program for patients with PVD. Standard risk factors for atherosclerosis should be controlled. Special attention should be paid to diabetes, which, in most cases, can be controlled by diet and exercise alone (49–51). Hyperlipidemia should also be controlled. Several studies (52–55) have reported some cases of regression of peripheral atherosclerosis with reductions in serum lipids. While most of these studies used drug therapy to reduce serum lipids, we have repeatedly shown that diet and exercise can produce major reductions in both serum cholesterol and triglycerides (24,28, 50,51,56). In addition to the importance of reducing serum lipids, Blankenhorn et al. (53) pointed out the importance of early treatment of the disease to obtain regression. This emphasizes the importance of Doppler exercise testing for early detection of the disease, especially in diabetic patients.

SUMMARY AND CONCLUSIONS

Peripheral vascular disease of the lower extremities is a major health problem that may lead to the development of gangrene and eventual amputation. Even patients without such drastic complications often experience a severe limitation in performance capacity. Diabetes mellitus is the primary risk factor associated with the development of PVD. Hyperlipidemia is also a major risk factor.

The clinical diagnosis of PVD has generally been made on the basis of subjective complaints of discomfort, fatigue, or pain in the legs with walking; diminished or nonpalpable distal pulses; and/or the presence of bruits at rest. When these walking symptoms develop or when resting pulses are diminished, atherosclerosis is well advanced and may be obstructing as much as 80% of the arterial lumen. Exercise stress testing using Doppler ultrasound to measure distal pressures is an effective method for detection of PVD in its early stages. At minimal walking speeds distal pressure measured in the posterior tibial artery will increase in normal individuals but will decrease in patients with PVD. Intermittent claudication is the only specific symptom of PVD. However, not everyone with PVD experiences claudication pain.

Regular exercise in the form of walking has been shown to significantly increase performance capacity in numerous studies and, in one report, to heal gangrenous feet. Patients should be encouraged to walk as long as possible, even to the point of severe pain, or to walk at a level adequate enough to create severe ischemia in the legs. Patients should walk to the point of severe pain, sit down and rest until the pain subsides, then get up and walk again until he or she has completed 20-30 min of exercise, twice per day. After 1 week the time is extended to 30-40 min per session. By 4 weeks major improvements are usually seen in performance capacity and the prescription is reduced to one 40-60-min bout of daily walking.

The exact mechanisms responsible for the increase in performance with regular exercise seen in PVD patients are not precisely known. An increase in collateral vessel formation to enhance blood flow and oxygen delivery to the muscle has been supported by some investigations. Actual measurements of blood flow to the lower leg, however, have been conflicting. A redistribution of blood away from inactive muscle has been suggested and has been supported by one animal study. An increase in oxidative capacity of muscle has been reported following training in both humans and animals. This adaptation might be important in fast-twitch glycolytic fibers but is relatively insignificant in other fiber types due to the normally high oxidative capacity and the limitation in oxygen delivery to the muscle.

Another important aspect in the rehabilitation of PVD patients is controlling diabetes and reducing serum lipids in an attempt to arrest or possibly reverse atherosclerotic PVD; this has been documented in some studies. Exercise can play a role in controlling these and other risk factors but diet is far more important. Obviously, a well-designed rehabilitation program would include both.

REFERENCES

1. Boyd AM: The natural course of arteriosclerosis of the lower extremities (Section of surgery: Obstruction of the lower limb arteries). *Proc R Soc Med* 55:591–593, 1962.
2. Kannel WB, Skinner JJ Jr, Schwartz MJ, et al.: Intermittent claudication incidence in the Framingham study. *Circulation* 41:875–883, 1970.
3. Friedman SA: Arteriosclerosis obliterans of the lower extremities. In *Vascular Diseases: A Concise*

Guide to Diagnosis, Management, Pathogenesis, and Prevention, Friedman SA (ed). Boston, J. Wright, PSG Inc., 1982, p 1–30.

4. Hagood CO Jr, Mozersky DJ, Tumblin RN, et al.: Practical office techniques for physiologic vascular testing. *South Med J* 68:17–21,1975.
5. Dry TJ, Hines EA Jr: The role of diabetes in the development of degenerative vascular disease: With special reference to the incidence of retinitis and peripheral neuritis. *Ann Intern Med* 14:1893–1902, 1941.
6. Bell ET: Incidence of gangrene of the extremities in nondiabetic and in diabetic persons. *Arch Pathol* 49:469–473, 1950.
7. Barnhorst DA, Barner HB: Prevalence of congenitally absent pedal pulses. *N Engl J Med* 278:264–265, 1968.
8. Franklin DL, Schlegel W, Rushmer RF: Blood flow measured by Doppler frequency shift of back scattered ultrasound. *Science* 134:564–565, 1961.
9. Watson NW, Rushmer RF: Ultrasonic blood flow meter transducers. *Proc San Diego Sympos Biomed Engineer* 3:87–91, 1963.
10. Yao ST, Hobbs JT, Irvine WT: Pulse examination by an ultrasonic method. *Br Med J* 4:555–557, 1968.
11. Colt JD: New Doppler pressure indexes plotted as curves: Curve configuration used to determine sites of arterial obstruction. *Am J Surg* 136:198–201, 1978.
12. Strandness DE Jr: *Peripheral arterial disease: A physiologic approach.* Boston, Little, Brown, and Co. 1969, p 1.
13. Campbell WB, Skidmore R, Woodcock JP, et al.: Detection of early arterial disease: A study using Doppler wave form analysis. *Cardiovasc Res* 19:206–211, 1985.
14. Carter SA: Response of ankle systolic pressure to leg exercise in mild or questionable arterial disease. *N Engl J Med* 287:578–582, 1972.
15. Crigui MH, Franek A, Barrett-Connor E, et al.: The prevalence of peripheral arterial disease in a defined population. *Circulation* 71:510–515, 1985.
16. Leary WV, Allen EV: Intermittent claudication as a result of arterial spasm induced by walking. *Am Heart J* 22:719–725, 1941.
17. Ejrup B: Tonoscillography after exercise. *Acta Med Scand* (Suppl) 211:54, 1948.
18. Winsor T: Influence of arterial disease on the systolic blood pressure gradients of the extremity. *Am J Med Sci* 220:117–126, 1950.
19. Carter SA: Indirect systolic pressures and pulse waves in arterial occlusive disease of the lower extremities. *Circulation* 37:624–637, 1968.
20. Yao ST, Hobbs JT, Irvine WT: Ankle systolic pressure measurements in arterial disease affecting the lower extremities. *Br J Surg* 56:676–679, 1969.
21. Carter SA: Clinical measurement of systolic pressures in limbs with arterial occlusive disease. *JAMA* 207:1869–1874, 1969.
22. May AG, DeWesse JA, Rob CG: Hemodynamic effects of arterial stenosis. *Surgery* 53:513–524, 1963.
23. Carter SA: Response of ankle systolic pressure to leg exercise in mild or questionable arterial disease. *N Engl J Med* 287:578–582, 1972.
24. Hall JA, Barnard RJ: The effects of an intensive 26-day program of diet and exercise on patients with peripheral vascular disease. *J Cardiac Rehabil* 2:569–574, 1982.
25. Berglund B, Eklund B: Reproducibility of treadmill exercise in patients with intermittent claudication. *Clin Physiol* 1:253–256, 1981.
26. Alpert J, Garcia del Rio H, Lassen NA: Diagnostic use of radioactive Xenon clearance and a standardized walking test in obliterative arterial disease of the legs. *Circulation* 34:849–855, 1966.
27. Lassen NA, Lindbjerg J, Munck O: Measurement of bloodflow through skeletal muscle by intramuscular injection of Xenon–133. *Lancet* 1:686–689, 1964.
28. Hall JA, Dixson GH, Barnard RJ, et al.: Effects of diet and exercise on peripheral vascular disease. *Phys Sportsmed* 10:90–101, 1982.
29. Scheel KW: The stimulus for coronary collateral growth: Ischemia or mechanical factors? *J Cardiac Rehabil* 1:149–153, 1981.
30. Schoop W: Bewegungstherapie bei peripheren durchblutungsstorungen. *Med Welt* 10:502–506, 1964.
31. Larsen OA, Lassen NA: Effect of daily muscular exercise in patients with intermittent claudication. *Scand J Clin Lab Invest* (Suppl) 99:168–171, 1966.
32. Skinner JS, Strandness DE: Exercise and intermittent claudication. II. Effect of physical training. *Circulation* 36:23–29, 1967.
33. Alpert JS, Larsen OA, Lassen NA: Exercise and intermittent claudication: Blood flow in the calf muscle during walking studied by the Xenon–133 clearance method. *Circulation* 39:353–359, 1969.
34. Ericsson B, Haeger K, Lindell SE: Effect of physical training on intermittent claudication. *Angiology* 21:188–192, 1970.
35. Zetterquist S: The effect of active training on the nutritive blood flow in exercising ischemic legs. *Scand J Clin Lab Invest* 25:101–111, 1970.
36. Dahllof AG, Bjorntorp P, Holm P, et al.: Metabolic activity of skeletal muscle in patients with peripheral arterial insufficiency. *Eur J Clin Invest* 4:9–15, 1974.
37. Ekroth R, Dahllof AG, Gunderall B, et al.: Physical training of patients with intermittent claudication: Indications, methods and results. *Surgery* 84:640–643, 1978.
38. Cachovan M, de Marees H, Kunitsch G: The effect of oxyfedrine and interval training in intermittent claudication. *Z Kardiol* 67:289–298, 1978.
39. Sorlie D, Myhre K: Effects of physical training in intermittent claudication. *Scand J Lab Clin Invest* 38:217–222, 1978.

40. Clifford PC, Davies PW, Hayne JA, et al.: Intermittent claudication: Is a supervised exercise class worthwhile? *Br Med J* 280:1503–1505, 1980.
41. Ruell PA, Imperial ES, Bonar FJ, et al.: Intermittent claudication: The effect of physical training on walking tolerance and venous lactate concentration. *Eur J Applied Physiol* 52:420–425, 1984.
42. Hutchinson K, O'Berle K, Crockford P, et al.: Effects of dietary manipulation on vascular status of patients with peripheral vascular disease. *JAMA* 249:3326–3356, 1983.
43. Sanne H, Sivertsson R: The effect of exercise on the development of collateral circulation after experimental occlusion of the femoral artery in the cat. *Acta Physiol Scand* 73:257–263, 1968.
44. Conrad MC: Effects of therapy on maximal walking time following femoral ligation in the rat. *Circ Res* 41:775–778, 1977.
45. Mathien GM, Terjung RL: Influence of training following bilateral stenosis of the femoral artery in rats. *Am J Physiol* 250:H1050–H1059, 1985.
46. Strandness DE Jr, Bell JW: Ankle responses after reconstructive surgery. *Surgery* 59: 514–516, 1966.
47. Holm J, Dahllof A, Schersten T: Metabolic activity of skeletal muscle in patients with peripheral vascular insufficiency: Effect of arterial reconstructive surgery. *Scand J Clin Lab Invest* 35:81–86, 1975.
48. Foley W: Treatment of gangrene of the feet and legs by walking. *Circulation* 15:689–700, 1957.
49. Anderson JW, Gustafson NJ, Bryant CA, et al.: Dietary fiber and diabetes: A comprehensive review and practical application. *J Am Diet Assoc* 87:1189–1197, 1987.
50. Barnard RJ, Lattimore L, Holly RG, et al.: Response of noninsulin-dependent diabetes mellitus patients to an intensive program of diet and exercise. *Diabetes Care* 5:370–374, 1982.
51. Barnard RJ, Massey MR, Cherny S, et al.: Long-term use of a high-complex carbohydrate, high-fiber, low-fat diet and exercise in the treatment of NIDDM patients. *Diabetes Care* 6:268–273, 1983.
52. Ost CR, Stenson S: Regression of peripheral atherosclerosis during therapy with high doses of nicotinic acid. *Scand J Clin Lab Invest* 19(Suppl):241–245, 1967.
53. Blankenhorn DH, Brooks SH, Selzer RH, et al.: The rate of atherosclerosis change during treatment of hyperlipoproteinemia.*Circulation* 57:355–361, 1978.
54. Olsson AG, Carlson LA, Erikson UA, et al.: Regression of computer-estimated femoral atherosclerosis after pronounced serum lipid lowering in patients with asymptomatic hyperlipidaemia. *Lancet* 1:1311, 1982.
55. Duffield RGM, Lewis B, Miller NE, et al.: Treatment of hyperlipidaemia retards progression of symptomatic femoral atherosclerosis: A randomized control trial. *Lancet* 2:639–642, 1983.
56. Barnard RJ, Guzy PM, Rosenberg JM, et al.: Effects of an intensive exercise and nutrition program on patients with coronary artery disease: Five-year follow-up. *J Cardiac Rehabil* 3:183–190, 1983.

CHAPTER 6

Patients with Diabetes Mellitus

Arthur S. Leon, M.D.

WHAT IS DIABETES MELLITUS?

Definition and Pathophysiology

Diabetes mellitus (DM) is one of the oldest known human diseases with the first recorded description appearing in 400 B.C. in India. Ancient Egyptian and Greek physicians also were aware of this disease. In fact, the term "diabetes" dates back to 2 A.D. and means in Greek "to run through a siphon," referring to the associated copious urination (polyuria) (1). "Mellitus," the Latin word for "honey," was added later when it was discovered that the sweetness of the urine provided a test for this disease.

In actuality, DM is a syndrome of heterogenous etiology in which symptoms and complications result from metabolic derangements, the most important of which is chronic elevation of blood glucose levels (hyperglycemia) stemming from an absolute or relative deficiency of insulin. Hyperglycemia ordinarily stimulates insulin secretion by specialized insulin-producing cells (beta cells) of the islets of Langerhans in the pancreas. Insulin exerts a glucose-lowering effect by stimulating glucose uptake in muscle, fat, and other tissues after binding to cell receptors. In addition, it suppresses glucose production and release by the liver (2). Insulin deficiency may result from either physical destruction of beta cells by several different processes, defective synthesis or release of insulin, or excessive levels of hormones antagonistic to insulin's actions (3). The resulting depletion or deficiency of insulin requires insulin replacement therapy.

A more common etiology of DM in our society is cellular insensitivity or resistance to insulin due to either decreased insulin binding to cell receptors or a postreceptor defect (2, 4). With this latter form of DM, circulating levels of insulin may be normal, moderately decreased, or even increased, but insufficient to compensate for the peripheral resistance. Delayed or abnormal islet beta cell responsiveness also may coexist with peripheral resistance (5–7). Although exogenous insulin may be required to help control hyperglycemia, patients with this form of DM do not develop ketoacidosis in the absence of insulin therapy (5).

Classification

Currently DM is commonly classified into two major categories: (a) insulin-dependent or type I DM (formerly juvenile-onset diabetes) and (b) noninsulin-dependent or type II DM (formerly maturity- or adult-onset diabetes). Type II diabetic individuals may during the course of their disease require insulin for control. This composite type is sometimes referred to as "insulin-requiring" rather than insulin-dependent diabetes. Other relatively minor categories of DM are "maturity-onset in the young," "secondary DM" (e.g., due to pancreatic disease, postpancreatectomy, or syndromes of excess hormones antagonistic to insulin, such as Cushing's syndrome), and DM associated with certain genetic syndromes (3, 4). Insulin-independent (type II) DM constitutes about 80% of all cases of the disease in our society as compared with 15% for the insulin-dependent (type I) and 5% for the remaining types (3).

Etiologic Factors

Predisposing factors for type I DM include heredity with a polygenic or multifactorial mode of inheritance, viral infections (mumps or Coxsackie B-4 viruses are suspect culprits), and an autoimmune process that destroys beta cells (3–6). Onset of type I DM most commonly occurs in early adolescence, although it may occur at any age (1,2).

For type II DM, a familial genetic predisposition also appears to be involved; however, epidemiologic studies suggest that the principal precipitating factor in our society is *obesity* (4). About 80% of type II diabetics are obese, while the incidence of disease is exceedingly low in lean individuals. Prevalence rates for the very obese are more than 20 times greater than for nonobese persons. Furthermore, experimentally-induced weight gain in both animals and humans has been demonstrated to cause insulin resistance due to loss of receptors in distended adipose cells (4, 8). This process can be reversed by weight loss.

A sedentary life-style appears to be another important risk factor for type II DM both because of its relationship to obesity and as an independent effect of physical inactivity on insulin sensitivity (4, 9). In fact, cellular resistance to insulin can be demonstrated within a few days of marked inactivity resulting from bed rest (9,10).

A decrease in glucose tolerance and an increased incidence of type II DM commonly occur during aging with the majority of individuals in our society over 40 years of age (4). It is likely that this is related to both a decrease in physical activity and weight gain that commonly occurs in adults following the attainment of physical maturity. A decrease in lean body mass during aging also may be a contributing factor.

Drugs such as thiazide diuretics, glucocorticoid steroids, and oral contraceptives also may precipitate diabetes in susceptible individuals, as can pregnancy (5).

There is a common misconception that DM is related to excess sugar ingestion. There now is strong supporting evidence that the principal dietary factor contributing to type II DM is an excess of calories from any source relative to energy requirements, culminating in obesity. The evidence also is overwhelming that a diet *high* in complex carbohydrate (starch and dietary fiber) improves glucose tolerance. In contrast, a high-fat diet may have opposite effects on glucose-insulin dynamics. Furthermore, a diet high in animal fat and cholesterol raises the blood cholesterol and low-density lipoprotein (LDL) concentrations and thereby accelerates atherosclerosis and contributes to vascular complications of DM (4, 11, 12).

Prevalence

DM affects 3 to 5% of the population with at least 5 million Americans having known disease and about an equal number undiagnosed DM (4). The disease is 50% more common in females than males although there is a slight male predominance in type I diabetes. The prevalence also is higher in blacks than whites, reaching a peak of 10.5% in those age 65 years and older.

DM ranked seventh in 1984 among the leading causes of mortality in the United States (13). It was the direct underlying cause of over 35,000 deaths or about 10 per 100,000. These data actually grossly underestimate the contribution of DM to mortality, since many people with diabetes die as a result of associated atherosclerotic complications (principally myocardial infarction or stroke). In addition to atherosclerotic complications, DM is a major cause of visual impairment, blindness (about 5,000 new cases per year), and renal disease in the United States (5). This includes 20% of all cases of end-stage renal failure. Furthermore, DM is responsible for 50% of lower limb amputations resulting from related peripheral vascular disease. Diabetic patients also account for 10% of all acute hospital days. The overall economic impact of this disease is probably over $10 billion a year.

Common Symptoms and Signs

The consequence of absolute or relative insulin insufficiency is an inability to transport glucose across cell membranes of most tissues (brain and blood cells are exceptions) for subsequent oxidation for fuel. The resulting hyperglycemia is the clinical hallmark of this disease and the basis for making the diagnosis (1–8, 14). The associated hyperosmolarity of the plasma is responsible for the symptom of excessive thirst (polydipsia), which leads to frequent urination (polyuria).

When the blood glucose concentration exceeds 160 to 180 mg/dl, it usually spills over into the urine (glycosuria). Glycosuria is accompanied by osmotic diuresis, further increasing the frequency of urination. The accompanying loss of large amounts of body water may result in dehydration. The loss of glucose calories in the urine contributes to weight loss. Symptoms from hyperglycemia generally occur only when elevation of blood sugar levels exceeds 300 mg/dl. Common symptoms include fatigue, weakness, weight loss, hunger, overeating (polyphagia), and blurring of vision.

In addition to the effect of insulin on glucose uptake and utilization, other metabolic actions include storage of glucose as glycogen in muscle and liver, fat (triglyceride) synthesis in adipose cells and inhibition of its breakdown (antilipolytic effect), and protein synthesis and storage (anabolic effect). Another consequence of insulin insufficiency is increased lipolysis of triglycerides in adipose tissues, which raises the concentration of free fatty acids (FFA) in the blood and their use for fuel. In type I diabetic individuals a limited capacity of the liver to utilize acetyl-coenzyme A generated from metabolism of FFA results in increased formation of so-called ketone bodies (acetoacetate, beta-hydroxybutyrate, and acetone). Ketone bodies accumulate in the blood and spill over into the urine, leading to acidosis and dehydration (ketoacidosis). This may terminate in coma which, prior to the discovery of insulin, was often fatal. Insulin replacement therapy helps correct the metabolic deficiency state, relieving symptoms and preventing ketoacidosis. Individuals with type II DM are generally ketosis-resistant. However, persons with both types of DM, including those who are asymptomatic with less severe insulin insufficiency and hyperglycemia, are likely to develop the late complications of the disease (4, 15).

DIAGNOSTIC CRITERIA

Symptoms and Signs

DM should be strongly suspected by the presence of the aforementioned symptoms or by demonstration on funduscopic examination of characteristic microaneurysms. Nevertheless, laboratory tests are essential for confirmation of the diagnosis as well as for management.

Laboratory Tests

Available biochemical tests include determination of urinary sugar and ketone content, blood glucose levels, glucose tolerance tests, glycosylated hemoglobin levels, plasma C-peptide levels, and radioimmunoassay for insulin. These will be briefly elaborated upon below:

Urinary Glucose and Ketone Determinations

Urinary glucose usually is measured by commercial test paper strips (e.g., Testape, Eli Lilly, Indianapolis, IN) that depend on the specific enzymatic reaction of glucose with glucose oxidase and peroxidase. The color on the paper strip gives an estimate of sugar concentration. This is useful information to help the diabetic person self-monitor responsiveness to therapy. Despite the relatively high sensitivity of paper strips, quantitative determination of urine sugar over a 24-hour period is recommended for a more precise evaluation of control of diabetes. However, a negative test for urine sugar by either method does not exclude the presence of diabetes since hyperglycemia may occur without glycosuria in the presence of either a high renal threshold for sugar or vascular disease. This also limits the usefulness of urinary glucose testing for self-monitoring purposes.

Qualitative testing of urine for ketone bodies can be carried out by using either test strips or tablets, and is of special importance in evaluating type I diabetic patients.

Blood Glucose Determination

The "normal" range of fasting blood glucose concentration varies with the type of blood specimen (capillary, venous whole blood, or plasma) and the mode of assay. The normal range for fasting "true glucose" in whole *venous* and *capillary* blood is 60 to 100 mg/dl, while levels of *plasma* glucose are about 15% higher (1, 5). Fasting plasma levels greater than 140 mg/dl are considered diagnostic of DM in nonpregnant patients (4, 13).

Since in mild cases of DM the results of urine and fasting blood glucose tests may be normal, there is general agreement that in screening for diabetes, a postprandial blood glucose analysis is a more sensitive test. This should be performed after a carbohydrate-rich meal, e.g., 2 slices of bread or a sweet roll. The upper limits of normal for postprandial plasma "true glucose" is about 180 mg/dl, and for capillary blood, about 190 mg/dl (1, 14).

A number of simple methods are now available for *self-monitoring* of blood sugar by the patient with reasonable accuracy. These require only a single drop of capillary blood, which can easily be obtained from a fingertip using an automatic spring-triggered lance (14). The basic ingredient required for measuring "true glucose" in capillary blood is a plastic strip impregnated with the glucose oxidase and other chemicals, which turn color when glucose reacts with this enzyme. The patient then either matches the color on the strip to that on a chart, or places the strips in a small meter that "reads" the glucose concentration colorimetrically. When properly performed, self-monitoring provides the type I diabetic patient reliable information for adjusting insulin dosage or food intake to maintain good diabetic control under varying conditions of physical activity. This represents a major "breakthrough" for the type I diabetic athlete.

Glucose Tolerance Test

An oral glucose tolerance test is commonly performed to confirm the diagnosis of subclinical DM in patients with "normal" or nondiagnostic elevations of fasting blood glucose. For the results of this test to be meaningful, the patient should discontinue drugs that adversely affect glucose tolerance for at least 3 days before the test, and consume during this period an unrestricted diet containing at least 250 gm of carbohydrate daily. Usual physical activity levels also should be maintained during this pretest period. After a sample of blood is taken for fasting blood sugar, 75 gm (or 1.75 gm/kg body weight up to 75 gm) of a glucose solution or a commercial test drink is administered and blood samples for glucose levels are commonly collected every 30 minutes for a least 120 minutes. The upper limit for 2-hour plasma glucose concentration is 200 mg/dl, and for capillary or venous whole blood, 180 mg/dl (5, 14).

Glycosylated Hemoglobin Determination

An indirect laboratory test for diagnosing DM and evaluating long-term blood sugar control has recently been developed. The level of glucose binding to species of hemoglobin known collectively as glycosylated hemoglobin or $HbgA_1$ is measured. This test is based on the observation that chronic high serum glucose levels are associated with increased nonenzymatic binding of glucose to body proteins including $HbgA_1$ (13, 16). The concentration of glycosylated hemoglobin reflects the individuals's usual serum glucose level over a period of weeks. Similar glucose-protein binding has been postulated to contribute to degenerative changes typically found in nerve fibers, the lens of the eye, capillary membranes, kidney glomeruli, and arterial linings in diabetic persons.

Currently the stable or ketoamine form of $HbgA_1$ is usually assayed rather than the less reliable total $HbgA_1$, which also is influenced by recent changes in glycemia. The ketoamine form reflects blood glucose levels for the previous 6 to 8 weeks and correlates well with fasting, postprandial, and mean daily blood glucose concentrations. The $HbgA_1$ determination should be considered as complementary to determination of blood glucose concentration in the diagnosis and management of DM; but it is not sensitive as a screening tool because of the overlap in $HbgA_1$ concentrations with those of nondiabetic individuals.

Plasma C-Peptide Determination

The diagnosis of insulin-dependent DM can be confirmed by measurement of plasma C-peptide response after intravenous administration of glucagon (3, 14). This is a test for residual pancreatic islets beta cell function. C-peptide is part of the proinsulin molecule, connecting the A and B chains of the insulin molecule. It is released along with insulin from the granules of the beta cell. Therefore, the C-peptide plasma concentration serves as an indirect measure of insulin secretion, and is useful to evaluate whether beta cells of insulin-requiring diabetic patients are still capable of producing insulin. DM patients still capable of producing some of their own insulin usually respond more easily to treatment.

Insulin Radioimmunoassay

Determination of plasma insulin levels by radioimmunoassay before and after a glucose challenge is of value when distinguishing diabetes due to insulin deficiency from the insulin resistance syndrome often found in obese type II diabetic individuals (17). There also is evidence that individuals with type II diabetes and insulin secretory deficiency are more likely to develop diabetic complications than those with normal levels (18). However, insulin levels cannot be measured directly in patients receiving exogenous insulin since antibodies against it interfere with the assay (14).

CLINICAL COURSE AND COMPLICATIONS

Natural History

The natural history or course of diabetes is extremely variable and difficult to predict for any given person. Many individuals even with severe type I disease are able to carry on active productive lives and remain free of complications. Several former outstanding athletes fall into this category. For example, major league baseball stars Jim (Catfish) Hunter and Ron Santo; Bobbie Clark, who played in the National Hockey League; and former famous tennis players, Bill Talbert and Hamilton Richardson. Others appear to be plagued with complications even if their diabetes is kept under good control (e.g., Jackie Robinson, famous outstanding college athlete and Brooklyn Dodger star). Diabetic complications may be classified as acute or chronic as discussed below.

Acute Problems

Acute situations may occur any time in the course of diabetes; these are usually temporary and remediable. These complications include diabetic ketoacidosis in type I diabetic persons. Before the discovery of insulin, 64% of diabetic patients died in diabetic coma due to ketoacidosis, compared with only 1% currently (19). Hyperosmolar coma may occur in type II patients due to severe dehydration that accompanies hyperglycemia without the development of ketoacidosis.

Chronic Problems

Late complications usually do not occur until diabetes has been present at least 1 year, and they increase in frequency with duration of the disease (19). These complications, the main causes of premature mortality in diabetic patients, are usually classified as microangiopathy (microvascular) and macroangiopathy (macrovascular or atherosclerotic) complications. The microangiopathies (4, 5, 19) and associated neuropathies are specific for DM with prevalence being more in the type I form than type II.

Microangiopathies

Retinopathy. Diabetic retinopathy, a form of microangiopathy, is the most common complication of diabetes and is found in 25 to 50% of the diabetic population. Microaneurysms in the area of the retinal capillaries are the characteristic early lesions and are referred to as "background or simple retinopathy." Although these early lesions are benign and do not interfere with vision, they may rupture, resulting in retinal hemorrhages, scarring, and formation of fragile new vessels. This advanced stage is referred to as *proliferative retinopathy* and can lead to retinal detachment, vitreous hemorrhages, progressive visual impairment, and blindness. Diabetic individuals also have an increased incidence of glaucoma and cataracts, which also can contribute to impaired vision. Although many patients with long-term diabetes have some degree of visual impairment, probably not more than 2% become completely blind (17).

Glomerulosclerosis. Diabetic glomerulosclerosis may lead to renal failure, a common cause of death in long-term type I diabetic patients. This condition is a less common cause of death in type II diabetic patients. There is a close pathophysiologic relationship between retinopathy and kidney disease in diabetic patients. The initial manifestation of kidney involvement is the finding of albumin in the urine (proteinuria) (1, 15). As this progresses, hypoalbuminemia may develop, causing peripheral edema. Other associated findings include an increase in blood pressure, blood cells, and casts in the urine, and a progressive rise in blood urea nitrogen and serum creatinine levels. Atherosclerosis of the renal vessels and chronic pyelonephritis may contribute to the progressive loss of renal function.

Neuropathy. Almost any nerve pathway, including peripheral motor and sensory, central, and autonomic nerves, can be affected by diabetes. Symptoms of neuropathy range in severity from mild to incapacitating. Common symptoms include numbness, tingling, pain in the lower extremities, muscle wasting and weakness, foot drop, absent ankle jerk reflex, gastrointestinal symptoms, postural hypotension, difficulty in emptying the bladder, and impotence (1, 5). The prevalence of neuropathy is higher in long-term type I diabetic patients compared with type II patients. The cause of the neuropathy is uncertain; both microangiopathy of blood vessels supplying the nerves and metabolic derangements are thought to be contributory (1).

Mechanism. A current controversial issue is the contribution of insulin deficiency to the pathogenesis of the microvascular complications. The specific metabolic events that lead to these complications is unknown, although possibilities include glycosylation of tissue proteins, which alters their structure or function; the accumulation of intracellular polyols (e.g., sorbitol) due to the metabolism of glucose by non-insulin-dependent pathways (the latter mechanism has been established as the cause of diabetic cataracts and is believed to be involved in diabetic neuropathy); excessive secretion of growth hormone; overproduction of insulin-like growth factors; and alterations in metabolism of prostaglandins and related tissue hormones, and, thereby, in platelet responsiveness (5). Currently available evidence strongly supports the hypothesis that these long-term complications related to diabetic microangiopathy, especially the retinopathy and nephropathy, are linked to metabolic control and are not independent genetically determined abnormalities (5). A large scale National Institutes of Health-sponsored 10-year multicenter trial (the Diabetes Control and Complications Trial) is currently underway to study the relationship between glycemic control and prevention of diabetic complications, especially retinopathy (5, 20). Although the results of this study will not be known for several years, it is encouraging that preliminary evidence seems to indicate that good glycemic control can prevent, attenuate, and perhaps reverse some of the long-term complications of DM (5). This has encouraged attempts to achieve near-normal glycemic control of patients with DM, especially type I patients.

Macroangiopathies (Atherosclerosis)

Frequency. Persons with all types of diabetes commonly have an accelerated form of atherosclerosis leading to cardiovascular disease. Typically, atherosclerotic complications appear after patients have had insulin-dependent diabetes for many years, and usually after evidence of microvascular disease is apparent. Type II diabetic subjects, however, may have atherosclerosis of the coronary and peripheral vessels relatively early in the course of known diabetes. This occurrence probably reflects atherosclerotic changes that begin during the subclinical phase of DM. In the Framingham study, the incidence of cardiovascular disease among diabetic men was about twice that of nondiabetic men (21). Among diabetic women, the incidence was about three times that of nondiabetic women. At least two-thirds of all deaths in diabetic individuals in Western countries are attributed to cardiovascular disease (4,5).

Mechanism. Some of the reasons for accelerated atherosclerosis in diabetic patients are now better understood (3, 12, 21–23). Multiple factors appear to be involved, in particular endothelial abnormalities, platelet malfunction, and lipid-lipoprotein disturbances (2, 12). Possible endothelial abnormalities include premature cellular aging, altered permeability to plasma proteins, and osmotic damage to the endothelium due to accumulation of abnormal metabolites. Endothelial damage may be accelerated by hypertension, which frequently accompanies diabetes. Platelet hyperaggregability and an associated diminished capacity of the body to counterregulate against platelet deposition on damaged endothelium have also been demonstrated in diabetic patients and may accelerate atherosclerosis and increase the possibility of thrombus formation.

Individuals with poorly controlled diabetes commonly have elevated plasma triglyceride levels and its principal carrier in the fasting state, very low-density lipoprotein (VLDL). VLDL is converted to low-density lipoprotein (LDL), which accelerates cholesterol deposition in the endothelial walls of arteries. In patients with high plasma triglyceride and VLDL levels, there commonly is found a coexisting depression of plasma levels of high-density lipoprotein (HDL). Reduced HDL cholesterol levels may also be found in diabetic individuals with normal triglyceride concentrations (21). HDL is a lipid scavenger that helps prevent or reverse atherosclerosis. A high LDL to HDL ratio favors the deposition of cholesterol in tissues. It has repeatedly been demonstrated in longitudinal epidemiologic studies that coronary heart disease (CHD) patients are likely to have high total and LDL cholesterol and/or low HDL cholesterol levels. These lipid and lipoprotein abnormalities are likely to be important contributors to accelerated atherosclerosis in diabetes. A low-carbohydrate, high-fat diet formerly favored for diabetic patients probably accelerates cholesterol deposition in the artery linings by raising total cholesterol and LDL levels (23). Obesity and physical inactivity also may contribute to an unfavorable blood lipid profile, since both conditions often are associated with increased plasma triglycerides (and VLDL) and reduced HDL cholesterol concentrations (4, 23).

There is also evidence that high blood insulin levels (hyperinsulinemia), common in obese individuals with or without type II diabetes, may promote the atherosclerotic process. Results of epidemiologic studies have shown a positive relationship between plasma insulin levels and CHD risk (24). Furthermore, experimental studies reveal that hyperinsulinemia increases lipid synthesis and deposition in the arterial wall as well as proliferation of arterial smooth muscle cells. Smooth muscle cells have a great affinity for cholesterol and become the characteristic "foam cells" of the atherosclerotic lesion. Elevated levels of circulating insulin also promote liver synthesis of triglycerides and VLDL, as evidenced by a high positive correlation between hyperinsulinemia and endogenous hypertriglyceridemia (23).

Clinical Manifestations. CHD is a major cause of death of diabetic patients. Another frequent heart problem is cardiac enlargement due to either hypertension and/or diabetic cardiomyopathy, both of which may result in congestive heart failure. About one-quarter of type I diabetic persons and one-half of type II diabetic persons die of heart disease (4, 19).

The cerebral arteries are other common sites of atherosclerosis in the diabetic population. Resulting cerebrovascular accidents (strokes) cause 6% and 15% of deaths in type I and type II diabetic patients, respectively (19).

Advanced atherosclerosis of peripheral arteries also frequently occurs with long-term DM, particularly in older adult diabetics who smoke. Associated circulatory impairment may lead to gangrene and amputation of the lower extremities. The prevalence of occlusive peripheral vascular disease in diabetic groups ranges from 16 to 58%, and gangrene at autopsy from 13 to 19%, which is 20 to 30 times more common compared with the general population (19).

MANAGEMENT OF DIABETES MELLITUS

General Guidelines

Secondary causes of, or contributing factors to, DM should be sought for and eliminated if possible. These include diabetogenic drugs, endocrine disorders, alcohol abuse, pancreatic and liver diseases, low carbohydrate intake, obesity, and marked physical inactivity. It also is extremely important in the diabetic patient to eliminate or control coexisting risk factors for atherosclerotic complications, especially cigarette smoking, hypertension, and elevated blood cholesterol levels.

The goal of treatment of DM is to restore the patient's metabolism and life-style as closely as possible to an optimal level, and to avoid acute and chronic complications. The therapeutic optimum is for the individual to have normal blood glucose levels and urine free of sugar (at least most of the time). The general consensus is that the plasma glucose range should be 70 to 100 mg/dl in the fasting and preprandial state, and 160 to 180 mg/dl 3 hours postprandially in nonpregnant patients with diabetes (1, 5, 14, 16). For pregnant women with diabetes, the goals are 60 to 90 mg/dl blood glucose levels preprandially, and 120 to 150 mg/dl 3 hours postprandially.

The discovery of insulin over 50 years ago has permitted persons with diabetes to lead successful lives. However, few remain free of complications over many decades. Possible reasons for failure include nonadherence to therapy, inadequate instructions by the physician and staff, or inadequacies in the conventional therapies. This sad picture has led to recent changes in the therapeutic approach. As previously mentioned, preliminary data suggest "tight diabetic control" is more effective in the prevention of microvascular and neurologic complications than those of macrovascular origin. It is hoped that application of the recent advances in the understanding of the atherosclerotic process and its risk factors, including diet, will reduce the toll of cardiovascular complications. A former logo of the American Diabetic Association, a triangle, represents the symbolic balance among the three essential elements of diabetic control—diet, medication, and exercise. These remain the bases for diabetic management, which will be the next topic of discussion.

Dietary Treatment

General Considerations

Diet has traditionally been the cornerstone in therapy of DM, and is generally the first step in therapy of the diabetic patient. For ketosis-resistant, asymptomatic, or only slightly symptomatic hyperglycemic patients, an attempt at the usual dietary treatment alone to control hyperglycemia is recommended for at least a month prior to the prescription, if necessary, of an oral hypoglycemic agent or insulin. More than one-third of ketosis-resistant patients with hyperglycemia can have their disease controlled with diet alone. In ketosis-prone patients for whom insulin therapy is required, an appropriate diet is first or simultaneously initiated, and the insulin dosage is adjusted to balance the glycemic effect of the diet. On the other hand, timing of the patient's meals and snacks, as well as exercise, strongly depends on the dosage and type of insulin or oral hypoglycemic agent prescribed.

The basic daily meal structure for the diabetic patient requiring insulin usually is three main meals plus snacks at midmorning, midafternoon, bedtime, and before exercising. A food exchange system developed through collaborative efforts of the American Diabetic Association, The American Dietetic Association, and the United States Public Health Service, generally is used for making dietary recommendations to the diabetic patient (1, 14). This is an excellent educational tool and allows considerable flexibility and variety in the diet. The food exchange system usually includes six lists of food types: (a) milk, (b) vegetable, (c) fruit, (d) bread, (e) meat, and (f) fat exchanges. A list also is available of foods that generally should be avoided unless specifically approved by the patient's physician and worked into the meal pattern, e.g., alcoholic beverages, as well as a list of foods permitted in unlimited amounts, e.g., raw vegetables. Foods also can be classified according to the *glycemic index*—the area under the blood glucose response curve for each food as expressed as a percentage of the area after ingestion of glucose (4, 5, 11).

Goals

Important goals of dietary therapy of DM include the following: (a) to meet all of the essential micronutrient requirements of the patient, i.e., vitamins and minerals, (b) to adjust calorie intake to establish or maintain proper body weight, and (c) to provide a proper blend of the macronutrients (carbohydrate, fat, and protein). The latter includes sufficient carbohydrate and dietary fiber to help glycemic control, sufficient protein to permit proper growth and development of diabetic children and adolescents, and a reduced intake of saturated fat and cholesterol to help prevent atherosclerotic complications.

Balanced Nutritional Intake. Selection of a proper number of items from each food exchange list allows the patient to meet energy and all essential micro- and macronutrient requirements (25).

Body-Weight Management. The initial consideration in prescribing a diet is to determine the appropriate daily energy requirements. Patients' calorie needs are dependent on a number of factors, including age, gender, height, weight, whether the patient's weight is appropriate for height, and usual physical activity habits. Type I diabetic patients generally are lean or underweight, particularly adolescents. In contrast, 70 to 90% of adults with type II diabetes are obese. Suggested desirable weights for heights and recommended energy intake levels have been published (25).

There are many approaches available for initially estimating daily caloric requirements. Davidson (14) proposes a simple method based on the patient's gender and desirable weight. For those who are at ideal weight, approximately 32 kcal/kg a day are needed to maintain this level. For the patient who needs to *lose* weight, daily caloric allowance is reduced to 22 kcal/kg. Forty-four kcal/kg a day are recommended for those who need to *gain* weight, for adolescents who need extra calories for growth, and for adults engaged in regular heavy physical activity. Caloric intake should be reduced 10% for each decade after the age of 50 years because of the decreases in the basal metabolic rate and in physical activity that commonly accompany aging. For adolescents, recommended energy intake ranges from 2000 to 3900 kcal/day for males, and from 1500 to 3000 kcal/day for females (25). The energy needs for men aged 19 to 50 years ranges from 2500 to 3300 kcal/day, and from 2000 to 2800 kcal/day for those aged 51 to 75 years. For women the ranges for the same age groups are 1700 to 2500 kcal/day and 1400 to 2200 kcal/day, respectively.

Carbohydrate Intake. The quantity and types of carbohydrate to recommend for diabetic individuals have been widely debated down through the ages. Until recent years, the prevailing view was that dietary carbohydrates should be restricted since diabetic patients have difficulty metabolizing them. Carbohydrate calories were replaced, primarily by calories from fat. However, the data are now clear that improved carbohydrate tolerance and diminished insulin requirements result from a diet high in complex carbohydrate (50 to 70% of calories) in the form of starchy, high-fiber foods (e.g., whole grain cereals and bread, fruits, starchy roots, legumes, and other vegetables). Conversely, severe restriction of carbohydrate intake even in nondiabetic individuals produces a temporary metabolic state similar to diabetes ("starvation diabetes"). High carbohydrate intake improves peripheral cellular sensitivity to insulin, promoting glucose utilization and metabolism without increasing insulin requirements. Meals high in fiber-rich food also reduce postprandial hyperglycemia and glycosuria in insulin-dependent diabetic patients, and may allow insulin doses to be reduced (15, 26). In addition, a high fat intake actually appears to diminish glucose tolerance (27).

Another area of controversy involves the influence of sucrose and other simple carbohydrates on blood glucose levels in diabetic patients. Traditionally there has been concern about the postprandial glycemic effect of rapidly absorbed simple carbohydrates, compared with less glycemia following more slowly absorbed complex carbohydrates. However, experimental data to substantiate this long held belief are lacking (11). In fact, recent studies indicate that the simple carbohydrates, sucrose and fructose, and the complex carbohydrate, starch, have similar glycemic effects in type I and type II diabetic individuals when consumed as part of a meal (14, 21). It, therefore, appears that total restriction of simple carbohydrates from natural sources may be unwarranted in diabetic diets. Enlightened current recommendations for carbohydrate intake are up to 50 to 60% of daily calories (with emphasis on complex carbohydrates).

Protein and Fat Intake. Protein intake should be between 15 and 20% of energy intake with an emphasis on vegetable sources because of concern over the associated fat and cholesterol content of animal sources. Fat should provide no more than 30% of the calories and the proportion of saturated, polyunsaturated, and monounsaturated fatty acids should be approximately equal. In addition, fish should be consumed several times a week to provide omega-3 polyunsaturated, fatty acids. These fatty acids have a potent lipid-lowering effect and antithrombotic activity, which may counteract abnormalities in these areas commonly present in diabetic individuals (28). These dietary recommendations are similar to the recommended United States dietary goals for the general public proposed by the Senate Select Committee on Nutrition (29) and the American Heart Association (30). Salt intake should also be restricted because of its relationship to blood pressure and the frequent association between diabetes and hypertension. It remains to be proven whether these dietary recommendations will reduce the toll of vascular complications in diabetic patients, but circumstantial evidence is strong that it should, and there are no known risks involved.

Pharmacologic Control

There are two general types of medication available to control diabetes if effective control cannot be accomplished by a comprehensive program of weight reduction, diet, and exercise; i.e., insulin administration and oral hypoglycemic agents. The use of these agents is discussed briefly, but more details are available elsewhere (1, 5, 6, 14–16, 31–34).

Insulin Therapy

Indications. Few developments in medicine have changed the course of a disease so drastically as the development of insulin by Banting and Best in 1921. The indications for insulin use are (a) to treat or avoid episodes of ketoacidosis in type I patients, (b) to control symptoms associated with the metabolic derangements that accompany marked hyperglycemia (greater than 180 mg/dl) and glycosuria in both type I or II diabetic patients not responding to nonpharmacologic treatment and/or maximal doses of oral hypoglycemic drugs, (c) achievement of approximately normal glycemia even in asymptomatic patients in an attempt to prevent diabetic complications ("tight or intensive control") (33), (d) when oral hypoglycemic agents are contraindicated in type II patients because of renal, hepatic, or allergic problems or as an alternative to hypoglycemic agents by preference of the clinician (31), and (e) for short-term use to control exacerbations of either type I or II diabetes because of infections, trauma, surgery, gestation, drugs, or myocardial infarction.

Goals. Goals of insulin therapy are to alleviate the patient's acute diabetic symptoms and to correct accompanying metabolic disorders, including returning the blood glucose concentration to as near-normal levels as possible while avoiding hypoglycemia. More specific criteria for optimal control will be discussed.

Initial insulin management usually is started in a hospital diabetic unit with the insulin dose(s) tailored in accordance with blood glucose responses. Subsequent management is based on home monitoring of capillary blood glucose levels in drops of blood obtained by fingersticks. In fact, successful management of insulin therapy is completely dependent on accurate assessment of blood glucose concentrations by the patient.

Conventional Regimen. In the United States and most of the world, insulin is usually obtained from the pancreas of cattle and pigs. Insulin from almost any animal is effective in humans, but slight variations in arrangements of the amino acids within the insulin molecule may lead to excessive antibody formation and render the insulin less effective. The recent synthesis of human insulin gives hope that this problem can be eliminated and that the effectiveness of insulin therapy can be improved.

To decrease the number of daily injections, certain materials have been added to prolong the action of insulin. These modified forms of insulin are generally classified by the duration of their action (i.e., fast- or short-acting, intermediate, or prolonged). Pharmacologic properties of common insulin preparations are summarized in Table 6.1.

An intermediate-acting insulin preparation, such as NPH or lente, generally is administered before breakfast as the sole or major source of insulin. Intermediate-acting insulins do not achieve their peak pharmacologic action until at least 6 hours after administration, and their effect is sustained for about 24 hours (Table 6.1). A potential problem with this pharmacologic profile is that hyperglycemia often occurs in the middle or late mornings before the maximal effect of the AM dose is achieved. To prevent such an occurrence, it is common practice to administer a mixture of short-acting insulin, such as regular insulin, with intermediate-acting insulin in the same syringe before breakfast (mixed-dosage regimen). Since regular insulin (CZI) generally achieves its peak effect in about 2 to 4 hours, this may abort the midmorning hyperglycemia common when intermediate-acting insulin is used alone. However, regular insulin should only be added after the appropriate dose of intermediate-acting insulin has been established.

Usually optimal control of hyperglycemia cannot be achieved with a single daily insulin injection, and two or more doses of intermediate insulin or the addition of regular insulin is required. If a twice-a-day regimen is required, two-thirds to three-quarters of the intermediate-acting insulin is usually given in the morning, and the remainder before supper. Also, if regular insulin is required, 5 to 10 units are administered in the same syringe with each dose of intermediate-acting insulin. If still more insulin is required to control postprandial hyperglycemia, regular insulin can be administered alone 30 minutes before

Table 6.1
Pharmacologic Characteristics of Various Insulin Preparations

Type	Preparation	Time to Onset of Action (hrs)	Time to Maximal Activity (hrs)	Duration of Action (hrs)
Rapid:	Regular (CZI) [a]	0.5–1	2–4	4–8
short-acting	Semilente	1–2	3–7	8–16
Intermediate-acting	NPH[b]	3–4	6–16	18–30
	Lente	3–4	6–16	18–30
Prolonged:	PZI[c]	6–8	14–24	24–36
long-acting	Ultra-Lente	5–8	14–26	32–>36

[a] CZI, crystalline zinc insulin.
[b] NPH, neutral protamine Hagedorn.
[c] PZI, protamine zinc insulin.

meals to allow the peak concentration of insulin to match the increase in blood glucose level induced by the meal.

An alternate method for stricter glycemic control is to administer a single dose of a long-acting form of insulin, such as Ultra-Lente, 30 minutes *before supper* or divided into two daily doses, with the second injection administered *before breakfast*. Regular insulin also can be added as required along with the Ultra-Lente doses and, if necessary, alone before lunch and dinner. It should be emphasized that each diabetic individual's regimen will be different depending on the patient's existing pathophysiology, eating and physical activity habits, and personal needs.

The target plasma or capillary glucose concentrations considered to reflect "excellent" diabetic control are 70 to 120 mg/dl in the fasting state or before meals, and 100 to 140 mg/dl 1 hour after meals (6). Control is considered poor if fasting and preprandial plasma glucose levels are greater than 150 mg/dl, and the 1 hour postprandial level is greater than 200 mg/dl.

Many physicians permit patients to administer extra regular insulin to lower elevated levels of blood glucose. One unit of regular insulin usually will lower blood glucose levels about 40 to 50 mg/dl when the glucose concentration is in the range of 150 to 200 mg/dl (14, 32, 33). For example, a blood glucose level of 200 mg/dl generally would require 2 units of regular insulin to reduce the blood glucose levels to 100 mg/dl. It generally is not recommended that a patient take more than 4 units of "corrective insulin" at a time without first checking with his or her physician.

Sites of Administration. Usual sites for subcutaneous administration of insulin include over the quadriceps muscle of the frontal thigh, the deltoid region of the upper extremities, and the abdominal and gluteal regions. Injection of insulin into a region of the body that will soon be involved in physical activity accelerates the absorption of insulin into the blood (35, 36). This leads to a more rapid onset of insulin action, a greater reduction in blood glucose, and a shorter duration of insulin action. For example, it would be inappropriate to administer insulin in the quadriceps region before walking or running, or in the deltoid region before weight lifting or swimming. In general the gluteal or abdominal regions seem more appropriate sites for insulin administration in physically active people since the rate of insulin absorption from these sites does not appear to be affected by exercise. Some diabetologists recommend limiting the injection sites to rotating positions on the abdomen (33).

Side Effects. Side effects of insulin therapy include local skin reactions at the site of injections, systemic allergic reactions, insulin resistance (>200 units of insulin required daily), decrease in subcutaneous fat at injection sites, and hypoglycemia ("insulin reaction") (1, 14).

Hypoglycemia is actually not a true side effect but an exaggerated therapeutic response. Occasional mild hypoglycemia is unavoidable during intensive insulin therapy (31). During a hypoglycemic reaction, the blood glucose usually is less than 60 mg/dl. However, signs and symptoms of hypoglycemia may occur in some diabetic patients with a rapid drop in blood glucose level even if the actual concentration is still elevated. Early symptoms and signs of hypoglycemia include hunger, anxiety, tremulousness, tachycardia, sweating, tingling of the lips or tongue, dizziness, and/or headache. Often only one or a few of these symptoms provide the patient an early warning system. These early symptoms and signs primarily result from sympathetic nervous system activation and may be masked in patients receiving beta-adrenergic drugs, such as propranolol. These symptoms/signs represent a true medical emergency since, if sugar is not administered quickly, the individual may experience more marked cerebral depression and dysfunction, including faintness, blurry or double vision, inability to concentrate, slurred speech, coordination problems, irritability, personality changes, drowsiness, or unconsciousness (coma). Because of the resemblance of these findings to alcohol or drug intoxication, it is imperative for the type I diabetic individual to wear a Medic Alert identification.

Hypoglycemic reactions may occur in well-controlled type I diabetic individuals because of an excess dose of insulin or, less commonly, oral hypoglycemic drugs, skipped meals, decreased food intake, or increased physical activity uncompensated for by extra food or a reduced insulin dose. Every type I diabetic individual must be trained to recognize these early warnings of hypoglycemia (confirmation now can easily be obtained by checking one's own capillary blood glucose levels) and to have an existing plan for combating low blood glucose levels. Food or snacks containing about 10 to 15 gm of a rapidly-absorbed form of simple carbohydrate, such as orange juice or hard candy, may be sufficient for treatment of mild insulin reactions. This should be repeated within 20 minutes if symptoms persist. This important topic of avoiding hypoglycemia will be discussed further later in this chapter from the perspective of the athlete with type I diabetes.

New Developments. Several recent developments should significantly improve metabolic control and make life easier and more normal for many insulin-dependent diabetic persons. These developments include various types of battery-powered portable or implantable insulin infusion devices or pumps (5, 14, 36, 37). Insulin pumps are refillable reservoirs, which administer short-acting insulin via a catheter to a needle under the skin or directly into a vein. A more sophisticated system, a "closed loop" pump or so-called "artificial endocrine pancreas," administers insulin "on demand" (37). Artificial pancreas-type of perfusion systems have a mechanical sensing device that monitors the blood glucose concentration. By means of a programmed algorithm, the required rate of insulin infusion is determined from the prevailing glucose concentration. The pump responds by infusing the appropriate amount of insulin. Prerequisites for insulin pump treatment have been published (5). Long-term use of the artificial pancreas-type insulin pump system currently is limited by its cumbersome size and the need for two patent intravenous lines. There also are potential serious risks with either type of insulin administration device associated with pump malfunction, catheter-related problems, and the potential for hypoglycemia or infections. However, as technology improves, these devices hold great promise for better control of diabetes and improved quality of life for the diabetic patient.

Another important development on the horizon is transplants of whole or partial pancreas or islet beta cells alone. Improved immunologic control since the advent of cyclosporin has made these viable options for the type I diabetic individual (38). Currently these procedures are limited primarily to patients with advanced eye, renal, or nerve damage. About 200 pancreas transplants a year currently are being performed, with the 1-year survival rate now 79%. The "rival" procedure of islet cell transplantation involves grafting donor islets in the liver using percutaneous intrahepatic catheterization of the portal vein. Implanted cells then act like those of the pancreas to provide the host with insulin in response to changes in blood glucose levels. The latter procedure has only been attempted in a few patients so far with limited success. Both procedures appear to offer a great deal of promise but require considerably more research before they become viable options for most diabetic patients.

Oral Hypoglycemic Agents

Oral agents are effective in controlling blood sugar levels in certain diabetic individuals; however, they require the presence of some insulin in the patient's beta cells to be effective (1, 6, 15, 34). The so-called sulfonylurea drugs first became available in 1955 and include Orinase, Diabinese, Dymelor, and Tolinase. Two "second-generation" sulfonylurea compounds recently have become available in the United States, glyburide and glipizide. As is the case with insulin, these preparations may be classified according to the duration of their action. Their apparent primary pharmacologic action is to stimulate pancreatic islet cells to release more insulin. They also appear to reduce glucose production and release by the liver, and potentiate insulin's action on glucose transport beyond the insulin receptor in muscle and adipose tissue, thereby increasing cellular uptake of glucose. The net result of these actions is increased effectiveness of available insulin.

The use of oral hypoglycemic drugs is

contraindicated in patients prone to ketoacidosis. These agents have been used primarily to treat persons with type II diabetes who are not responding to diet, or persons with mild stable type I diabetes capable of insulin production and requiring less than 20 units of insulin per day for control. The drugs currently are being used in 30 to 50% of all diabetic patients.

Possible side effects of the sulfonylurea drugs include an "insulin-like" hypoglycemic reaction resulting from unusual amounts of exercise or other stresses, skin rashes, loss of appetite, gastrointestinal upset, and serious interaction with other drugs and certain nutrients. Hyponatremia and mild intolerance to alcohol also have been reported (15). Generally, however, these agents are well tolerated, with an overall incidence of side effects of only 3 to 5%.

The use of these agents has become a subject of much controversy, based on the interpretation of a large multicenter research study, the University Group Diabetes Program. In this study, mild, type II, ketoacidosis-resistant diabetic patients or adults with glucose intolerance were treated with a prescribed dietary regimen in combination with oral hypoglycemic agents, tolbutamide or phenformin, insulin, or a placebo. The major conclusions drawn from the study were: (a) the combination of dietary change and tolbutamide was no more effective than dietary change alone in prolonging life; and (b) cardiovascular mortality was *higher* in the groups receiving tolbutamide therapy than in those treated with diet alone or diet plus insulin therapy (39). Controversy exists over criteria for patient selection and various other aspects of the study design, and the results are not universally accepted (6). Therefore, the exact role of the oral hypoglycemic agents cannot be clearly defined at this time, and their use probably should be limited, especially in younger diabetic patients.

EXERCISE EFFECTS

Acute Effects

An appreciation of the metabolic effects of acute exercise is required for an understanding of some of the potential benefits and hazards of exercise for patients with DM. This topic has previously been reviewed (27, 32, 36, 40, 41).

During exercise, increased requirements for fuels and oxygen to the contracting skeletal muscles and for the maintenance of an adequate supply of nutrients to vital organs are met by major metabolic, hormonal, and cardiovascular adjustments. The principal fuels are carbohydrates (in the form of glycogen stored in the muscles and blood-borne glucose) and blood-borne free fatty acids (FFA) derived primarily from triglycerides in adipose tissue. The relative contribution of carbohydrate and FFA to oxidative energy production depends both on the intensity and duration of muscular exertion. The more strenuous the exercise, i.e., the greater the percentage of maximal oxygen uptake ($\dot{V}O_2max$) achieved, the greater the dependence of the participating muscles on carbohydrates for fuel. With light- or moderate-intensity dynamic or aerobic exercises, such as walking, running, cycling, and swimming, an orderly sequence of fuel utilization takes place. During the first few minutes, muscle glycogen is the primary source of fuel. After about 5 to 10 minutes, blood glucose and FFA become increasingly more important substrates. Glucose utilization may increase 20-fold over the basal rate and contribute 25 to 40% of the total oxidative fuel requirements. An increase in blood flow to the exercising muscle contributes to the increased glucose uptake.

Despite increased utilization, the blood glucose level remains unchanged or shows only a slight decrease even after hours of exercise. What makes this possible is a continuous replenishment of the blood glucose pool through an increase in rate of glucose production and release by the liver. For at least the first 40 minutes of dynamic exercise, increased liver glucose production is derived primarily from the breakdown of hepatic glycogen (glycogenolysis); however, glycogen stores are limited, particularly in diabetic individuals. During more prolonged exercise, the formation of *new* hepatic glycogen and glucose becomes an increasingly more important contributor to glucose released by the liver (gluconeogenesis). Substrates for gluconeogenesis include blood-borne lactate, pyruvate, glycerol, and certain amino acids. Eventually even this process begins to fail, and blood glucose levels fall. However, this is accompanied by a progressive shift from dependence on carbohydrate to FFA for oxidative metabolism as a compensatory mechanism. Diabetic individuals show an increased efficiency for utilization of FFA as fuels, compared with nondiabetics. Exercise conditioning also improves the ability to use FFA as a fuel, thereby having a carbohydrate-sparing effect. Despite this shift during prolonged exercise to the increased use of FFA for fuel, muscle glycogen utilization remains essential for maintaining muscle contractions, and initial stored levels are a limiting factor for performing prolonged dynamic exercise.

A reduction of depletion of muscle and liver glycogen stores stimulates activity of an enzyme essential for glycogen synthesis (glycogen synthetase). Increased activity of this enzyme appears to be associated with an accelerated, noninsulin-dependent uptake of glucose by muscle and the liver, which persists for 24 to 48 hours following prolonged exercise while glycogen stores continue to be replenished. During this recovery period, there is a temporary improvement of glucose tolerance and insulin sensitivity in both diabetic and nondiabetic individuals.

A number of hormones contribute to regulation of fuel availability, rate of utilization, and homeostasis during exercise. Insulin levels play a key role. Insulin is essential for glucose uptake by muscle. As an adaptation to prolonged exercise, endogenous levels fall, apparently due to both an increase in tissue insulin receptor activity and increased noninsulin-dependent cell uptake of glucose. Reduction in endogenous plasma insulin levels and improved insulin sensitivity may persist for several days after prolonged exercise. For the insulin-dependent diabetic person this translates to a reduction in exogenous insulin requirements or an increased need for carbohydrates.

Another consequence of reduced levels of endogenous insulin is stimulation of hepatic glycogenolysis and gluconeogenesis and glucose release. In addition, reduced circulating insulin levels promote adipose fat hydrolysis and FFA release. Exercise also stimulates the release of hormones whose effect on carbohydrate and lipid availability is the opposite of that associated with insulin. These so-called "counterregulatory" hormones include catecholamines, glucagon, growth hormone, and cortisol, all of which promote hepatic glucose production and FFA release from adipose tissue in both diabetic and nondiabetic individuals.

In type I diabetes the metabolic response to acute exercise is profoundly influenced by the adequacy of diabetic control by exogenous insulin. When insulin levels are sufficient to control diabetes adequately, or if only mild or moderate hyperglycemia without ketosis is present, acute exercise can reduce blood glucose levels and insulin requirements for as long as 24 to 48 hours. In this situation acute exercise has a temporary ameliorating effect on control of diabetes.

If exercise is performed at the time of peak effect of insulin administration (e.g., within 2 hours after an injection of regular insulin) or if excess insulin is administered, the decline in blood glucose is accentuated during exercise for two reasons: (a) insulin-enhanced glucose uptake and utilization by muscle, and (b) insulin suppression of hepatic glucose production and release. A hypoglycemic reaction may result.

In contrast, when insulin deficiency is severe and metabolic control is poor (e.g., a fasting plasma glucose level over 300 mg/dl with or without ketoacidosis), the diabetic state may be worsened during exercise with an increase in hyperglycemia and ketoacidosis resulting. Mechanisms for this paradoxical response include elevated blood levels of the "counterregulatory" hormones, increased hepatic glucose production and release, and elevated blood FFA levels and their increased conversion by the liver to ketone bodies. This possible adverse effect of exercise underscores the importance of adequate control of diabetes prior to initiating any vigorous exercise program.

Potential Health Benefits of Exercise Training

Regular exercise is generally considered to be beneficial for most diabetic patients.

Potential health benefits are summarized in Table 6.2 and the current status of scientific evidence for each of the possible benefits is briefly reviewed below:

Improved Physical Fitness

Physical fitness has been defined as the ability to carry out daily tasks with vigor, with alertness, and without fatigue, with ample reserve energy to enjoy leisure-time pursuits and to meet unforeseen emergencies, and to respond to physical and emotional stress without an excessive increase in heart rate and blood pressure (42, 43). The measurable components of physical fitness may be divided into two groups: One related to *health* and the other related to *skills*, which primarily pertain to athletic performance (43). The health-related components are (a) cardiorespiratory endurance, (b) muscular endurance, (c) body composition and (d) flexibility. Skill-related fitness components are agility, balance, coordination, speed, power, and reaction time.

Cardiorespiratory endurance or aerobic capacity relates to the maximal ability of the circulatory and respiratory systems to supply oxygen and fuel to the skeletal muscles and other organs and to eliminate metabolic waste products (e.g., CO_2, lactic acid) (43). It is determined by measuring the aerobic capacity or $\dot{V}O_2$max during all-out exercise on the treadmill or cycle ergometer. An improvement in this component by endurance exercise training usually is accompanied by beneficial effects on carbohydrate and lipid metabolism and favorable body composition changes (reduced body fat with no change or a small increase in lean body mass) in both nondiabetic and diabetic individuals. An increase in $\dot{V}O_2$max not only enhances maximal capacity for endurance types of physical exertion, but reduces fatigue and the level of perceived exertion during performance of sustained more-moderate intensity activities.

In order to increase $\dot{V}O_2$max, it is necessary to perform dynamic endurance-type physical activities regularly, such as walking, running, bicycling, or swimming, which increase the heart and respiratory rates. It has been repeatedly demonstrated that to obtain significant improvement in $\dot{V}O_2$max (typically 5 to 30%), 20 to 60 minutes of training activities are required at least three times a week at an intensity of 50 to 85% of a person's baseline $\dot{V}O_2$max. This level of exercise corresponds to about 60 to 90% of maximal heart rate (39, 43). An inverse relationship exists between the intensity of exercise and the duration necessary for improving $\dot{V}O_2$max. In other words, if you perform moderate intensity exercise (50 to 60% of $\dot{V}O_2$max), a longer duration and/or frequency of exercise sessions is required than is necessary with higher intensity exercise. A trade-off is that the more moderate exercise is less likely to result in musculoskeletal injury as compared with high-intensity exercise, and adherence is generally better. It should also be emphasized that the relative improvement (%) in aerobic capacity after a training program is inversely related to baseline $\dot{V}O_2$ max levels. An improvement in $\dot{V}O_2$max results from increases in the maximal arteriovenous oxygen difference, the maximal stroke volume of the heart, or both. To maintain one's existing level of $\dot{V}O_2$max, only twice a week exercise is usually required.

Table 6.2
Potential Health Benefits Accompanying Exercise Conditioning for the Patient with Diabetes Mellitus

1. Improved physical fitness
2. Prevention or reduction of obesity
3. Improved metabolic control
4. Improved blood lipid profile
5. Reduced risk of coronary heart disease
6. Psychosocial benefits

Prevention or Reduction of Obesity

The role of obesity in insulin resistance and in the etiology of type II DM has been previously discussed. Physical inactivity is often a major contributor to obesity. Regular exercise can reduce susceptibility to diabetes by weight maintenance in addition to the metabolic and endocrinologic adaptations discussed previously. Regular walking is the most popular form of physical activity for people of all ages in the United States. Its value for normalizing body weight and mobilizing adipose stores in obese women and men has been demonstrated even in the absence of dietary changes. The loss of lean body mass commonly observed during dieting does not occur during weight reduction associated with exercise alone or when exercise is employed in combination with mild-to-moderate caloric restriction in obese individuals (44–47). Moreover, weight loss through exercise may slightly exceed levels anticipated through direct expenditure of calories alone (44). Two mechanisms may play a role; appetite suppression for at least 30 to 90 minutes after exercise and an increase in resting metabolic rate for 1 or more hours.

Improved Metabolic Control

The common recommendation of regular exercise as part of the therapy for control of DM is based on the following data: (a) the enhanced glucose uptake by the exercising muscle in both nondiabetic and diabetic individuals previously described, (b) the well-known blood glucose-lowering effect of an acute exercise session in diabetic patients first reported prior to the discovery of insulin (48), (c) reduction in exogenous insulin requirements of type I diabetic individuals observed on days in which vigorous exercise is performed, which was initially demonstrated over 60 years ago (49), (d) improved insulin sensitivity with exercise training in nondiabetic subjects, particularly in obese people with hyperinsulinemia or glucose intolerance (50), and (e) a reversible adverse effect on insulin sensitivity and glucose tolerance of physical inactivity resulting from a few days of bed rest in nondiabetic men (9, 10).

However, despite these observations, there is a paucity of controlled studies to determine if chronic exercise training has *independent* metabolic benefits for either type I or type II diabetic individuals beyond that due to repeated "bursts" of acute exercise or to accompanying weight loss.

Contradictory results have been obtained from the few controlled chronic exercise studies involving type I diabetic individuals. Most studies involving children or adolescents have demonstrated substantial increases in $\dot{V}O_2$max and improved metabolic control with regular vigorous exercise performed for at least 30 minutes three times a week for up to 12 weeks. Exercised subjects, compared with physically inactive control subjects, have been able to reduce their daily insulin requirements significantly (51, 52), lower fasting blood glucose and glycosylated hemoglobin concentrations (53), or improve insulin sensitivity as measured by the euglycemic clamp technique (54). However, differences in the type of metabolic response in these studies may be related to how well the DM was controlled prior to the exercise program, changes in caloric intake during the exercise program, extent of improvement in $\dot{V}O_2$max with training, and whether there was an accompanying increase in lean body mass.

In one of the few controlled studies involving *adult* type I diabetic patients, Zinman et al. (55) evaluated the metabolic effects of stationary cycle ergometer exercise training, including 45-minute sessions three times a week for 12 weeks. An *acute glucose-lowering effect was confirmed with each exercise session*, and $\dot{V}O_2$max was significantly improved with training; however, the subjects failed to demonstrate an associated improvement in blood glucose control, $HbgA_1$ levels, or insulin requirements. Increased caloric intake, primarily as carbohydrate on exercise days, was considered to be a likely cause of the failure to improve glycemic control with training. Wallberg-Henriksson et al. (56) likewise failed to find a change in glycemic control in a group of 13 type I diabetic women performing daily cycle ergometer exercise for 5 months. The same investigators had previously reported increased peripheral insulin sensitivity but unchanged blood glucose control following exercise training in type I diabetic men (57). Yski-Järvinen et al. (58) studied the metabolic effects of a four times a week cycle ergometer exercise program in type I diabetic patients after achieving near-normal glycemic control using a portable insulin infusion pump for continuous subcutaneous insulin infusion (CSII). Patients were randomly assigned to a sedentary control group continuing on CSII or to receive repeated self-administered insulin doses while continuing the exercise program. A 6% reduction was demonstrated in insulin requirements (2 units/day) in the exercise group after 6 weeks of training. Insulin sensitivity as determined by the euglycemic clamp technique was found to be significantly greater in the exercise compared with the sedentary control group. This was accompanied by a 60% increase in rate of glucose uptake. However, basal hepatic glucose production remained elevated (but could be suppressed by insulin administration), and plasma C-peptide levels remained low in both groups.

It is concluded from these controlled studies that exercise three or four times a week in type I DM will not significantly improve glycemic control, especially if food intake is significantly increased on exercise days. However, daily exercise will probably improve blood glucose control through overlapping effects of acute exercise sessions. Furthermore, insulin sensitivity usually can be improved by exercise training programs. This most likely results from exercise conditioning effects on skeletal muscle involved in the regular exercise, including increased muscle mass, augmented muscle blood flow and capillary density, enhanced mitochondrial oxidative enzyme activity, activation of the glucose transport system, and increased glycogen synthesis (41, 54).

There have been even fewer controlled studies evaluating the effects of exercise alone on metabolic control of noninsulin-dependent (type II) DM. These also have yielded contradictory results. In a study in the author's laboratory (59), the metabolic effects of moderate intensity treadmill walking for 30 or 60 minutes per session two to four times a week for 12 weeks were studied in 48 overweight, previously sedentary middle-aged men with uncontrolled mild or moderate type II DM or glucose intolerance. Body weight was kept constant in an attempt to distinguish the effects of exercise from weight reduction. The exercise regimen resulted in a small increase in $\dot{V}O_2$max (5.5%) and a significant reduction in skinfold thickness despite the constant body weight. However, there was no associated improvement in either fasting glucose or glycosylated hemoglobin levels, glucose tolerance, basal plasma insulin levels, or in the insulin response to oral glucose. These findings agree with the data of Ruderman et al. (60). The latter study also involved middle-aged, moderately obese type II subjects (N = 6) who performed progressive cycle ergometer exercise 5 days per week for 6 weeks. The training program resulted in a 15% improvement in $\dot{V}O_2$max although body weight remained unchanged.

In contrast, several studies have reported improvement in glucose homeostasis with exercise training in diabetic men and women. Saltin et al. (61) subjected 11 sedentary, nonobese, middle-aged men with glucose intolerance to twice weekly 60-minute sessions of vigorous exercise for 12 weeks and demonstrated a 20% increase in $\dot{V}O_2$max with body weight remaining constant. These investigators reported an associated improvement in glucose tolerance, but not in insulin sensitivity. Another group of 25 men, also with impaired glucose tolerance, received a similar exercise conditioning program along with a weight-reduction diet, and experienced a 4.5 kg weight loss. This latter group demonstrated both an improvement in glucose tolerance and a reduction in plasma insulin levels, which were reversed after 2 weeks of detraining. An additive metabolic effect of weight loss and exercise also has been demonstrated in the author's laboratory as well as by others in nondiabetic obese people (46).

Schneider et al. (62) exercised 14 patients with type II DM for 6 to 10 weeks with a resulting significant decline in fasting plasma glucose and in glycosylated hemoglobin levels, but no improvement in glucose tolerance or insulin sensitivity. A recent well-controlled study by Reitman et al. (63) involved six obese men and women with recent-onset type II DM who were hospitalized on a clinical research ward. The subjects were given a vigorous exercise program employing an intensity of 60 to 90% of $\dot{V}O_2$ max. The program involved intermittent exercise on a cycle ergometer for 20 to 40 minutes, 5 or 6 days a week. A significant decline in fasting plasma glucose occurred in all subjects, body weight remained unchanged, and oral glucose tolerance improved in five of the six subjects. Individual improvement in plasma glucose was proportional to the level of hyperglycemia prior to training. However, the effect on insulin sensitivity during euglycemic clamp studies was extremely variable and an observed increase in mean insulin-induced glucose disposal rate for the group did not reach statistical significance. Recently, Krotkiewski et al. (64) subjected a group of 46 type II diabetic men and women to a 3-month, three times a week program combining walking, jogging, calisthenics, and cycle ergometer exercise. Aerobic capacity increased by 14%, but body weight remained constant. Although fasting blood glucose and insulin levels were unchanged, exercise training improved both glucose tolerance and insulin sensitivity.

There appear to be a number of factors contributing to the inconsistencies observed in the aforementioned studies. These include: (a) the heterogeneity of study populations, (b) baseline differences in disease severity, (c) differences in relative weight, body fatness, and initial physical fitness of study subjects, (d) presence or absence of weight changes during training, (e) the type, intensity, frequency, and duration of exercise and (f) the magnitude of the resulting improvement in $\dot{V}O_2max$ achieved. Exercise training programs in nondiabetic individuals also have yielded inconsistent effects on glucose-insulin metabolism, probably for some of the same reasons mentioned above. Additional research is needed to clarify these discrepancies. However, encouraging results on metabolic control by type II diabetics have been demonstrated with a combined program of treadmill walking; a high complex carbohydrate, high-fiber, low-fat diet; and associated weight reduction (65). Thus, based on the available evidence it appears that moderate, regular endurance exercise has a modest independent effect on glucose homeostasis, and that an exercise program is appropriately viewed as an adjunct to other modes of treatment for control of both type I and type II DM.

Improved Blood Lipid Profile

The effects of exercise training on blood lipids and lipoprotein levels have been recently extensively reviewed (66, 67). The relevance of the blood lipid profile to the diabetic individual is through its relationship to atherosclerotic diseases. Elevated blood levels of total and LDL cholesterol and, perhaps, triglycerides and VLDL cholesterol increase the risk of CHD and other macrovascular diseases, while HDL cholesterol levels show an inverse relationship to these diseases (66, 67). It is well-known that endurance-trained men and women athletes have favorable blood lipid and lipoprotein profiles. More specifically, they generally have lower plasma levels of triglycerides (and of its principal carrier in the fasting state, VLDL) and higher levels of HDL cholesterol, compared with sedentary controls. Endurance exercise training requiring an energy expenditure of 1000 kcal/week or more usually produces favorable blood lipid-lipoprotein alterations in nondiabetic men, especially if accompanied by weight loss (46, 66–69). These changes include increases in plasma HDL cholesterol and the ratio of HDL cholesterol to total cholesterol, and reductions in plasma triglycerides and VLDL cholesterol with a less consistent decrease in plasma LDL cholesterol. Exercise conditioning appears less likely to significantly alter the blood lipid profiles of women than men, perhaps due to more favorable baseline levels among women (67).

The effect of exercise training on the blood lipid profile of diabetic men and women has not been extensively studied. Several studies in type I diabetic men have reported a favorable increase in the ratio of HDL cholesterol to total cholesterol, but no significant changes in absolute concentrations of plasma HDL cholesterol, total cholesterol, or triglycerides (57, 58). However, Wallberg-Henriksson et al. (56) reported no change in the postconditioning lipid profile in type I diabetic women. Similarly, type II diabetic subjects in the author's laboratory showed no changes in blood lipids following an exercise training program (59). These findings are in agreement with those of Krotkiewski et al. (64). In contrast, Ruderman et al. (60) found significant decreases in plasma total cholesterol and triglyceride levels after exercise training in type II diabetic patients in the absence of weight loss. Unfortunately, the investigators did not measure HDL cholesterol levels. It should be noted, however, that improved control of diabetes alone may raise HDL cholesterol levels and normalize the blood lipid profile (70).

A proposed mechanism for favorable alterations in blood lipid and lipoprotein levels by exercise is through the induction of enzymes involved in lipid metabolism including lipoprotein lipase, hepatic lipase, adipose tissue lipase, and lecithin: cholesterol acyltransferase (LCAT) (65, 67).

Reduced Risk of Coronary Heart Disease

An inverse relationship between physical activity levels and the incidence of CHD and associated mortality has repeatedly been demonstrated in epidemiologic studies (71, 72). This has also been demonstrated to be true even in middle-aged men at high risk of CHD because of levels of blood cholesterol, blood pressure, and cigarette smoking (73). In addition, epidemiologic studies show that a below average level of physical fitness (aerobic capacity) is independently associated with an unfavorable coronary risk factor profile and an increased risk of CHD.

Reduced risk of CHD appears to be optimally afforded by 2000 kcal per week of physical activity, and some protection by at least 500 kcal per week (71–72). Possible physiologic mechanisms by which exercise reduces CHD risk include the blood lipid changes described above, improved glucose-insulin metabolism, lower body weight, reduced blood pressure and heart rate, decreased myocardial oxygen requirements (as a result of decreased systolic blood pressure and heart rate) and, perhaps, increased myocardial vascularity, reduced blood coagulability, and decreased vulnerability to serious cardiac rhythm disturbances. Moreover, studies in monkeys on atherogenic diets have demonstrated that exercise reduces the severity of atherosclerosis; however, no confirmation of this is available in humans. A definitive clinical trial proving the protective effects of regular exercise against CHD or other atherosclerotic manifestations has not been done in either nondiabetic or diabetic individuals. Nevertheless, the author feels the available evidence is sufficient to include exercise as part of a CHD prevention program for both groups.

Psychosocial Benefits

It is widely believed among health professionals that regular exercise provides psychosocial benefits that improve the quality of life; however, this is difficult to substantiate by controlled studies (74). Physical activities should be selected that are fun and enjoyable. Improved feelings of well-being, health consciousness, self-confidence, self-control, and self-esteem are especially important for patients with diabetes. Exercise may also prove helpful in relieving muscular tension and mental depression, and in promoting sound sleep.

Exercise Hazards and Precautions

There are special problems and hazards associated with exercise for diabetic individuals, particularly for those requiring insulin for metabolic control (see Table 6.3). Detractors who feel that exercise is merely a "perturbation that makes treatment of diabetes difficult," agree that the "present knowledge and technology allow the well-informed and cooperative patient with insulin dependent diabetes to exercise and even to reach the elite level" (75). Potential problems for the exercising diabetic individual include:

Worsening of Metabolic State

Individuals with type I diabetes should not perform vigorous or prolonged exercise if ketoacidosis is present or their fasting

Table 6.3
Health Hazards Associated with Exercise in Persons with Diabetes Mellitus

1. Worsening of metabolic state
2. Hypoglycemia
3. Aggravation of retinopathy
4. Musculoskeletal and soft-tissue injuries
5. Complications from foot injuries
6. Myocardial infarction or sudden death

plasma glucose level exceeds 250 to 300 mg/dl. In such persons, exercise training may actually worsen the metabolic state. Consequently, a formal exercise regimen should be proscribed until improved metabolic control is obtained using diet and/or insulin or an oral hypoglycemic agent.

Hypoglycemia

For the diabetic on insulin therapy, the principal risk associated with exercise is an insulin reaction or hypoglycemia. This problem is of less magnitude in patients on oral hypoglycemic drugs. The risk of hypoglycemia is most marked in individuals receiving intensive multidose insulin therapy or continuous insulin infusion delivery by pump. Even if hypoglycemia does not occur during the exercise itself, the possibility remains for a delayed episode of hypoglycemia after exercise due to a fall in blood glucose as depleted muscle and liver glycogen stores are being replenished. Certain precautions are required to avoid or minimize hypoglycemic reactions. These are summarized in Table 6.4 and discussed below.

First, it is important for all diabetic individuals receiving insulin to try to maintain as much *consistency* in life habits as possible. This is particularly important for those who are participating in exercise programs or in organized sports. This includes keeping as constant as possible the time of day for getting up, going to bed, for meals and snacks, for administration of insulin, the dose(s) and form(s) of insulin, the caloric content of meals and snacks, and the usual amount and intensity of exercise. Such consistency simplifies the process of regulating blood glucose levels. It also helps with the decision-making for adjusting food intake and insulin dose to changes in physical activity levels as the need arises. Quantifiable or reproducible forms of exercise, such as walking, jogging, bicycling, and lap swimming, are more easily regulated by adjustments in food intake and/or insulin dosage to avoid hypoglycemia.

A major breakthrough for improving metabolic control as well as for avoiding hypoglycemia during or following exercise is the general availability of techniques for self-monitoring blood glucose levels. Blood glucose levels should be checked by an insulin-dependent diabetic several times during the day; for example, upon arising, before meals, 90 minutes following meals, at bedtime, perhaps at 3 AM for those on intensive therapy, and before, during, and after exercise. For those participating in team sports, it is now even possible to measure capillary blood glucose levels between quarters or at half-time or whenever an insulin reaction is suspected.

When a type I diabetic first begins an exercise program or sports participation, it is advisable, at least initially, to reduce the basal insulin requirements by 20 to 40% to avoid hypoglycemia until a new balance between food intake, physical activity, and insulin levels is established (25, 32). An alternative in the well-controlled diabetic person is to increase food intake to compensate for the increased physical activity. Another approach to compensate for anticipated unusually prolonged physical ac-

Table 6.4
Special Precautions and Procedures to Prevent Exercise-induced Hypoglycemia for the Insulin-dependent Diabetic Individual

1. Maintain consistency in life habits
2. Careful self-monitoring of capillary blood glucose levels
3. Use injection sites for insulin other than the extremities involved in exercise
4. Avoid exercising during time of peak insulin activity or take special precautions
5. Exercise after a light meal or carbohydrate snack
6. Inform others about diabetic condition, symptoms of hypoglycemia and what to do in the event of an insulin reaction
7. Prompt cessation of exercise upon experiencing hypoglycemia with administration of a carbohydrate snack

tivity is to base the estimate of extra carbohydrate needs on the approximate energy cost of the activity (14). This is determined by the type of physical activity, its intensity and duration, and the body weight of the individual (42, 76). For activities considered light or moderate (5 kcal/min or 300 kcal/hr or less), no additional preexercise food is recommended unless the activity will exceed 30 minutes; and, if so, a snack containing 5 gm of glucose for every 30 minutes of exercise should be sufficient (14). For heavier activities, one-half of the estimated caloric expenditure should be taken in advance of the exercise.

Insulin should not be administered in extremities that are directly participating in the activity because of an accelerated rate of absorption. The abdominal wall and gluteal region are the preferred sites for most exercisers.

Exercise should be avoided, if possible, during the peak action of the form of insulin used; e.g., the peak action for NPH or Lente insulin is approximately 6 to 16 hours after injection, and for regular insulin 2 to 4 hours after administration (Table 6.1). A particularly good time to exercise in terms of glycemic control is about 1 to 2 hours after a light meal or carbohydrate snack since the postprandial blood glucose level peaks at this time. Extra food (in addition to the previous meal or snack) should be consumed before exercising if it is necessary to exercise when insulin activity is at its peak. This can be determined by self-monitoring of blood glucose levels 30 minutes prior to the physical exertion. Extra carbohydrates (15 to 30 gm) should then be ingested 15 to 20 minutes before the anticipated activity. In addition, extra carbohydrate snacks should be readily available to replenish the body's glucose supply during prolonged exercise. The carbohydrate content of snacks commonly used by diabetic athletes is shown in Table 6.5. A snack containing 5 to 10 gm of carbohydrate is recommended every 30 to 45 minutes of exercise in order to avoid hypoglycemia. Some diabetic individuals also require additional food immediately after vigorous activities.

Exercise should be promptly discontinued at the first suspicion of an insulin reaction. An athlete participating in team sports should also make certain that his or her teammates, coaches, and trainer are aware of the diabetic state, usual symptoms and signs of hypoglycemia, the remedy provided for its management, and the location of the athlete's reserve carbohydrate snack supply. Management of hypoglycemic reaction has previously been discussed.

Sports should be avoided if the diabetic athlete and/or the public would be placed in great jeopardy by the onset of hypoglycemia, e.g., scuba diving, parachute jumping, hang gliding, or automobile racing. Guidelines have been published for avoiding hypoglycemia during exercise for type I diabetic individuals using portable continuous subcutaneous insulin injection systems (36, 37, 77). Zinman and Vramic (36) report that it is possible to regulate the rate

Table 6.5
Commonly Available Sources of Simple Carbohydrate (CHO) (10–15 gm per serving) for Management or Prevention of Hypoglycemia during Prolonged Exercise [a]

Source	Serving to Provide 10–15 gm CHO	
	Commom Measure	gm
Fruit/Juice		
Apple (3 per lb)	3/4	113
Apple juice	1/4 cup [b]	63
Cranberry juice cocktail	1/4 cup [b]	63
Fig	1	21
Grape juice	1/4 cup [b]	63
Lemonade	1/2 cup [b]	124
Orange	1	180
Peach	2	228
Pear	1/2	94
Raisin	1/4 oz package	14
Soft Drinks		
Ginger ale	3/4 cup [b]	185
Cola type	1/2 cup [b]	123
Candy/Sugar		
Chocolate	1 oz	28
"Glucotabs"	2	
Honey	1 tbsp	21
Life savers	8	
Sugar (table)	1 tbsp	11
Sugar (cube)	2	

[a] From *Book of Health,* New York, Franklin Watts, 1981, pp. 60–96.
[b] 1 cup = 8 fl oz.

of insulin administration using these pumps to provide excellent glycemic control during exercise. Nevertheless, prior to prolonged postprandial exercise, it is prudent to reduce both the basal insulin infusion rate as well as the usual premeal bolus of insulin 20 to 50%. Furthermore, the catheter infusion sites are susceptible to disruption during exercise. Implantable pumps as they become more widely available will eliminate this problem. An alternative approach is to remove the portable pump prior to exercise and use a small dose of regular insulin instead for glycemic control. This approach is not feasible with the "closed loop" pumps, which have intravenous lines. These latter pumps also are too large and cumbersome to use during vigorous exercise.

Complications From Proliferative Retinopathy

Simple or background retinopathy with microaneurysms of the small arteries of the retina and associated small retinal exudates or hemorrhages is not considered a contraindication to exercise, although contact sports probably should be avoided (14). In a minority of diabetic individuals, this condition progresses to proliferative retinopathy with formation of new retinal vessels. These new vessels are friable and often rupture, causing large retinal and vitreous hemorrhages, retinal detachment, and sometimes blindness (14). Since blood flow and blood pressure increase during exercise, there is concern that vigorous exercise may promote retinal hemorrhage in such individuals. Therefore, strenuous exercise is discouraged in patients with active proliferative retinopathy, at least until the condition has been controlled or treated with photocoagulation (25, 27). Recent vitreous or major retinal hemorrhages are absolute contraindications to exercise.

Musculoskeletal and Soft-Tissue Injuries

There is no evidence that diabetic individuals are more prone to injuries of muscle and joints and their attaching structures. To reduce the possibility of such injuries, similar precautions as for nondiabetic individuals are advised. These include warm-up and cool-down periods incorporating flexibility exercises; initiating a physical conditioning program at a relatively low intensity, duration, and frequency of exercise; and progressing gradually (42, 44).

Contact sports were formerly prohibited for diabetic individuals because of fear that soft-tissue injuries would not heal well. This is generally not true in diabetic persons whose diabetes is under reasonably good control, and such sports are now permitted for young diabetic individuals.

Complications from Foot Injuries

Proper foot care is extremely important for all diabetic individuals and athletes in particular, since infections and ulcerations of the feet are a major cause of morbidity. Gangrene, amputation, and death may result. This is of particular concern to those over age 40, who are more likely to have coexisting macrovascular circulatory problems. In general, serious foot problems are related to three factors: (a) neuropathy, which decreases the ability to perceive pressure and pain, making the diabetic individual unaware of repeated trauma, (b) impaired circulation in the feet due to peripheral vascular disease, which delays healing, and (c) poorly controlled diabetes, which reduces resistance to infection.

It is especially important that the feet of diabetic individuals over the age of 40 and those who have had diabetes 10 years or more be examined regularly by a physician or podiatrist. The presence of calluses and corns are important signs of potential serious problems since most foot ulcers start under these pressure areas. These lesions should be pared off routinely by a physician or podiatrist. The source of the pressure causing their formation (e.g., ill-fitting shoes, foot deformities, or flat feet) also should be identified and corrective measures taken. Preventive measures may include softer and better fitting shoes or prosthetic inserts for dress and sport shoes, and prophylactic surgery to correct foot defects.

Other important foot hygiene measures include careful trimming of the toenails, seeking professional help for ingrown or thickened toenails, proper care of the skin including talcum powder to remove excess moisture and special powders to treat fungus infections between the toes (athlete's feet), and lanolin or other similar ointments to lubricate dry skin.

Myocardial Infarction or Sudden Death: The Value of Exercise Testing in Detecting Susceptible Individuals

Coronary heart disease is the most common cause of death in diabetic adults. Even asymptomatic diabetic individuals over the age of 35 are likely to have underlying coronary atherosclerosis (including possible significant left main coronary artery disease), particularly if they have an abnormal blood lipid profile, elevated blood pressure, and/or smoke cigarettes (4, 22). Medical evaluation before embarking on an exercise program, therefore, is imperative in diabetic individuals over age 35 or even for those younger who have significant coronary risk factors. Selected clinical studies in such persons may help rule out silent myocardial ischemia and serve as a basis for prescribing safe levels of exercise.

The evaluation should include a standard multistage exercise ECG test (44) and/or thallium scintigraphy (78) using a treadmill or cycle ergometer protocol. In a study in the author's laboratory (59) involving 48 men aged 33 to 69 years with type II diabetes or glucose intolerance, 11 (22.9%) had ischemic ECG changes during a symptom-limited treadmill exercise test (Bruce protocol). The exercise test results also provide objective information for prescription of exercise intensity and training heart rate levels. If ischemia is uncovered on exercise ECG and/or thallium scanning, the training heart rate should be kept at least 10 to 20 bpm below the level resulting in ischemic changes during the exercise test. All of the diabetic men in the above-mentioned study who had ischemic exercise ECG changes were able to complete a 12-week supervised treadmill walking program successfully by taking such precautions (59).

SUMMARY AND CONCLUSION

Classification of the two major types of diabetes mellitus is based on whether the patient requires insulin to reduce hyperglycemia and avoid ketoacidosis, i.e., type I or insulin-dependent, and type II or non-insulin-dependent diabetes. These two types differ in their pathophysiology. Type I diabetes is caused by conditions destroying beta cells of the pancreatic islets and is accompanied by an actual deficiency of insulin. It usually manifests during childhood or adolescence. Type II, the more prevalent form, is caused primarily by a resistance to insulin action due to insulin receptor and/or postreceptor defects in skeletal muscle, fat, and other tissues; however, beta cell dysfunction also may be present. The type II variety usually occurs in individuals over age 30 who are obese and physically inactive. Strategies for prevention of type II diabetes include maintaining proper weight and remaining physically active.

Late complications of both types of diabetes result from microvascular disorders and/or macrovascular (atherosclerotic) diseases. A large-scale study is in progress to determine if intensive control of hyperglycemia helps prevent these late complications, particularly the common microvascular complications, diabetic retinopathy and glomerulosclerosis, that may result in visual impairment and renal failure.

Prevention of atherosclerotic complications is believed to require, in addition to control of diabetes, the reduction of other coronary risk factors commonly associated with diabetes, including obesity and physical inactivity with type II diabetes, and an abnormal blood lipid profile and elevated blood pressure with both types.

Effective treatment of diabetes mellitus begins with dietary intervention. This includes caloric manipulation to achieve normal weight, and a high intake of complex carbohydrate and a reduced intake of saturated fat in accordance with recent health recommendations for the general public. Both loss of excess weight and a high intake of complex carbohydrate help improve peripheral insulin sensitivity. A reduced intake of saturated fat and associated dietary cholesterol helps lower total and LDL cholesterol and, hopefully, will reduce the possibility of atherosclerotic complications.

Pharmacologic intervention with insulin

injections or oral hypoglycemic agents is required for symptomatic severe hyperglycemia, ketoacidosis, or in the event of failure of milder hyperglycemia to respond to a diet and exercise program. The currently recommended therapeutic approach is to use multiple subcutaneous injections of a combination of a moderate or long-acting insulin preparation with short-acting regular insulin for "tight" diabetic control. Battery-operated portable insulin pumps for continuous subcutaneous administration are being increasingly employed for insulin delivery as an alternative to multiple-dose injections.

Endurance-type exercise clearly has an acute blood glucose-lowering effect by promoting increased glucose uptake by active muscle, which persists for several days into the recovery period while muscle and liver glycogen stores are being replenished. Chronic exercise training of sufficient intensity, duration, and frequency to increase maximal oxygen uptake by 15% or more generally increases insulin sensitivity, particularly in type I diabetic individuals, and if not compensated by an excessive increase in caloric intake, also may improve glycemic control and reduce insulin requirements. On the other hand, exercise may aggravate uncontrolled diabetes when blood glucose levels are ≥ 250-300 mg/dl and/or when ketoacidosis is present. Other possible beneficial adaptations to chronic exercise training are loss of body fat, improvement in the blood lipid profile, reduced risk of coronary heart disease, and psychological benefits.

In diabetic patients receiving insulin, a major concern during exercise is prevention of hypoglycemia or insulin reaction. Consistency in eating, exercise, insulin administration, and other habits reduces this possibility. Frequent self-monitoring of blood glucose levels is crucial to help the diabetic athlete or recreational exerciser adjust insulin dosage and food intake. A type I diabetic individual initiating a vigorous exercise program either must reduce his or her insulin dosage or increase food intake to avoid insulin reactions. The blood glucose concentration before, during, and after prolonged exercise serves as an important guide. It generally is advised that a light meal or snack be ingested 60 to 90 minutes prior to prolonged exercise. This should be supplemented every 30 to 45 minutes during prolonged exercise with a beverage or snack high in simple carbohydrate. Following exercise, blood glucose levels should continue to be monitored because of the possibility of delayed hypoglycemia as liver and the muscles replenish their carbohydrate (glycogen) stores.

Vigorous exercise and particularly contact sports should be avoided in the presence of uncontrolled proliferative retinopathy because of the danger of inducing retinal or vitreous hemorrhages or retinal separation. Proper fitting footwear and careful foot care and hygiene are crucial to the diabetic exerciser to avoid foot ulcers, blisters, corns, calluses, and other problems that may lead to serious complications, including infections, gangrene, and amputations. This is a particular problem for the diabetic individual with neuropathy, peripheral vascular disease, and increased susceptibility to infections due to elevated blood sugar.

Before diabetic individuals embark on an exercise program that is more strenuous than brisk walking, a careful medical evaluation is necessary to rule out contraindications and to prescribe safe levels of exercise. A multistage exercise electrocardiographic or thallium imaging test should be included for all diabetic individuals over age 35 and for younger ones who have other risk factors for coronary heart disease to rule out manifestations of significant latent coronary heart disease and to establish a baseline fitness level. The prescribed exercise should be commensurate with the severity of diabetes, fitness status, and recreational interests of the individual, as well as the availability of exercise facilities. To minimize the risk of musculoskeletal problems, the initial starting level of programs should be of short duration and gradually progress. Warm-up and cool-down periods should also be included. Finally, for most middle-aged or older adults with diabetes, competitive and isometric activities should be avoided because of the possibility of excessive cardiovascular stress.

ACKNOWLEDGMENT

The author wishes to express his appreciation to Marilyn Borkon for her assistance in the preparation of this manuscript.

REFERENCES

1. Kral PL (ed): *Joslin Diabetes Manual*, ed 11. Philadelphia, Lea and Febiger, 1978, p 1.
2. Radder JK: Pathogenesis of diabetes mellitus. Type I. Diabetes mellitus. In Radder JK, Lemkes HHPJ, Kraus HMJ (eds): *Pathogenesis and Treatment of Diabetes Mellitus*. Boston, Martinus Nijhoff Publisher, 1986, p 1.
3. Gerich JE: Insulin-dependent diabetes mellitus: Pathophysiology. *Mayo Clin Proc* 61:787–791, 1986.
4. West KM: *Epidemiology of Diabetes and Its Vascular Lesions*. New York, Elsevier, 1978, p 1.
5. Saudek CD: Diabetes Mellitus. In Harvey AM, Johns R, McKusick VA (eds): *The Principle and Practice of Medicine*, ed 21. Norwalk, CT., Appleton-Century-Crofts, 1984, p 889.
6. Skyler JS: Non-insulin-dependent diabetes mellitus: A clinical strategy. *Diabetes Care* 7 [Suppl]:118–129, 1984.
7. Raskin P: Islet-cell abnormalities in non-insulin dependent diabetes mellitus. *Am J Med* 79[Suppl]:2–5, 1985.
8. Truglia JA, Livingston JN, Lockwood DH: Insulin resistance: Receptor and post-binding defects in human obesity and non-insulin-dependent diabetes mellitus. *Am J Med* 79[Suppl]:13–22, 1985
9. Lipman RL, Schnure JJ, Bradley EM, et al.: Impairment of peripheral glucose utilization in normal subjects by prolonged bed rest. *J Lab Clin Med* 76:221–230, 1970.
10. Lipman RL, Raskin P, Love T, et al.: Glucose intolerance during decreased physical activity in man. *Diabetes* 21:101–107, 1972.
11. Arky RA: Diet and diabetes. In Alberti KGMM, Krall LP (eds): *The Diabetes Annual, Part 2*. New York, Elsevier, 1986, p 49.
12. Bierman EL, Brumzell JD: Interaction of atherosclerosis, abnormal lipid metabolism, and diabetes mellitus. In Katzen HM, Mahler RJ (eds): *Diabetes, Obesity, and Vascular Disease—Part I*. New York, John Wiley and Sons, 1978, p 187.
13. U.S. Dept. Health and Human Services: *Health United States 1985*. Hyattsville, MD, Dec 1985, OHHS Pub No (PHS) 86–232; p 416.
14. Davidson MB: *Diabetes Mellitus, Diagnosis and Treatment*, ed 2. New York, John Wiley and Sons, 1986, p 1.
15. Boden G: Treatment strategies for patients with non-insulin-dependent diabetes mellitus. *Am J Med* 79[Suppl 2B]:23–26, 1985.
16. Service FJ: What is "tight control" of diabetes? Goals, limitations and evaluation of therapy. *Mayo Clin Proc* 61:792–795, 1980.
17. Hales CM, Randle PJ: Immunoassay of insulin with insulin antibody precipitate. *Biochem J* 88:737–746, 1973.
18. Turkington RW, Weindling HK: Insulin secretion in the diagnosis of adult-onset diabetes mellitus. *JAMA* 240:833–836, 1978.
19. Davidson MB: The continuing changing natural history of diabetes. *J Chronic Dis* 34:5–10, 1981.
20. Anonymous: Tight control trial needs more diabetics. *World News* 24:6, Feb 23, 1987.
21. Kannel WB, McGee DL: Diabetes and glucose tolerance as risk factors for cardiovascular disease: The Framingham Study. *Diabetes Care* 2:120–126, 1979.
22. Cowell JA: Atherosclerosis in diabetes mellitus. *J Chronic Dis* 34:1–4, 1981.
23. Saudek CD, Edler HA: Lipid metabolism in diabetes mellitus. *Am J Med* 66:843–852, 1979.
24. Pyöräla K: Relationship of glucose tolerance and plasma insulin to the incidence of coronary heart disease. Results from two population studies in Finland. *Diabetes Care* 2:131–141, 1979.
25. Committee on Dietary Allowances, Food and Nutrition Board: *Recommended Dietary Allowances*, ed 9. Washington, DC, National Academy of Science, 1980, p 1.
26. Anderson JW, Gustafson NJ: A guide for intensive nutrition management of obesity in diabetes mellitus. *Intern Med Specialist* 7:100–117, 1987.
27. Jensen MD: The roles of diet and exercise in the management of patients with insulin-dependent diabetes. *Mayo Clin Proc* 61:813–819, 1986.
28. Mehta JJ, Lopez LM, Wargovich T: Eicosapentaenoic acid: Its relevance in atherosclerosis and coronary artery disease. *Am J Cardiol* 59:155–159, 1987.
29. Select Committee on Nutrition and Human Needs, U.S. Senate: *Eating in America. Dietary Goals for the United States*. Cambridge, MA, MIT Press, 1977, p 1.
30. Nutrition Committee and the Council on Atherosclerosis: *Recommendation for Treatment of Hyperlipidemia in Adults*. Dallas, American Heart Association, 1984, p 1065A–1090A.
31. Moffitt PS: Guidelines for the proper use of insulin in non-insulin dependent diabetes mellitus. *Intern Med Specialist* 7:109–124, 1986.
32. Berg KE: *Diabetic's Guide to Health and Fitness. An Authoritative Approach to Leading an Active Life*. Champaign, IL, Life Enhancement Publications, 1986, p 1.
33. Zimmermann B: Practical aspects of intensive insulin therapy. *Mayo Clin Proc* 61:806–812, 1986.
34. Owens, DR: Effects of oral sulfonylureas on the

spectrum of defects in non-insulin-dependent diabetes mellitus. *Am J Med* 79[Suppl]:27–32, 1983.
35. Ryan A: Diabetes and exercise. *Phys Sportsmed* 7:49–60, 1979.
36. Zinman B, Vramic M: Diabetes and exercise. *Med Clin North Am* 69:145–157, 1985.
37. Rizza RA: Treatment options for insulin-dependent diabetes mellitus: A comparison of the artificial endocrine pancreas, continuous subcutaneous insulin infusion and multiple daily insulin injections. *Mayo Clin Proc* 61:796–805, 1986.
38. Anonymous: Pancreatic grafts grow in number. *Med World News* 24:21–22, 1987.
39. University Group Diabetes Program: A study of the effects of hypoglycemic agents on vascular complications in patients with adult-onset diabetes. II. Mortality results. *Diabetes* 19[Suppl]:785–830, 1970.
40. Felig P, Koivisto V: The metabolic response to exercise: Implications for diabetes. In Lowenthal DT, Bhardwaja K, Oaks WW (eds): *Therapeutics Through Exercise.* New York, Grune and Stratton, 1979, p 3.
41. Koivisto VA, Groop L: Physical training in juvenile diabetics. *Ann Clin Res* 14[Suppl]:74–79, 1982.
42. Leon AS, Fox SM III: Physical fitness. In Wynder EL (ed): *The Book of Health. A Complete Guide to Making Health Last a Lifetime*. New York, Franklin Watts, 1981, p 283.
43. Caspersen CJ, Powell KE, Christenson GM: Physical activity, exercise, and physical fitness: Definitions and distinctions for health related researches. *Public Health Reports* 100:126–131, 1985.
44. Pollock ML, Wilmore JH, Fox SM III: *Exercise in Health and Disease. Evaluation and Prescription for Prevention and Rehabilitation*. Philadelphia, WB Saunders, 1984, p 51.
45. Gwinup G: Effect of exercise alone on the weight of obese women. *Arch Intern Med* 135:676–680, 1975.
46. Leon AS, Conrad J, Hunninghake DB, et al.: Effects of a vigorous walking program on body composition, and carbohydrate and lipid metabolism of obese young men. *Am J Clin Nutr* 32:1776–1787, 1979.
47. Brownell KD, Stunkard AJ: Physical activity in the development and control of obesity. In Stunkard AJ (ed): *Obesity*. Philadelphia, WB Saunders Co, 1980, p 300.
48. Allen FM: Notes concerning exercise in the treatment of severe diabetes. *Boston Med Surg J* 173:743–744, 1915.
49. Lawrence RD: Effects of exercise on insulin action in diabetes. *Br Med J* 1:648–650, 1920.
50. Rauramaa R: Relationship of physical activity, glucose tolerance, and weight management. *Prev Med* 13:37–46, 1984.
51. Struwe FE: Stoffwechselfuhrung Diabetischer Kinder Unter Korperlicher Belastung. In Jahnke K, Mehnet H, Reis HD (eds): *Muskelstoffwechsel, Korperliche-Leistungsfahigheit and Diabetes Mellitus.* Stuttgart, Schattauer, 1977, p 513.
52. Akerblom HK, Koivukangas T, Ilkka J: Experience from a winter camp for teenage diabetics. *Acta Paediatr Scand* 283[Suppl]:50–52, 1979.
53. Campaigne BN, Gilliam TB, Spencer ML, et al.: Effects of a physical activity program on metabolic control and cardiovascular fitness in children with insulin-dependent diabetes mellitus. *Diabetes Care* 7:57–62, 1984.
54. Landt KW, Campaigne BN, James FW, et al.: Effects of exercise training on insulin sensitivity in adolescents with type I diabetes. *Diabetes Care* 8:461–465, 1985.
55. Zinman B, Zuniga-Guajardo S, Kelly D: Comparison of the acute and long-term effect of exercise on glucose control in type I diabetes. *Diabetes Care* 7:515–519, 1984.
56. Wallberg-Henriksson H, Gunnarsson R, Rössner S, et al.: Long-term physical training in female type I (insulin-dependent) diabetic patients: Absence of significant effects on glycemic control and lipoprotein levels. *Diabetologia* 29:53–57, 1986.
57. Wallberg-Henriksson H, Gunnarsson R, Henriksson J, et al.: Increased peripheral insulin sensitivity and muscle mitochondrial enzymes but unchanged glucose control in type I diabetics after physical training. *Diabetes* 31:1044–1050, 1982.
58. Yski-Järvinen H, DeFronzo R, Koivisto VA: Normalization of insulin sensitivity in type I diabetic subjects by physical training during insulin pump therapy. *Diabetes Care* 7:520–527, 1984.
59. Leon AS, Conrad J, Casal DE, et al.: Exercise in diabetics: Effects of conditioning at constant body weight. *J Cardiac Rehabil* 4:278–286, 1984.
60. Ruderman NB, Ganda OP, Johansen K: The effect of physical training on glucose tolerance and plasma lipids in maturity-onset diabetes. *Diabetes* 28[Suppl]:89–92, 1978.
61. Saltin B, Lingarde F, Houston M, et al.: Physical training and glucose tolerance in middle-aged men with chemical diabetes. *Diabetes* 28[Suppl]:30–42, 1979.
62. Schneider SH, Ruderman NR, Amorosa LF et al.: Physical training of non-insulin dependent diabetes (abst). *Diabetes* 30[Suppl]:74A, 1981.
63. Reitman JS, Vasquez B, Klimes I, et al.: Improvement of glucose homeostatis after exercise training in non-insulin-dependent diabetes. *Diabetes Care* 7:434–441, 1984.
64. Krotkiewski M, Lonnroth P, Mandroukas K, et al.: The effects of physical training on insulin secretion and effectiveness and on glucose metabolism in obesity and type 2 (non-insulin-dependent) diabetes mellitus. *Diabetologia* 28:881–890, 1985.
65. Barnard RJ, Lattimore L, Holly RG, et al.: Re-

sponse of noninsulin dependent diabetes patients to an intense program of diet and exercise. *Diabetes Care* 5:370–374, 1982.

66. Haskell WL: The influence of exercise training on plasma lipids and lipoproteins in health and disease. *Acta Med Scand* 711[Suppl]:25–37, 1986.
67. Goldberg L, Elliot DL: The effects of physical activity on lipid and lipoprotein levels. *Med Clin North Am* 69:41–55, 1985.
68. Sopko G, Leon A, Jacobs DR Jr: Effects of exercise and weight loss on plasma lipids in young obese men. *Metabolism* 34:227–236, 1985.
69. Lampman RM, Santinga JT, Savage PJ, et al.: Effect of exercise training on glucose tolerance, in vivo insulin sensitivity, lipid and lipoprotein concentrations in middle-aged men with mild hypertriglyceridemia. *Metabolism* 34:205–211, 1985.
70. Calvert GD, Mannik T, Graham JJ, et al.: Effect of therapy on plasma-high-density-lipoprotein concentration in diabetes mellitus. *Lancet* 2:66–68, 1978.
71. Leon AS: Physical activity levels and coronary heart disease. Analysis of epidemiologic and supporting studies. *Med Clin North Am* 69:3–20, 1985.
72. Paffenbarger RS, Hyde RT: Exercise in the prevention of coronary heart disease. *Prev Med* 13:3–22, 1984.
73. Leon AS: Exercise and coronary heart disease. *Hosp Med* 4:38–57, 1983.
74. Hughes JR: Psychologic effects of habitual aerobic exercise. A critical review. *Prev Med* 13:66–78, 1984.
75. Richter EA, Galbo H: Diabetes, insulin and exercise. *Sports Med (New Zealand)* 3:275–288, 1986.
76. Katch FI, McArdle WD: *Nutrition, Weight Control and Exercise*, ed 2. Philadelphia, Lea and Febiger, 1983, p 308.
77. Trovati M, Carta Q, Cavalot F, et al.: Continuous subcutaneous insulin infusion and postprandial exercise in tightly controlled type I (insulin-dependent) diabetic patients. *Diabetes Care* 7:327–330, 1984.
78. Iskandrian AS, Hakki AH: Thallium-201 myocardial scintigraphy. *Am Heart J* 109:113–129, 1985.

CHAPTER 7

Patients with End-Stage Renal Disease

James M. Hagberg, Ph.D.

Since the advent of extracorporeal hemodialysis 40 years ago for the treatment of the uremia associated with end-stage renal failure, dialysis procedures have undergone dramatic medical and bioengineering improvements. In addition, only 20 years ago improvements in vascular access made long-term dialysis a possibility (1). However, the prolongation of life brought about by dialysis has been associated with numerous medical complications secondary to renal failure and dialysis that predispose these patients to various chronic progressive diseases (1–11). Thus, while a substantial number of patients succumb to infections resulting from suppressed immune defense mechanisms, most reports indicate that a majority of dialysis patients will eventually die from diseases related to the cardiovascular system (3, 8–11).

It is hardly surprising that heart disease is epidemic in these patients since many of them are glucose intolerant, insulin resistant, and hypertriglyceridemic and have low high-density lipoprotein (HDL) cholesterol levels, hypertension, and a sedentary lifestyle (1–19). Thus, these patients have many of the known risk factors for coronary artery disease. Recent surveys also indicate that dialysis populations have generally undergone very little rehabilitation, and that only 60% of those without diabetes and less than one-quarter of those with diabetes are able to take part in any daily activities beyond those of basic living (12, 13).

In addition to heart disease risk factors, patients with end-stage renal disease requiring dialysis often have numerous other medical complications secondary to their renal failure, including anemia, infections, pericarditis, chemical abnormalities, peripheral neuropathies, encephalopathies, and generally rather severe psychiatric, emotional, and social problems (1, 12, 13, 20, 21). Thus, this population is especially prone to heart disease, has numerous other medical complications, and is excessively, and often needlessly, sedentary. The appeal of exercise training as a potential rehabilitative modality in these patients is largely due to the fact that many of the heart disease risk factors prevalent in this population are improved with exercise training in otherwise healthy individuals (22–25).

EXERCISE TESTING

The first concern relative to exercise testing of dialysis patients is the stability of their treatment regimen. It is recommended that patients with heart disease not be subjected to exercise testing when any recent or uncontrolled cardiovascular or pulmonary abnormalities are evident (26). This is somewhat more of a problem in dialysis patients because of their numerous attendant medical problems and the difficulty in stabilizing them with respect to diet, dialysis, and medical management for prolonged periods of time. In addition, a physical and cardiovascular examination are necessary for each patient prior to each exercise test, primarily because of their sometimes huge fluid and blood pressure shifts, and the potential for congestive heart failure.

Serum potassium (K^+) levels must be measured in dialysis patients prior to exercise testing, especially if it is their initial exercise test. Exercise causes a K^+ efflux from exercising muscle in both healthy individuals (27–29) and dialysis patients (30). The K^+ shift appears to be of the same magnitude during exercise in both dialysis patients and healthy individuals; however, the patients' serum K^+ levels may already be elevated prior to the start of exercise. When the exercise-induced shift in K^+ occurs on top of these already elevated K^+ levels, serum K^+ levels may become elevated to the point where myocardial conduction and possibly rhythm abnormalities may occur. The effect of hyperkalemia may be evident in the ECG recorded at rest prior to exercise. Predictors of an elevated serum K^+ level include tall and/or peaked T waves and widening of the QRS complex; an absence of P waves may also occur, but only during a serious, life-threatening hyperkalemia (31). This ECG evidence of hyperkalemia would be present only at serum K^+ levels in excess of 5.0–5.5 mEq/liter if all other electrolyte levels are within normal ranges; however, alterations in other electrolyte levels, especially sodium and calcium, modify the ECG responses at a given serum K^+ level (31). *Our general rule has been to avoid exercise-testing a patient whose pretest K^+ levels are in excess of 5 mEq/liter.* We believe these safety precautions have been one reason that we have not had any medical complications during maximal exercise testing in these patients.

History and physical examination prior to exercise also will alert staff to potential problems that might become evident during the exercise test, and may provide evidence of absolute or relative contraindications for the test. It is important to determine if the patient has experienced any recent symptoms of ischemic heart disease or cardiac decompensation, such as angina, dyspnea, or excessive weight gain. The possibility of pericardial and pleural rubs should also be assessed. Moreover, a third heart sound on the cardiovascular examination, especially if of recent onset and in association with pulmonary rales and jugular venous distention, suggests the occurrence of congestive failure, which would be a relative contraindication for exercise testing.

Blood pressure should be checked carefully in the arm opposite the arteriovenous shunt at rest prior to exercise, and the test should not be performed if pressures exceed 200/120. Left ventricular hypertrophy (LVH) is present in many dialysis patients and is suggested by a forceful to heaving cardiac impulse and a fourth heart sound. The presence of LVH is of importance when assessing the exercise ECG, since it can alter the interpretation of exercise-induced ST-segment depression, particularly when resting repolarization abnormalities of the ST-segment and T wave, characteristic of left ventricular strain, are present. However, in the absence of left ventricular outflow obstruction or other contraindications to exercise, LVH itself does not prohibitively increase the risk of exercise testing. One must be alert for new or subtle ST changes on the resting ECG that suggest the occurrence of recent myocardial ischemia or pericarditis, since the history and physical examination may not always provide evidence of these clinical problems.

Pericarditis may be diagnosed by auscultation of a pericardial friction rub. However, some patients with large pericardial effusions, having the potential for dangerous hemodynamic compromise, will have no pericardial friction rub and little if any evidence of a compressive cardiac disorder including a pulsus paradoxus. Pulmonary hypertension frequently exists in patients with chronic renal disease and is suggested by a pulmonic ejection sound, a loud pulmonic component of the second heart sound, and/or a murmur of pulmonary insufficiency. The latter finding may appear with fluid retention and may simulate aortic insufficiency. Thus, the information gained during the cardiovascular examination, when considered along with the ECG at rest and the patient's recent history, may indicate that exercise is contraindicated and/or may alert the testing personnel evaluating this patient to the potential for certain cardiovascular signs or symptoms.

Another consideration for exercise testing is when to test patients relative to their dialysis session. Following dialysis the blood chemistries of the patients are probably at their optimum, but many are extremely fatigued from the procedure itself. Conversely, immediately prior to dialysis the patients' blood chemistries and cardiovascular status may be the most compromised. Nevertheless, the maximal exercise tests in our studies have taken place at the end of the patients' longest interdialytic interval, which for our patients was 3 days; and with close attention to the safety precautions presented above, we have experienced no complications associated with these tests. Barnea and coworkers (32) indicated that the physical work capacity of dialysis patients is, on average, not different before and after dialysis, though blood pressure and rate-pressure product at maximal exercise were somewhat lower after dialysis.

Thus, it appears that exercise tests in these patients either before or after dialysis can be used to prescribe exercise intensity for training sessions that either precede or follow dialysis sessions. Exercise testing while the patient is dialyzing has also been shown to be feasible since only 100–200 ml of blood is extracorporeal during the dialysis procedure. However, maximal oxygen consumption ($\dot{V}O_2max$) is reduced by approximately 20% during dialysis (33), probably as a result of a reduction in stroke volume and cardiac output as blood volume is contracted by the dialysis procedure (34–37).

It is critical to consider the very low exercise capacities of the large majority of these patients when subjecting them to maximal exercise tests. Virtually all studies have found that the physical work capacity or $\dot{V}O_2max$ of these patients is approximately one-half of that in age- and sex-matched healthy sedentary individuals (14–18, 38–46). This corresponds to $\dot{V}O_2max$ values between 15 and 20 $ml \cdot kg^{-1} \cdot min^{-1}$ for the majority of these patients. For exercise test protocols to yield useful cardiovascular information, they must start at intensities that are within the submaximal capacities of the patients being tested; therefore, because of the very low capacities of these patients, the initial work rate or power output in their test protocols must elicit $\dot{V}O_2$ values in the range of 5–8 $ml \cdot kg^{-1} \cdot min^{-1}$.

Two protocols used to test patients with ischemic heart disease—the Bruce and Ellestad protocols—have estimated $\dot{V}O_2$ requirements in the range of 16–18 $ml \cdot kg^{-1} \cdot min^{-1}$ in the third minute of exercise (26, 47); such a work rate would require essentially 100% of an average dialysis patient's $\dot{V}O_2max$ and would yield little useful or valid cardiovascular information relative to heart rate, blood pressure, and ECG responses to progressively increasing work rates. The Balke and the standard Naughton protocol, which require a $\dot{V}O_2$ of 12 and 10 $ml \cdot kg^{-1} \cdot min^{-1}$, respectively, in the third minute of exercise, would be more appropriate for these patients (26, 47). However, the modified Naughton protocol starting at 1 $mi \cdot h^{-1}$ would be much better since it requires an estimated $\dot{V}O_2$ of 6–7 $ml \cdot kg^{-1} \cdot min^{-1}$ during the first stage of exercise (26, 47). We have used a modified Bruce treadmill test protocol starting at 1.7 $mi \cdot h^{-1}$ on a level grade, which requires an estimated $\dot{V}O_2$ of 8 $ml \cdot kg^{-1} \cdot min^{-1}$ during the first stage (26, 48). Painter and coworkers (44, 45) used a protocol that first determined a comfortable walking speed on the treadmill for each subject; this speed was kept constant for the remainder of the test while the grade was increased to elicit increments in $\dot{V}O_2$ of approximately 3.5 $ml \cdot kg^{-1} \cdot min^{-1}$ every 2 minutes until the subject was unable to continue. During cycle ergometer tests, the initial work rate for dialysis patients has generally been in the range of 10 to 20 Watts, whereas maximal power outputs are generally 75 to 100 Watts. Therefore, the increments between stages must also be very small to ensure adequate exercise time to assess the heart rate, blood pressure, and ECG responses to progressive levels of submaximal exercise.

EXERCISE PRESCRIPTION

Conventional exercise prescriptions for both healthy individuals and patients generally attempt to achieve a training intensity between 60 and 75% of the person's $\dot{V}O_2max$ (47). The goal of such training programs is to stress the aerobic systems involved in efficient energy production over fairly prolonged periods of time. Sixty to 75% of $\dot{V}O_2max$ has been selected as the appropriate exercise intensity because training programs at this intensity have been shown to elicit significant increases in $\dot{V}O_2$max and because the intensity is, in most individuals, below the point where significant sustained elevations in blood lactate levels occur. Two recent reports have indicated that dialysis patients have higher blood lactate levels, compared with healthy individuals when studied at similar low level absolute work rates (49, 50). However, this difference appears to be a function of these patients' low $\dot{V}O_2$max values since it has been shown that dialysis patients have the same blood lactate responses as healthy individuals to 1 hour of submaximal exercise and to a progressive cycle ergometer $\dot{V}O_2$max test when the work rates are compared on a relative basis, i.e., as a percentage of each individual's $\dot{V}O_2$max (42, 51).

Our recent study of these patients' hemodynamic and metabolic responses to 1 hour of submaximal exercise indicates that they have no markedly abnormal substrate metabolism or glucose homeostasis responses that would be contraindications for this type of exercise on a regular basis in a training program (42). Thus, if the exercise prescription is indexed to the hemodialysis patients' markedly reduced $\dot{V}O_2$max, there is little reason to expect that their acute responses to exercise will differ from those of healthy individuals. However, much more information is necessary regarding the basic exercise physiology of these patients before this statement can be made without reservation.

Virtually all exercise rehabilitation programs base their training prescriptions on heart rate as a result of the well-known linear relationship between heart rate and relative exercise intensity (47). When applying this principle to hemodialysis patients, a number of potential confounding variables have to be kept in mind to ensure the validity of a heart rate-based training prescription. The first point is that the maximal heart rates of hemodialysis and peritoneal dialysis patients are much lower than those of healthy men and women of the same age (32, 44, 45). This reduction in maximal heart rate may be as much as 20 to 40 beats·min^{-1} and is believed to be due to abnormalities within their sympathetic nervous system. Thus, in dialysis patients, it is not possible to base exercise prescriptions on a maximal heart rate estimated from age using the available equations.

Another point to be considered in establishing heart rate-based training prescriptions in these patients is that their heart rate responses to exercise and other cardiovascular challenges are somewhat abnormal (42, 52–55). This is attributed to the autonomic dysfunction known to exist in these patients (1, 21). We found that at exercise intensities below 70% of $\dot{V}O_2$max, dialysis patients increased their heart rate less relative to maximal heart rate reserve than did healthy individuals (42). This reduced heart rate response occurred along with an attenuated rise in systolic blood pressure despite markedly elevated plasma norepinephrine levels in these patients (42). Thus, more work needs to be done to investigate the heart rate–$\dot{V}O_2$ relationship in these patients during submaximal exercise to ensure that heart rate-based exercise training prescriptions are achieving the desired exercise training intensities.

For a number of reasons it appears that cycle ergometer training may be the best mode of exercise for dialysis patients, especially in the initial stages of their training. The major reason is that work rates can be set quite accurately and, since efficiency varies only minimally between individuals during cycling, this allows the $\dot{V}O_2$ cost and relative intensity of the exercise to be estimated accurately. This is critical in these patients because of their low maximal capacities. The variations in efficiency among individuals while walking or jogging are enough to cause major errors in the relative intensity of these types of prescribed exercise in dialysis patients, since a 2 ml·kg^{-1}·min^{-1} error in estimated $\dot{V}O_2$ requirement is equal to 10% of the average dialysis patient's $\dot{V}O_2$max.

Secondly, cycle ergometry may be best for these patients because it is a nonweight bearing exercise. Since most dialysis patients have osteoporosis, osteomalacia, and osteitis fibrosa associated with nephrogenic osteodystrophy, they have an increased prevalence of fractures, bone pain, and skeletal deformities (56). Thus, cycle ergometry, as a nonweight bearing mode of exercise and one in which energy demands can be estimated accurately, may be the exercise of choice for these patients, especially at the initiation of an exercise program. We have found that once these patients have increased their exercise capacities after the initial months of training and are familiar with heart rate palpation and the rationale underlying exercise prescription, it is safe to proceed to walking and later to walk/jogging.

CHRONIC ADAPTATIONS TO TRAINING

Exercise training as a rehabilitative modality for dialysis patients has only been studied for the past 8 to 10 years (14–18, 38, 40, 41, 43, 44, 46). At the time of our initial studies (17, 18) there was only a single case report available of a dialysis patient who underwent exercise training (38). There now have been a number of studies that have assessed various aspects of the responses of these patients to physical conditioning.

The one consistent finding in these patients is that $\dot{V}O_2max$ can be increased by 20–30% with exercise training (14–18, 41, 43, 44). Such an increase with training is similar to what would be expected on a relative basis in a healthy individual subjected to an appropriate exercise training program (47). Thus it appears that the trainability of these patients, at least with respect to relative increases in $\dot{V}O_2max$, is not different from that of healthy men and women. However, it is important to remember that this 20–30% increase in $\dot{V}O_2max$ occurs from a very low initial value; therefore, the training-induced increase in absolute terms is very low in these patients. In fact, a 20–30% increase in $\dot{V}O_2max$ may amount to only 3–4 $ml \cdot kg^{-1} \cdot min^{-1}$ which, for some of the smaller patients, may be just barely outside the measurement error for repeat $\dot{V}O_2max$ determinations.

The majority of dialysis patients are anemic, with hemoglobin levels and hematocrits approximately 50% of normal; the reduced hemoglobin levels are the result of both enhanced red blood cell destruction caused by an unknown uremic toxin and depressed erythropoiesis because of the lack of erythropoietin production by the nonfunctioning kidney (1, 20).

Exercise training in our dialysis patients resulted in a 16 to 34% increase in hematocrit and a 27 to 37% increase in hemoglobin levels (15–18); the increases in hemoglobin concentration and hematocrit were the result of increased red blood cell survival times and an increased red blood cell synthesis, as indicated by increased reticulocyte counts (16). Plasma volume did not change in these patients; therefore, total red blood cell mass increased with training, and the increase in hemoglobin concentration was not due to hemoconcentration (16).

One other study also reported an increase in hematocrit with training in these patients (46). In contrast, a number of other studies in dialysis patients failed to find increases in hematocrit or hemoglobin levels with exercise training (38, 40, 41, 43, 44).

The low levels of hemoglobin in the majority of dialysis patients contribute to their low $\dot{V}O_2max$ values since most studies in these patients have reported that hemoglobin levels are directly correlated with their $\dot{V}O_2max$ values (39, 41, 45). It is also possible that an increased hemoglobin concentration may help elicit the increase in $\dot{V}O_2max$ that occurs with training in these patients, since anemic but otherwise healthy individuals increase their $\dot{V}O_2max$ when their hemoglobin levels are brought within normal ranges (57). In our training studies in these patients, the relative increase in $\dot{V}O_2max$ was similar to that in hematocrit and hemoglobin levels (15–18). However, the one other study that reported an increase in hematocrit in dialysis patients with training did not find an increase in $\dot{V}O_2max$ (46).

The remaining training studies in these patients reported increases in $\dot{V}O_2max$ despite unchanged hemoglobin levels (41, 43, 44); these studies, however, did not measure total red blood cell mass and/or plasma volume. Therefore, it is still not known whether the increase in $\dot{V}O_2max$ elicited by exercise training is contingent upon an increase in red blood cell mass and hemoglobin levels.

Most renal failure patients have hypertension that can be controlled by ultrafiltration; however, 10 to 30% of dialysis patients with hypertension have hormonal abnormalities that result in increased blood pressure when the excess fluid volume is removed by dialysis (4–6). Those patients whose blood pressures are not reduced by ultrafiltration generally have been found to have an abnormality in the sodium-renin-angiotensin system characterized by high circulating renin levels (4–6). The presence of hypertension in this population helps to account for their increased mortality and morbidity due to coronary artery disease (3, 8–10).

Exercise training has been reported to lower the systolic and diastolic blood pressures of otherwise healthy individuals with essential hypertension, but the reduction averages only 11 mm Hg and the interpretation of the data is confounded by numerous design deficiencies (25). However, in dialysis patients whose pressures are not controlled by ultrafiltration, we have found dramatic reductions in blood pressure that averaged 31 and 19 mm Hg for systolic and diastolic pressures, respectively, after 14 ± 5 months of exercise training (14). These reductions in blood pressure were also accompanied by substantial decreases in required antihypertensive medications (14). No significant changes in plasma volume or interdialytic weight gain occurred in these patients; thus, these changes in blood pressure were not a function of improved ultrafiltration (16).

Painter and coworkers (44) also reported that exercise training improved blood pressure control in five of eight hypertensive dialysis patients as evidenced by reduced resting and exercise blood pressures and reductions in antihypertensive medications. Thus it appears that exercise training may have the capacity to improve blood pressure control in dialysis patients and to reduce their need for antihypertensive medications.

Hypertriglyceridemia is present in 30 to 50% of hemodialysis patients (7, 11, 15–18, 58) and, though most of these patients have normal total cholesterol levels, their high-density lipoprotein (HDL) cholesterol levels are below normal (7, 11, 15–18, 58). In fact, HDL cholesterol levels in hemodialysis patients are only 50% of those of healthy age- and sex-matched individuals (7, 11, 15–18, 58). Both of these lipid abnormalities may contribute to the high incidence of coronary artery disease in dialysis populations. It has also been proposed that the higher HDL cholesterol levels in black male dialysis patients may be a reason for their enhanced survival compared with white males (58).

In our studies of dialysis patients, plasma triglyceride levels decreased by 29 to 41% with training, and very-low-density lipoprotein triglyceride levels decreased by 30 to 47% (15–18). Plasma total cholesterol and low-density lipoprotein cholesterol levels did not change with training; however, HDL cholesterol levels increased by 16 to 23% (15–18). These patients also increased their plasma apoprotein A-I and HDL_2 levels with training (16). In contrast, Painter and coworkers (44) found no change in HDL cholesterol levels in their dialysis patients with training; however, their subjects were not fasted when blood samples for the lipid analyses were drawn, which may confound interpretation of their results.

Dialysis patients also are glucose intolerant and insulin resistant, which contributes to their plasma lipid abnormalities and increased risk for coronary artery disease (3, 8–10, 19). We have recently shown that the insulin resistance and glucose intolerance of Type II diabetics can be nearly normalized with a prolonged, intense exercise training program without changing body weight and body composition (24). Exercise training in our dialysis patients reduced their fasting plasma insulin levels by 20 to 40%, and increased their glucose disappearance rate during an intravenous glucose tolerance test by 20 to 42% (15–18). These patients also demonstrated a 25% increase in the amount of insulin bound to mononuclear cells and had a nearly 75% reduction in the amount of insulin required to inhibit 50% of tracer binding to mononuclear cell insulin receptors after training (15, 16).

These are the only studies of the effect of exercise training on glucose metabolism in dialysis patients. Therefore, they need to be confirmed by other investigators. However, these initial results appear to offer great promise concerning the effects of exercise training on the abnormal glucose metabolism of dialysis patients.

Because of the lack of control of their own medical status and the medical complications that accompany renal failure, these patients generally have been reported to have depression, poor levels of social adjustment, elevated levels of hysteria, and hypochondriasis (12, 13, 59, 60). There is some evidence that exercise training can improve the psychological profile of individuals with subclinical levels of these psychological constructs, but the preponderance of existing evidence applies to populations that do not have the severity of underlying medical problems that exist in dialysis patients (22, 61).

We have reported that, cross-sectionally, in dialysis patients, $\dot{V}O_2$max is closely correlated with levels of depression on both the Beck Inventory and MMPI (60). In our longitudinal studies of dialysis patients, we also found significant psychological benefits associated with the exercise training program that were not evident in age- and sex-matched control patients (59). The training program resulted in a decrease in depression and hostility, and improved anxiety scores on the Multiple Affect Adjective Check List. Increased participation in and enjoyment of pleasant events also were evident (59).

Thus, it appears that many of the medical complications that result either directly or indirectly from renal failure and from the dialysis process itself can be improved, and in many cases quite dramatically, by a prolonged program of endurance exercise training. However, as reviewed above, training studies in these patients have consistently shown only an increase in $\dot{V}O_2$max. Reports of improved blood pressure control, increased hematocrits and hemoglobin levels, improved lipoprotein-lipid profiles, improved glucose metabolism, and improved psychological status have not been systematically confirmed and have been studied only infrequently. Additional studies are necessary to attempt to replicate these initial findings, assess the possibility of additional beneficial training adaptations that may occur in these patients, and provide information as to the mechanisms underlying these adaptations.

SPECIAL EXERCISE PRECAUTIONS, LIMITATIONS, AND PROBLEMS

Most special precautions and limitations that exist in dialysis patients relative to exercise testing and training have been discussed in the two preceding sections. However, a few points bear repeating. The first of these is the lability concerning the medical status of most dialysis patients. They are intermittently ill or infected because of their general debilitated state and their compromised ability to fend off immune challenges. Thus a patient who may be in excellent health for a training session might be very sick by the next visit, even if it is only 2 days later. Personnel involved in exercise training must keep this in mind so that they are constantly alert for signs or symptoms of impending diseases that would be contraindications for exercise in these patients.

The second point to consider is one already made relative to exercise testing, but one that can play a critical role in determining the safety of the training sessions. Many patients in our dialysis training projects began to feel much better after the start of exercise training, and this caused them to be less stringent about their dietary restrictions. The one cardiovascular incident during our 5 years of training dialysis patients occurred when a patient ingested too much K^+ during a Thanksgiving dinner. He developed ventricular fibrillation and arrested during his exercise session the next day; fortunately he was resuscitated without residual effects. Thus, it is important to monitor directly serum K^+ levels even during training sessions, especially in patients whose serum K^+ varies markedly from day to day. Changes in the T wave on the patient's resting ECG, while helpful, are less reliable. Additional cardiovascular signs and symptoms to be aware of are those caused by congestive heart failure. It is also important to monitor insulin requirements in insulin-dependent hemodialysis patients to minimize the risk of exercise-induced hypoglycemia.

SUMMARY AND CONCLUSION

Dialysis patients have numerous medical complications that are either a direct or indirect result of renal failure and the dialysis process. Exercise *testing* in this population can be safe and yield useful cardiovascular information. Exercise *training* is also feasible; however, because of their increased likelihood of developing complications, the majority of dialysis patients may not be appropriate candidates for long-term exercise training programs (43). While exercise programs may be beneficial for selected dialysis patients, particularly with regard to augmenting aerobic capacity, the cardiorespiratory and metabolic adaptations to long-term exercise training remain unclear. Thus, the need for additional training studies is apparent. Further studies are also necessary to describe the basic exercise physiology of this population so that accurate and valid exercise prescriptions can be derived that will result in the institution of safe exercise training programs.

REFERENCES

1. Drukker W: Hemodialysis: A historical review. In Drukker W, Parsons FM, Maher JF (eds): *Replacement of Renal Function by Dialysis*. The Hague, Martinus Nijhoff Medical Division, 1978, p 3.
2. Bullock RE, Amer HA, Simpson I, et al.: Cardiac abnormalities and exercise tolerance in patients receiving renal replacement therapy. *Br Med J* 289: 1479–1484, 1984.
3. Rostand SG, Gretes JC, Kirk KA, et al.: Ischemic heart disease in patients with uremia undergoing maintenance hemodialysis. *Kidney Int* 16:600–611, 1979.
4. Lazarus JM, Hampers CL, Merrill JP: Hypertension in chronic renal failure. *Arch Intern Med* 133:1059–1066, 1974.
5. Mitas JA, O'Connor DT, Stone RA: Hypertension in renal insufficiency. *Postgrad Med* 64:113–120, 1978.
6. Del Greco F, Davies WA, Simon NM, et al.: Hypertension of chronic renal failure: Role of sodium and the renal pressor system. *Kidney Int* 7(Suppl):S176–S183, 1975.
7. Rapoport J, Aviram M, Chaimovitz C, et al.: Defective high-density lipoprotein composition in patients on chronic hemodialysis. *N Engl J Med* 299:1326–1329, 1978.
8. Nicholls AJ, Edward N, Catto GRD, et al.: Accelerated atherosclerosis in long-term dialysis and renal-transplant patients: Fact or fiction? *Lancet* 1:276–278, 1980.
9. Lazarus JM, Lowrie EG, Hampers CL, et al.: Cardiovascular disease in uremic patients on hemodialysis. *Kidney Int* 7(Suppl):S167–S175, 1975.
10. Scharf S, Wexler J, Longnecker RE, et al.: Cardiovascular disease in patients on chronic hemodialysis therapy. *Prog Cardiovasc Dis* 22:343–356, 1980.
11. Bagdade JD: Hyperlipidemia and atherosclerosis in chronic dialysis patients. In Drukker W, Parsons FM, Maher JF (eds): *Replacement of Renal Function by Dialysis*. The Hague, Martinus Nijhoff Medical Division, 1978, p 538.
12. Gutman RA, Stead WW, Robinson RR: Physical activity and employment status of patients on maintenance dialysis. *N Engl J Med* 304:309–313, 1981.
13. Evans RW, Manninen DL, Garrison LP, et al.: The quality of life of patients with end-stage renal disease. *N Engl J Med* 312:553–559, 1985.
14. Hagberg JM, Goldberg AP, Ehsani AA, et al.: Exercise training improves hypertension in hemodialysis patients. *Am J Nephrol* 3:209–212, 1983.
15. Goldberg AP, Geltman EM, Hagberg JM, et al.: Therapeutic benefits of exercise training for hemodialysis patients. *Kidney Int* 24 (Suppl):S303–S309, 1983.
16. Harter HR, Goldberg AP: Endurance exercise training: An effective therapeutic modality for hemodialysis patients. *Med Clin North Am* 69:159–175, 1985.
17. Goldberg AP, Hagberg JM, Delmez JA, et al.: The metabolic and psychological effects of exercise training in hemodialysis patients. *Am J Clin Nutr* 33:1620–1628, 1980.
18. Goldberg AP, Hagberg JM, Delmez JA, et al.: Metabolic effects of exercise training in hemodialysis patients. *Kidney Int* 18:754–761, 1980.
19. Knochel JP: Endocrine changes in patients on chronic dialysis. In Drukker W, Parsons FM, Maher JF (eds): *Replacement of Renal Function by Dialysis*. The Hague, Martinus Nijhoff Medical Division, 1978, p 546.
20. Eschbach JW: Hematologic problems of dialysis patients. In Drukker W, Parsons FM, Maher JF (eds): *Replacement of Renal Function by Dialysis*. The Hague, Martinus Nijhoff Medical Division, 1978, p 557.
21. Tyler HR: Neurological aspects of dialysis pa-

tients. In Drukker W, Parsons FM, Maher JF (eds): *Replacement of Renal Function by Dialysis*. The Hague, Martinus Nijhoff Medical Division, 1978, p 601.

22. Greist J, Klein M, Eichers R, et al.: Running as a treatment for depression. *Behav Med* 5:19–24, 1978.
23. Haskell WL: The influence of exercise training on plasma lipids and lipoproteins in health and disease. *Acta Med Scand* 711(Suppl):25–38, 1986.
24. Holloszy JO, Schultz J, Kusnierkiewicz J, et al.: Effects of exercise on glucose tolerance and insulin resistance. *Acta Med Scand* 711(Suppl):55–66, 1986.
25. Hagberg JM, Seals DR: Exercise training and hypertension. *Acta Med Scand* 711(Suppl):131–136, 1986.
26. American College of Sports Medicine: *Guidelines for Exercise Testing and Prescription*. Philadelphia, Lea and Febiger, 1986, p 9.
27. Laurell H, Pernow B: Effect of exercise on plasma potassium in man. *Acta Physiol Scand* 66:241–242, 1966.
28. Hnik P, Holas M, Krekule I, et al.: Work-induced potassium changes in skeletal muscle and effluent venous blood assessed by liquid ion-exchanger microelectrodes. *Pflugers Arch* 362:85–94, 1976.
29. Bergstrom J, Guarnieri G, Hultman E: Carbohydrate metabolism and electrolyte changes in human muscle tissue during heavy work. *J Appl Physiol* 30:122–125, 1971.
30. Huber W, Marquard E: Plasma potassium and blood pH following physical exercise in dialysis patients. *Nephron* 40:383–384, 1985.
31. Littman, D: The electrocardiogram in specific disorders. *Textbook of Electrocardiography*. New York, Harper and Row, 1972, p 482.
32. Barnea N, Drory Y, Iaina A, et al.: Exercise tolerance in patients on chronic hemodialysis. *Isr J Med Sci* 16:17–21, 1980.
33. Burke E, Germain M, Fitzgibbons J, et al.: Maximal exercise during hemodialysis. *Med Sci Sports Exerc* 17:183, 1985.
34. Bornstein A, Zambrano SS, Morrison RS, et al.: Cardiac effects of hemodialysis: Noninvasive monitoring of systolic time intervals. *Am J Med Sci* 269:189–192, 1975.
35. Chaignon M, Chen W-T, Tarazi RC, et al.: Effect of hemodialysis on blood volume and cardiac output. *Hypertension* 3:327–332, 1981.
36. Chaignon M, Chen W-T, Tarazi RC, et al.: Blood pressure response to hemodialysis. *Hypertension* 3:333–339, 1981.
37. Chaignon M, Chen W-T, Tarazi RC, et al.: Acute effects of hemodialysis on echocardiographic-determined cardiac performance: Improved contractility resulting from serum increased calcium with reduced potassium despite hypovolemic-reduced cardiac output. *Am Heart J* 103:374–378, 1982.
38. Jette M, Posen G, Cardarelli C: Effects of an exercise program in a patient undergoing hemodialysis treatment. *J Sports Med Phys Fitness* 17: 181–186, 1977.
39. Ulmer HE, Greiner H, Schuler HW, et al.: Cardiovascular and physical working capacity in children with chronic renal failure. *Acta Paediatr Scand* 67:43–48, 1978.
40. Roseler E, Aurisch R, Precht K, et al.: Hemodynamic and metabolic responses to physical training in chronic renal failure. *Proc Eur Dial Transplant Assoc* 17:702–706, 1980.
41. Zabetakis PM, Gleim GW, Pasternack FL, et al.: Long-duration submaximal exercise conditioning in hemodialysis patients. *Clin Nephrol* 18:17–22, 1982.
42. Kettner A, Goldberg AP, Hagberg JM, et al.: Cardiovascular and metabolic responses to submaximal exercise in hemodialysis patients. *Kidney Int* 26:66–71, 1984.
43. Shalom R, Blumenthal JA, Williams RS, et al.: Feasibility and benefits of exercise training in patients on maintenance dialysis. *Kidney Int* 25:958–963, 1984.
44. Painter PL, Nelson-Worel JN, Hill MM, et al.: Effects of exercise training during hemodialysis. *Nephron* 43:87–92, 1986.
45. Painter PL, Messer-Rehak D, Hanson P, et al.: Exercise capacity in hemodialysis, CAPD, and renal transplant patients. *Nephron* 42:47–51, 1986.
46. Mist BA, Short CD, White JA, et al.: Cardiovascular responses to exercise in patients on regular hemodialysis therapy. In Watkins J, Reilly T, Burwitz L (eds): *Sport Science: Proceedings of the Eighth Commonwealth and International Conference on Sport, Physical Education, Dance, Recreation, and Health*. London, EFN Spon, 1986, p 30.
47. Pollock ML, Wilmore JH, Fox SM: *Exercise in Health and Disease: Evaluation and Prescription for Prevention and Rehabilitation*. Philadelphia, WB Saunders, 1984, p 244.
48. Schwartz KM, Turner JD, Sheffield LT, et al.: Limited exercise testing soon after myocardial infarction: Correlation with early coronary and left ventricular angiography. *Ann Intern Med* 94:727–734, 1981.
49. Parrish AE: The effect of minimal exercise on blood lactate in azotemic subjects. *Clin Nephrol* 16:35–39, 1981.
50. Parrish AE, Zikria M, Kenney RA: Oxygen uptake in exercising subjects with minimal renal disease. *Nephron* 40:455–457, 1985.
51. Wolfe GA, Dwyer HJ, Feinstein EI, et al.: Anaerobic threshold in hemodialysis patients. *Med Sci Sports Exerc* 17:183, 1985.
52. Pickering TG, Gribbin B, Oliver DO: Baroreflex sensitivity in patients on long-term hemodialysis. *Clin Sci* 43:645–647, 1972.
53. Kersh ES, Kronfield SJ, Unger A, et al.: Auto-

nomic insufficiency in uremia as a cause of hemodialysis-induced hypotension. *N Engl J Med* 290:650–653, 1974.

54. Lilley JJ, Golden J, Stone RA: Adrenergic regulation of blood pressure in chronic renal failure. *J Clin Invest* 57:1190–1200, 1976.
55. Naik RB, Mathias CJ, Wilson CA, et al.: Cardiovascular and autonomic reflexes in hemodialysis patients. *Clin Sci* 60:165–170, 1981.
56. Coburn JW, Llach F: Renal osteodystrophy and maintenance dialysis. In Drukker W, Parsons FM, Maher JF (eds): *Replacement of Renal Function by Dialysis*. The Hague, Martinus Nijhoff Medical Division, 1978, p 571.
57. Gardner GW, Edgerton VR, Barnard RJ, et al.: Cardiorespiratory, hematological, and physical performance responses of anemic subjects to iron treatment. *Am J Clin Nutr* 28:982–988, 1975.
58. Goldberg AP, Harter HR, Patsch W: Racial differences in plasma high-density lipoproteins in patients receiving hemodialysis: A possible mechanism for accelerated atherosclerosis in white men. *N Engl J Med* 308:1345–1353, 1983.
59. Carney RM, McKevitt PM, Goldberg AP, et al.: Psychological effects of exercise training in hemodialysis patients. *Nephron* 33:179–181, 1983.
60. Carney RM, Wetzel RD, Hagberg JM, et al.: The relationship between depression and aerobic capacity in hemodialysis patients. *Psychosom Med* 48:143–147, 1986.
61. Carr DB, Bullen BA, Skrinar GS, et al.: Physical conditioning facilitates the exercise-induced secretion of beta-endorphin and beta-lipotropin in women. *N Engl J Med* 305:560–563, 1981.

CHAPTER 8

Moderate and Extreme Obesity

Richard M. Lampman, Ph.D.
David E. Schteingart, M.D.

INTRODUCTION

According to the National Health and Nutrition Examination survey (NHANES II), approximately 40 million people in the United States are 20% or more overweight (1). Of these, more than 13 million are more than 40% overweight. Individuals who are 41-100% overweight are considered to be moderately obese, while those more than 100% overweight suffer from severe or morbid obesity.

At a Consensus Development Conference of the National Institutes of Health in February 1985, it was concluded that obesity is a medical condition that causes significant morbidity and decreased life expectancy (1–3). There is a positive correlation between an increase in body mass index as an expression of fatness and excess mortality. The medical significance of obesity is seen in the frequent association between obesity and noninsulin-dependent diabetes mellitus, hypertension, hyperlipidemia, osteoarthritis, psoriasis, respiratory insufficiency (including sleep apnea), gallstones, and biliary tract disease (4). Obese women suffer from menstrual irregularity and excessive body hair growth. Also, there is an increased incidence of cancer of the colon in obese men and of the reproductive tract in obese women (5).

While a direct relationship between obesity and cardiovascular disease is still debatable (6), it is clear that diabetes, hypertension, and hyperlipidemia, well-known atherogenic factors, are frequently associated with obesity (4, 6–19). Weight reduction effectively reduces the complications associated with obesity, lowers the risk of atherogenesis, restores health, and increases life expectancy. This may result in major savings in health-care costs by eliminating the need for costly treatment of the complications associated with obesity.

In obesity, an intake of calories in excess of caloric requirements leads to the increased accumulation of fat. While the causes of obesity are not always easy to define, it is generally agreed that the condition is of multifactorial origin, with genetic, metabolic, biobehavioral, and psychosocial factors contributing to a disruption in the control of energy balance (4, 20–27). The mechanism that regulates food intake is complex and involves an interplay between cognitive and biochemical signals that modulate the initiation and cessation of eating behavior. It is possible that psychosocial factors, together with abnormal hormonal and neurochemical secretion, increase food intake. In addition, defective thermogenesis may cause a decrease in energy expenditure and explain why some individuals seem to gain weight with relatively low caloric intake.

In view of the lack of a clear understanding of the mechanisms that cause obesity (28), it is not surprising that treatment is frequently unsatisfactory. *Less than 5% of patients who lose weight by traditional medical approaches keep their weight off indefinitely.* A high incidence of recidivism is characteristic of obese people, particularly those severely overweight who require chronic, ongoing treatment for their condition.

Single treatment techniques, such as weight-reduction diets, exercise, and hypnosis, are usually ineffective in inducing sustained weight loss. In contrast, a combination of treatment techniques administered by a specialized professional team offers the best chance for effective weight reduction and maintenance.

The combination of diet and exercise has long been considered the treatment of choice for people with severe obesity (29, 30). A possible beneficial effect of exercise on insulin sensitivity and glucose levels has also made exercise a recommended treatment for people with glucose intolerance. Support for the notion that exercise can help obese people comes from reports of the effect of strenuous exercise and physical training in nonobese, sedentary people, athletes, and patients with mild or moderate degrees of obesity. Similar studies have not been frequently performed in people with severe or morbid obesity.

A review of these data (31–37) reveals a rather wide variety of experimental protocols applied to diverse groups of people for whom exercise was prescribed at different levels of intensity and variable duration. Most of these studies have been done under strict supervision in a laboratory setting. Some have used control groups; in others, the patients were studied before and after exercise and served as their own controls.

Physical exercise may induce weight loss by increasing caloric expenditure. Although intense, prolonged exercise may have a daily calorie cost close to 1,000 kilocalories (kcal), more moderate exercise, as practiced by nonathletes, is usually in the 200-400 kcal range. When exercise is used alone, without a calorie-restricted diet, no significant weight loss and, occasionally, actual weight gain have been described (38, 39). This may in part be due to compensatory increases in food consumption with mild-to-moderate exercise; only more strenuous physical activity is capable of suppressing appetite. If physical exercise is added to a very-low-calorie diet, weight reduction still primarily results from the diet. In this situation the small calorie deficit induced by exercise (200 kcal) would hardly be noted in the context of the larger deficit induced by dietary restriction (3200 kcal).

It has been suggested that physical training can change body composition by decreasing adiposity and increasing muscle mass. Studies to show this effect, however, have not been consistent. In slightly obese individuals who were studied while on a maintenance diet, this has been noted to occur only with intense, prolonged exercise (38). In severely obese patients ($\bar{x} \pm SD = 112 \pm 10$ kg) who were told not to restrict their diet during strenuous physical training, Bjorntorp et al. (38) found that body weight, body cell mass, and body fat showed no significant changes after 3 or 6 months of training. When physical exercise was added to a calorie-restricted diet, the enhancement of loss of fat has not been consistently supported (34, 35, 40). From these studies, it appears that changes in body composition occur only when there is intense physical training performed on a regular basis for periods of 3 or more months.

It appears that insulin resistance is a common finding in obesity (41–44) and that strenuous exercise and physical training can increase insulin sensitivity. Insulin-mediated glucose uptake is more efficient in athletes and well-trained people, and this correlates with an increase in muscle enzymes after physical training (39, 45, 46). Studies in nonobese, untrained individuals also show that strenuous exercise and physical training enhance peripheral tissue sensitivity to insulin (31, 47, 48). The augmentation of insulin sensitivity appears to be directly proportional to the improvement in physical fitness. Other studies, however, have suggested that the effect of physical training on insulin sensitivity may be related to the effect of exercise on adiposity (49). In fact, when maximum aerobic power and adiposity were compared independently of each other with plasma glucose, plasma insulin, and percent of ^{125}I-insulin binding, a significant correlation was found only with adiposity.

In obese subjects, Fahlen et al. (50) found that plasma insulin levels and the insulin/glucose ratio in response to an oral glucose challenge decreased the day following strenuous exercise, indicating increased insulin sensitivity. This effect persisted for 4–6 days after exercise. Koivisto and coworkers (51) found that acute exercise decreased glucose and insulin levels and increased receptor affinity without increasing receptor concentration. Bjorntorp and associates

(31) trained 10 obese patients over an 8-week period using a cycle ergometer supplemented with static and dynamic exercises in arm, abdominal, back, and leg muscles. They observed a decrease in insulin concentration response to an oral glucose challenge without changes in glucose levels. These changes appeared to be mediated by alterations in muscle enzymes.

The addition of exercise to a low-calorie diet may enhance insulin action or prevent the impairment that results from starvation. For example, Krotkiewski et al. (35) found that glucose tolerance deteriorated in patients on diet alone but did not change in a group that combined diet and exercise. In contrast, Bogardus et al. (33) failed to find a difference in the degree to which fasting insulin and glucose levels decreased in obese patients who dieted and exercised as compared with those who only dieted.

From the information available in the literature, it appears that strenuous exercise and prolonged physical training lower plasma insulin and, probably, glucose levels, and that they increase the sensitivity of the peripheral tissues to insulin.

Physical exercise has been used for its possible beneficial psychological effects. It has been shown that physical training can hasten recovery from psychosocial manifestations of stress. Sinyor et al. (52) studied 15 highly trained subjects at various points before, during, and following exposure to a series of psychosocial stresses. They were compared with 15 untrained matched control subjects. The trained subjects showed higher levels of norepinephrine and prolactin early in the stress period, but a more rapid heart rate recovery following the stressors and lower levels of anxiety at the conclusion of the session. These studies suggest that aerobically trained individuals may be capable of faster recovery in both physiological and subjective dimensions of emotionality. Rindskopf and Gratch (53) studied the effect of running in conjunction with psychotherapy as treatment for anxiety and depression. The patients were divided into groups in which running alone or running and psychotherapy were administered. These subjects were tested using the Symptoms Check List-90 Revised (SCL-90-R) in addition to the Trait version of the State-Trait Anxiety Inventory and the Cognitive-Somatic Anxiety Questionnaire. The investigators found that both groups reported reduced anxiety and depression at the end of the treatment period and significant improvement in interpersonal functioning. Although the change in interpersonal functioning seemed to be greater for the running/therapy group, it was apparent that exercise training alone can significantly decrease anxiety and depression.

Pauly et al. (54) studied the psychological effects of a 14-week exercise program, including 20-minute continuous aerobic activity sessions three times weekly, in 73 male and female nonobese individuals. Significant improvements were noted in self-concept (physical, personal, and social) and trait anxiety.

It is clear from the foregoing comments that exercise plays a beneficial role in the treatment of obesity and that its physiological and metabolic effects may help reverse some of the complications observed in people with moderate or severe obesity.

This chapter will focus on the special needs of moderate and severely obese patients undergoing physical training as part of a weight-reduction program, and will emphasize the methodological adjustments required for these people to exercise safely and effectively.

EXERCISE TOLERANCE TESTING

Medical Evaluation

A thorough medical evaluation, including a comprehensive history and detailed physical examination, should disclose the presence of medical conditions that may contraindicate a vigorous exercise program (55). These conditions include cardiovascular disease, uncontrolled diabetes, respiratory insufficiency, and musculoskeletal disease. Since physical training has the potential to interact with medications, all drugs that the patient is taking should be reviewed and altered, if necessary, at any stage of the exercise training program. For example, if a patient is taking insulin, the dose, type, and time of administration may need to be changed to prevent the development of hypoglycemia. Patients on β blockers for hypertension may need to reduce the dose and adjust the exercise program to the maximal heart rate achievable under β-blockade.

During this initial evaluation, patients complete a physical activity assessment questionnaire to establish their leisure time activity preference and the extent to which they routinely participate in vigorous exercise. Obese patients often overestimate both their daily physical activity levels as well as their ability to perform strenuous physical work.

Exercise Testing: Considerations and Special Concerns

Following completion of the medical examination and history, the patients are told of the exercise testing procedure, what preparations should be made for eating prior to the test, and what attire should be worn during the test. In most cases the patients are somewhat apprehensive about the procedure, especially about the prospect that they will need to walk to exhaustion on a motorized treadmill; usually, the test turns out to be beneficial since it demonstrates that they will be able to exercise safely. While the graded exercise test helps to determine the presence of latent coronary artery disease and evaluate current cardiovascular status (56), the results can be used to prescribe an individualized, progressive exercise training program (57). If at all possible, laboratory $\dot{V}O_2$max determinations should be included as part of the exercise testing procedure, since the information will be useful in assessing changes in functional capacity that occur with endurance training.

Special problems due to the size and weight of the patients, such as adequacy of testing devices, electrocardiographic (ECG) lead stability, and accuracy of blood pressure readings, are frequently encountered and need to be resolved to obtain meaningful measurements (Table 8.1; Figs. 8.1 and 8.2). For example: 1) Testing should be performed on a motor driven heavy duty treadmill, preferably with a 220-volt motor. If the obese individual lacks physical conditioning or coordination, a sturdy cycle ergometer, a hand-crank ergometer, or a combination of both is an adequate alternative testing method.

2) Recording of ECG tracings during the test may be difficult because of excessive skin mobility over the chest; thus, the patient's chest may need to be strapped with an elastic bandage to secure lead stability and stability of the tracing (Fig. 8.3).

3) Blood pressure recording may be made difficult by a large-sized conical-shaped arm, requiring that the cuff be taped to the skin to insure stability (Fig. 8.4). Electronic blood pressure devices usually produce inaccurate blood pressure determinations in the obese patient.

Test Performance

A testing protocol should be selected after it is determined how strenuously the patient can exercise. Certain protocols are too difficult for many obese patients and may cause local muscle fatigue, resulting in premature test termination. A routinely used treadmill test protocol in our laboratory is a modification of the method described by Montoye et al. (58). This works well for patients with varying walking speeds and abilities (Fig. 8.5). The initial speed of the treadmill is set at 1.0 $mi \cdot h^{-1}$ for 1 minute to provide a brief adjustment period to treadmill walking. During the actual test, this speed is maintained or is adjusted and held constant at 1.5, 2.0, 2.5, or 3.0 $mi \cdot h^{-1}$, depending on the patient's ability to maintain a comfortable walking gait. The grade is initially set at 0% and is increased by increments of 3% every 3 minutes throughout the test. Heart rate and blood pressure measurements by auscultatory methods are recorded at rest and at 2.5-minute intervals (Fig. 8.6).

ECG leads aVF, V_2, and V_5 are continuously monitored and recorded at designated times. Resting and exercise oxygen consumption are determined using open circuit spirometry (Fig. 8.6). The composition of expired gases is determined using an Applied Electrochemistry (Model #S-3A) oxygen analyzer and a Beckman (Model #LB_2) carbon dioxide analyzer. Minute in-

Table 8.1
Common Problems Encountered During Exercise Tolerance Testing of Moderately and Severely Obese Patients

	Problem	Special Procedure or Solution
Testing Device		
Treadmill	Massive weight slows belt speed	Heavy duty treadmill motor (220 volts)
	Difficulty of foot placement on narrow belt	Wide belt (Fig. 8.1)
Cycle ergometer	Massive weight of patient has the potential to break cycle frame or parts	Sturdy cycle ergometer with at least a 40-lb flywheel
	Discomfort of seat	Padded seat
Weighing scale	Patient's weight exceeds range of most scales	Special scale with the capacity to weigh up to 700 lb
Examination table	Patient is usually too large to fit on most tables—results in muscle artifact in baseline ECG	Extralarge table or take ECG while patient is lying on floor mat or in standing position, if necessary
ECG		
Rest	Difficulty in ECG electrode placement	Carefully palpating for anatomical landmarks through the patient's massive tissue (Fig. 8.2)
Exercise	Excessive skin movement	Chest area strapped with a wide flexible elastic bandage (Fig. 8.3)
Blood Pressure		
Rest	Extra large arm	Use a large, wide (20.3 × 81.3 cm) occluding cuff; secure by adhesive taping the cuff to the arm
Exercise	Inability to consistently find the brachial pulse	Marking skin over which the brachial pulse can be found
Start of Test	Large body size prevents visualization of foot placement on the treadmill	Patient stands in center of belt on one foot while preparing to step on the belt when it starts to move at 1 $mi \cdot h^{-1}$
Oxygen Consumption		
Respiratory valve	Patient is unable to communicate the degree of muscle or chest discomfort	Use of hand signals indicating the discomfort area and severity of pain on a scale of 1 to 5

spired ventilation is measured using a Parkinson-Cowan Dry gas meter (Model #CD-4).

Metabolic variables are calculated by standard formulas (59). Since the patient is unable to communicate while breathing through the respiratory valve, he/she uses hand signals to indicate muscular or chest discomfort and when he/she is ready to stop the test. If pain develops, the patient points to the afflicted area and holds up one to five fingers to indicate slight to severe pain. A raised thumb indicates the test is to continue; a thumbs down, the test is to terminate.

To facilitate maximal testing, patients are encouraged to walk until exhausted. Guidance for these decisions is obtained by noting the patient's heart rate response as well as the overall performance. Medical reasons for prematurely terminating an exercise test are given in Table 8.2.

Following the test, an immediate post-exercise three-lead ECG tracing is recorded, a blood pressure measure obtained, and the respiratory valve removed. ECG rhythm is continuously monitored and ECG tracings are recorded at 2-minute intervals for 6 to 8 minutes. If the patient displayed ST-T changes and/or arrhythmias or marked hyper- or hypotension, ECG tracings and/or blood pressure measures are continually recorded at 2-minute intervals until the ECG pattern returns to normal and/or the blood

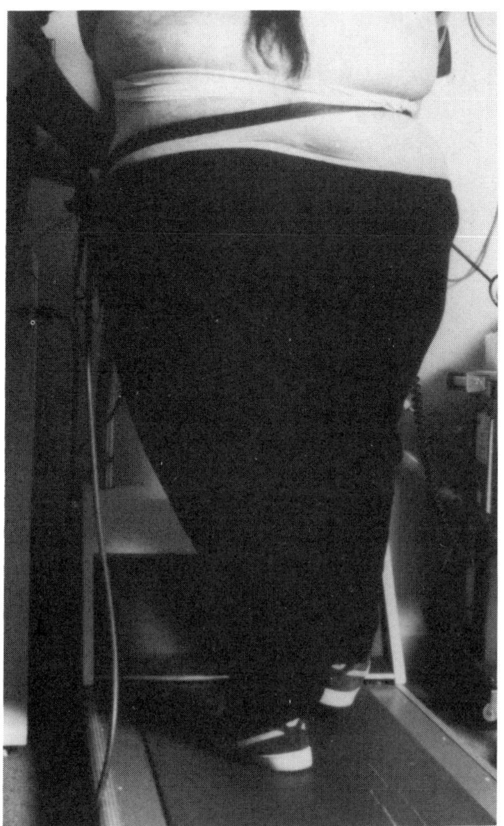

Figure 8.1. Foot placement on treadmill belt.

pressure recovers within 10–20 mm Hg of the patient's resting value.

Even though these patients are of excessive size and weight, the exercise test is safe (55). In most cases, patients have the coordination and balance to walk without difficulty on the treadmill. After their initial fear and anxiety over taking the test are overcome, patients quickly realize they have the ability to exercise strenuously and will be able to participate successfully in a progressive physical conditioning program.

EXERCISE PRESCRIPTION FOR MODERATELY AND SEVERELY OBESE PATIENTS

Since the moderately and severely obese patient has special needs when embarking on a vigorous exercise training program, information obtained by exercise tolerance testing is helpful in developing general approaches to exercise training. Test results are also valuable for tailoring the exercise program to each patient's needs. This individualized approach improves motivation and reinforces compliance, thus furthering the difficult goal of losing weight successfully.

Severely obese individuals usually lead very inactive lives, and as a result of their excessive body size, often experience difficulties in performing simple daily activities. These patients perceive even mild activities as being difficult because of their reduced functional capacity as assessed by low $\dot{V}O_2max$, expressed as $ml \cdot kg^{-1} \cdot min^{-1}$. Foss (60, 65) lists several potential problems, such as heat intolerance, hyperpnea-dyspnea, movement restriction, musculoskeletal pain, local muscular weakness, and anxiety over lack of balance, that may limit the exercise performance of severely obese patients. While exercise testing and training precautions for the severely obese should be recognized, our experience, and that of others, is that these patients can safely participate in progressive intensity exercise programs and should be encouraged to do so by medical personnel (30, 35, 61–65).

Historical Perspective

In the early 1970s when our multidisciplinary approach to the treatment of obesity was being initiated, we were concerned about the safety of including exercise training in the treatment of severely obese patients. While Alexander (66) suggested that severely obese patients had a high incidence of systemic and/or pulmonary arterial hypertension and cardiac failure, Kenrick and associates (67) showed that severely obese patients could safely participate in vigorous exercise training. We therefore undertook a study to measure these patients' work tolerance and fitness levels, and used them to construct reasonable and safe protocols.

Our initial findings were that patients with severe obesity had reduced work tolerance and extreme variability in their initial physical fitness levels (62). $\dot{V}O_2max$ ranged from 12.9 to 22.3 $ml \cdot kg^{-1} \cdot min^{-1}$,

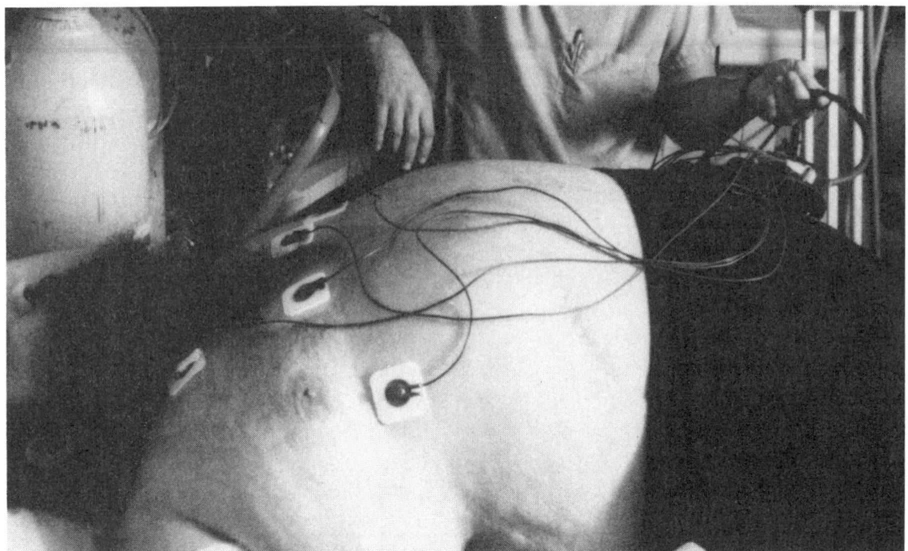

Figure 8.2. Placement of ECG.

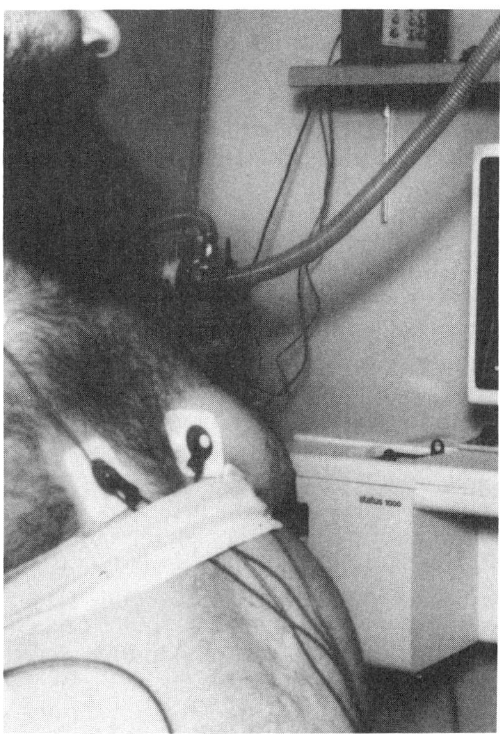

Figure 8.3. Securement of ECG leads with elastic bandage.

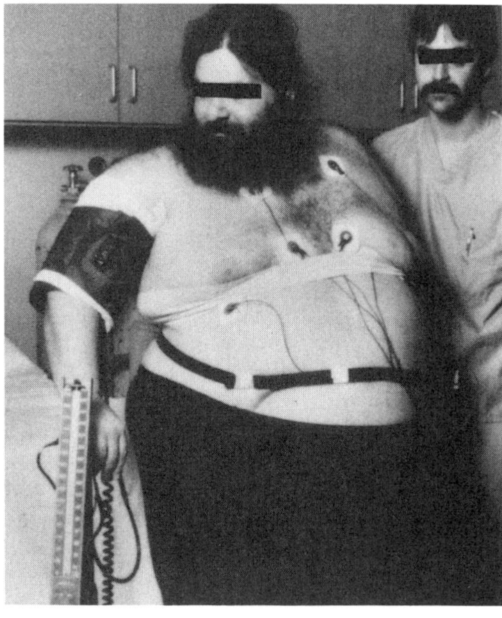

Figure 8.4. Securement of blood pressure cuff.

and only weak correlations were found between the patients' initial fitness level and their age, body weight, or sex. Based on these observations we concluded that an individualized but flexible training protocol was most desirable for optimal training.

To devise a training program that could be adjusted as patients gained in physical

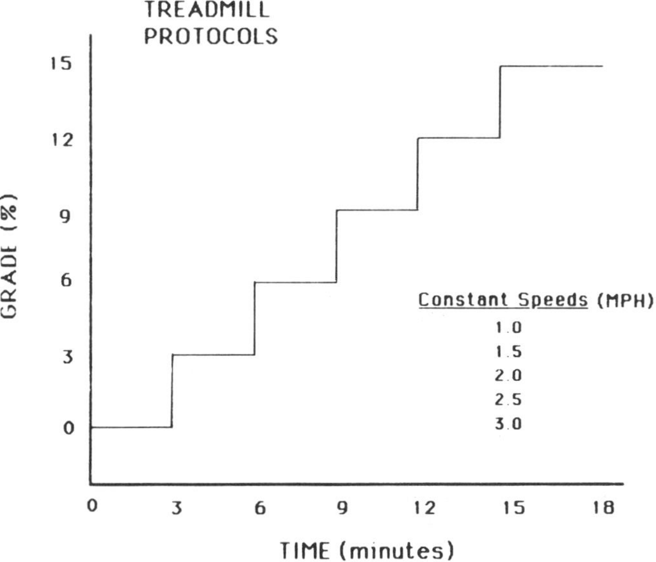

Figure 8.5. Treadmill protocol for exercise testing moderately and severely obese patients.

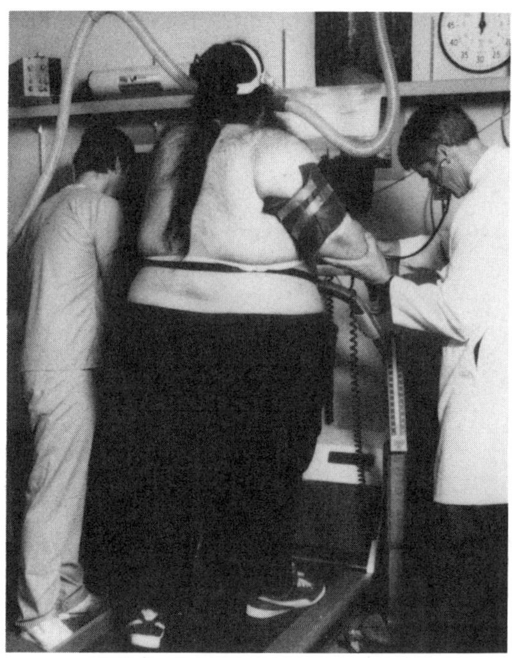

Figure 8.6. Treadmill testing of severely obese patient.

work capacity, we gave a second treadmill test 2 to 3 days following their initial test to determine the length of time they were able to sustain a fixed walking pace. This test involved walking to voluntary exhaustion at an arbitrarily set treadmill speed of 1.0, 1.5, 2.0, or 2.5 $mi \cdot h^{-1}$ at a grade of 0%. The speed was predetermined, based on the patients' initial graded exercise test and their ability to walk comfortably at a given speed.

Results from both tests were subsequently used to determine a reasonable intensity and duration of effort for an exercise training program involving slow-to-brisk walking and, occasionally, jogging. On the basis of these testing data, we designed the initial training protocol. Subsequent progression of effort was established on the basis of the patients' response and tolerance. *The ultimate goal for each obese patient was to raise the fitness level to the point at which he or she could walk 2 miles continuously at the fastest pace possible.* This approach was tested on 22 obese people who participated in a multidisciplinary weight-reduction program consisting of a hypocaloric diet, physical training, and psychotherapy. Results from this work showed that the heavier patients (159-236 kg) required from 1 to 2 months of progressive exercise training before they were able to walk 2 miles continuously, while the less obese patients (132-159 kg) were capable upon entering the program of walking 2 miles in 35 to 40 minutes (63).

Table 8.2
Reasons for Prematurely Stopping Exercise Tolerance Testing

ST-T segment depression or elevation ≥ 2 mm	Diastolic blood pressure ≥ 120 mm Hg
Premature ventricular beats—runs of 3 or more	Hypotensive response—drop in systolic blood pressure ≥ 20 mm Hg
Atrial tachycardia	Lightheadedness
Atrial fibrillation	Dyspnea
2nd or 3rd degree heart block	Severe muscular pain
Chest discomfort	Exhaustion
Systolic blood pressure ≥ 250 mm Hg	

Based on their performance records, three progressive patterns for accomplishing the goal of 2 miles of walking continuously were developed. These programs consisted of 3-, 5-, or 7-week protocols having various rates of progression (Fig. 8.7). Shown in Table 8.3 are the criteria used for assignment of obese patients to one of the three protocols. Table 8.4 describes the three protocols, showing the initial starting distance and the expected increases per week.

Obese people get easily frustrated with their weight-reduction effort and are prone to becoming lax with their exercise and diet program after short intervals. These protocols established goals and expectations and helped eliminate attempts by patients to decrease the intensity and/or duration of exercise per session. By determining in advance specific training protocols in terms of initial walk/jog distances and increases in distance covered per week, patients were able to quickly achieve their optimal walking or jogging pace and obtain good train-

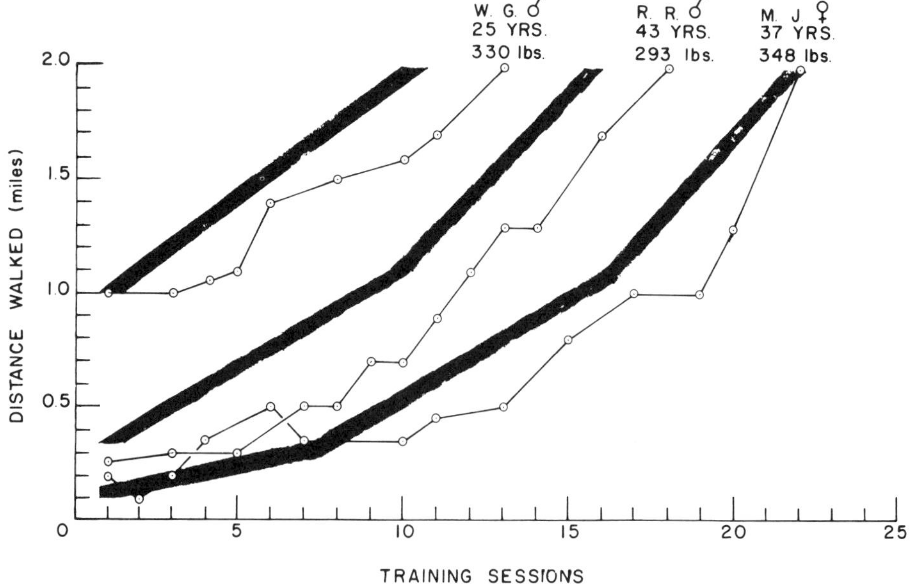

Figure 8.7. Progression of three selected obese patients having different patterns of accomplishing a goal of walking 2 miles. The heavy lines depict three general progressive patterns for reaching a goal of walking 2 miles continuously over a 3-, 5-, or 7-week period. (From Foss ML, Lampman RM, Schteingart DE: Physical training program for rehabilitating extremely obese patients. *Arch Phys Med Rehabil* 57:428, 1976.)

Table 8.3
Criteria for Assignment into One of Three Progressive Training Protocols

Initial fitness level	Balance and coordination
Body weight	Attitude
Age and sex	Level of anxiety
Physical handicaps	

ing effects. While other investigators (68, 69) have found it necessary to constantly supervise and direct obese patients to maintain good adherence to exercise training programs, we have found that the protocols themselves provide motivation by enhancing the patients' interest, enthusiasm, and cooperation in the early phases of their program.

Traditional Concepts

Once obese patients are able to accomplish the goal of walking or jogging 2 miles continuously, their fitness level reaches a point at which a more traditional approach (57) to exercise training can begin. During this period, rhythmic dynamic activity is the best form of exercise, with the intensity and duration of effort periodically adjusted as the patient loses weight and gains in fitness level.

Mode of Activity

Physical activities best suited for moderately to extremely obese people are those involving rhythmic dynamic action of large muscle groups, such as walking, dancing, cycling, swimming, and, in some cases, jogging. Low-impact activities, such as those involving the use of stationary cycle ergometers, are recommended to prevent excessive jarring on the patients' joints. Dancing and ball-bouncing activities are excellent for exercising many muscle groups, but should also involve low-impact gliding steps. Swimming exercises are good for obese patients since they prevent excessive impact on joints.

Swimming, however, poses some problems and limitations. First, obese patients are frequently embarrassed to be seen in a swimsuit. Second, due to the low density of body fat, which causes increased buoyancy, the effort to stay afloat is reduced, making it more difficult to reach an optimal training intensity. Third, many obese patients have never learned to swim. Another excellent water activity is to have the pa-

Table 8.4
Three General Training Protocols Used for Progressing Extremely Obese Patients to Accomplish a Goal of Walking 2 Miles Continuously [a]

Progressive Protocols
3-Week Protocol [b]
Start .8–1.0 mile (initially)
Increase .15 mile/walk session for 3 weeks
5-Week Protocol [b]
Start .1–.4 mile (initially)
Increase .125 mile/walk session for 3 weeks
Increase .25 mile/walk session for the next 2 weeks
7-Week Protocol [b]
Start .05–.2 mile (after orientation)
Increase .05 mile/walk session for 1–2 weeks
Increase .125 mile/walk session for the next 3 weeks
Increase .25 mile/walk session for the next 2 weeks

[a] From Foss ML, Lampman RM, Schteingart DE: Physical training program for rehabilitating extremely obese patients. *Arch Phys Med Rehabil* 57:425–429, 1976.
[b] Protocols based on 2 walking + 1 recreation session/week.

tient perform a running motion in the deep end of the pool where the feet cannot touch bottom. Since this can be a very strenuous activity, patients should be carefully supervised and paced.

Weight-lifting activities have not been generally employed in physical conditioning programs for the obese. However, as part of the obese patient's overall exercise program, weight-lifting activities should be performed at least two to three times per week following a period of moderate-intensity rhythmic exercise, preferably involving the legs. Weight-lifting should be done with light to moderately heavy weights lifted over the full range of the muscle or muscle group.

Recreational activities such as badminton, volleyball, basketball, paddleball, and racketball should also be included in a well-balanced program. The advantage of these activities is that they allow the patient to become proficient in a variety of activities that can be performed in social settings and continued following completion of the formal program.

Intensity and Duration of Effort

Results of the patients' exercise tolerance test should be used to determine the intensity of effort required to improve aerobic capacity. The usually recommended intensity of effort designed to elicit an exercise heart rate between 70 to 85% of the maximal attainable rate (57) is applicable to obese patients. A prudent approach for most obese people is to exercise initially at even lower intensities, with emphasis placed on duration of effort. Obese patients in our programs typically exercise at a training heart rate between 120 to 140 beats·min^{-1} for durations of 30 to 60 minutes per session (30). During the initial phase of training, workouts can be accomplished by interspersing periods of vigorous exercise with periods of reduced intensity within the same activity. The total time of peak intensity should be 30 to 60 minutes.

The progression of total work effort should be slow during the first 3 to 5 weeks of training, more rapid from 6 to 16 weeks, and reach a maintenance level of 30 to 60 minutes of continuous exercise by 17 to 24 weeks. As an example of progression, during the first week of training patients perform short periods of work lasting 5 to 10 minutes at an intensity designed to reach the exercise target heart rate response. Interspersed between these 5- to 10-minute bouts of vigorous activity are 1 to 2 minutes of reduced intensity effort, referred to as recovery time. Three to six bouts per session are necessary to accomplish at least 30 minutes of vigorous exercise.

During the following 3 to 5 weeks of training, the intermittent bouts of vigorous exercise are lengthened by 1 minute per bout. The number of bouts is decreased to compensate for this increase, but, again, the goal is to accomplish at least 30 minutes of vigorous exercise. At 6 weeks, the bouts of exercise are increased by 2 to 4 minutes per week until 30 to 60 minutes of vigorous activity is performed continuously. At this time, the intensity of effort can be raised by conducting the protocol described at a 5% higher heart rate response.

For example, patients may begin their training at 70% or lower and increase by 5% increments until they reach 85% of maximum heart rate response. To establish this response, patients are taught to measure their pulse rates, using either the brachial or carotid pulse, while walking slowly. The first pulse detected is counted as "zero" and the count continues for ten seconds. Rather than having the patient multiply by six, it is easier just to inform them as to what value should be obtained for ten seconds.

Frequency of Exercise

To achieve optimal training effects and take advantage of both the cardiovascular and metabolic effects of exercise, patients should be expected to exercise on a daily basis. This can be accomplished by different training protocols:

1. Supervised, vigorous walking 3–4 times weekly alternating with unsupervised milder intensity walking;
2. Supervised vigorous walking 3–4 times weekly alternating with recreational activity as described;
3. Daily high-intensity exercise, making

sure that the mode of activity varies from day to day (walking, jogging, biking, swimming, etc).

Vigorous programs practiced on a daily basis should commence, however, only after several weeks or months of muscle strengthening and considerable weight loss. Daily logs are kept for review with the team staff during their weekly clinical sessions.

A Modern Approach to Exercise Training for Total Body Fitness

Obese patients currently engaged in our multidisciplinary rehabilitation program follow exercise protocols consisting of a combination of aerobic conditioning and circuit training. These activities are designed to a) improve cardiovascular status and b) enhance muscle strength of both the upper and lower extremities. This total body fitness program for moderately and severely obese patients is as follows:

Stage 1. Warm-up for 4 to 6 minutes at a moderate intensity level by walking/jogging on a track or treadmill, or pedalling on a stationary cycle ergometer.

Stage 2. Flexibility, range of motion, and isometric stretching activities for 5 to 10 minutes. Each stretch should be held just short of discomfort (i.e., 15 to 30 seconds), and the muscle being stretched should be totally relaxed. Examples of muscles that should be stretched and range-of-motion exercises are as follows:

Muscles to Stretch	Range of Motion Exercises
• Soleus	• Arm circles
• Gastrocnemius	• Trunk rotation
• Hamstrings	• Side bends
• Quadriceps	• Arm rotations
• Deltoids	• Back flexion and extension

Stage 3. Rhythmic, dynamic activities such as walking, cycling, low-impact aerobic dancing for 10 to 15 minutes, performed at the prescribed target exercise heart rate.

Stage 4. Muscular strengthening activities involving weight-lifting and calisthenics performed in a circuit training sequence for 15 to 20 minutes. Patients are instructed to choose a weight they can lift at least 10 to 15 times. As the patient becomes stronger, more emphasis is placed on muscle strengthening activities involving eccentric contractions. Routinely performed activities are:

- One-arm barbell curl
- Abdominal curl
- Bench press
- Quadriceps contraction
- Military press
- Lateral pulldown
- Leg press
- Shoulder elevator press
- Underhand wrist curls
- Waist bent row

Stage 5. Repeat of aerobic exercises for 10 to 12 minutes.

Stage 6. Muscular endurance exercises for the upper extremities, such as activities performed on a rowing machine or hand crank ergometer for 4 to 6 minutes.

Stage 7. Cool-down activities involving slow walking, flexibility, range of motion, and isometric stretching for 10 to 12 minutes.

This program is supervised by exercise physiologists and is performed thrice weekly. Each day following this total body fitness training procedure, obese patients exercise on their own by brisk walking, jogging, or cycling for at least 30 minutes.

Safety Tips and Special Considerations

Most obese patients are extremely concerned about their appearance, and some individuals express a desire to exercise in seclusion. It is best to have the patients exercise in an area that is also used by others to counteract their tendency to isolation and reinforce socialization with people outside the program. If this is done, patients become accustomed to performing physical exercise in the presence of others, and their initial concern diminishes.

Many obese patients lack appropriate dress for exercising, and appropriate personal hygiene. Patients should be encouraged to purchase good running shoes so as to provide maximum stability and control. When used by obese people, running shoes break down rapidly and should be replaced as often as necessary. Clothing needs depend on activities selected and the environmental conditions under which the patient participates. Showering after training should be mandatory.

Excessive sweating causing dehydration is a major problem for obese people. Water should be taken before, during, and following exercise training.

Abrupt increases in the intensity and/or duration of exercise could lead to muscular or skeletal injuries. If the patient follows the program described, however, musculoskeletal injuries are minor and rarely occur.

A major problem following weight loss is loose and hanging skin, especially in the thigh, abdominal, and triceps areas. As fitness improves and patients start jogging, their flapping skin may reduce their mechanical efficiency. Excessive movement of redundant skin in these areas can be restricted by wrapping with a wide elastic bandage or removed with cosmetic surgery.

BENEFITS OF PHYSICAL TRAINING AS A COMPONENT OF A MULTIDISCIPLINARY TREATMENT PROGRAM FOR MODERATELY AND SEVERELY OBESE PATIENTS

Obesity is a condition of multifactorial etiology in which excessive food intake and decreased caloric expenditure contribute to a positive caloric balance with increased accumulation of fat. It has been suggested that a combination of treatment approaches that include a hypocaloric diet, exercise, and psychotherapy has a greater possibility of inducing long-lasting weight loss than any of these interventions alone. Since 1972 at the University of Michigan, we have developed a multidisciplinary treatment program for patients with moderate and severe obesity.

This program has both an ambulatory and a residential component. Patients are admitted to the program for periods of 6 months during which they participate in a variety of treatment activities that are administered and supervised by a treatment team composed of an internist-endocrinologist, an exercise physiologist, an exercise therapist, a nurse, a dietitian, a psychiatrist, a social worker, and a vocational rehabilitation counselor. The treatment includes a 600-kcal·d^{-1} diet containing 45 g of carbohydrate and 55 g of protein, and supplemented by multivitamins, minerals, and calcium in sufficient amounts to meet the Recommended Dietary Allowance. Daily sodium and potassium intake are kept constant at approximately 120 and 100 mEq, respectively. In addition, patients receive physical exercise training sessions three times weekly for 60 minutes per session, occupational therapy, diet counseling, and group psychotherapy once a week.

Fig. 8.8 shows a typical weight loss pattern from a study of 50 extremely obese patients who underwent both caloric restriction and exercise training for 9 months (30). Patients were restricted to 400-600 kcal·d^{-1}, vigorously exercised three times per week, and participated in recreational activities during a fourth exercise session. Weight losses ranged between 45 to 127 kg, with the most rapid weight loss occurring during the first 2 months. Substantial weight losses continued over the next 3 to

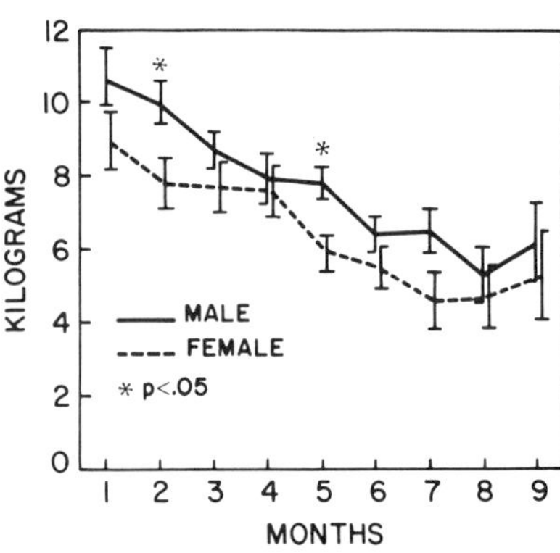

Figure 8.8. Typical weight loss pattern per month for moderately and severely obese patients in response to a 9-month hypocaloric diet and exercise program. (From Lampman RM, Schteingart DE, Foss ML: Exercise as a partial therapy for the extremely obese. *Med Sci Sports Exerc* 18:19–24, 1985.)

7 months, but at a slower rate in both males and females.

At the time of admission to the program, women were 288.8 ± 14.5% ($\bar{x}$ ± SEM) of ideal body weight while men were 269.7 ± 10.9%. During the first month in the program, average weight loss for all patients was 9.7 ± 0.55 kg (8.8 kg for the females and 10.5 kg for males). While body weights for both groups continued to decline with therapy, the female patients showed greater weight losses during the second and fifth months. The goal of the program was to have the patient lose weight to the point of feeling both physically and psychologically improved and able to maintain socioeconomic independence. Most patients did not reach ideal body weight but significantly improved their appearance and fitness level (Figs. 8.9 and 8.10). Upon leaving the program, patients were given information about diet and exercise programs they could continue at home, as well as about suitable support agencies in their communities.

The exercise training program used in this study significantly ($p<0.01$) reduced resting heart rates over a 9-month period (Fig. 8.11). Treatment periods 1, 2, and 3 corresponded to measurements taken at 3-month intervals. Initially, resting heart rates were 85 ± 3.44 ($\bar{x}$ ± SEM) beats·min^{-1}.

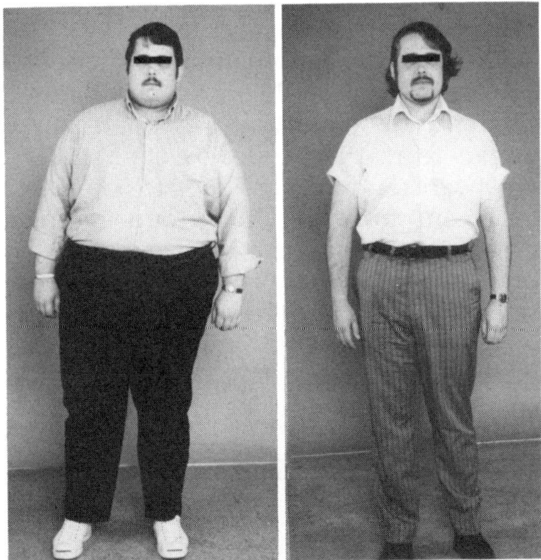

Figure 8.9. Improved appearance of an obese patient following 9 months of diet and exercise.

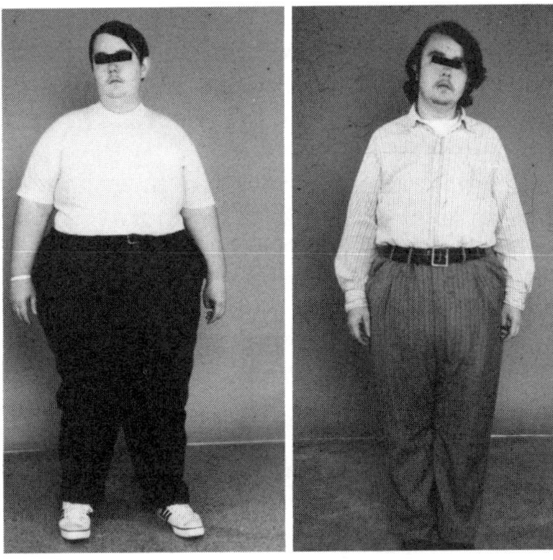

Figure 8.10. Improved appearance of an obese patient following 9 months of diet and exercise.

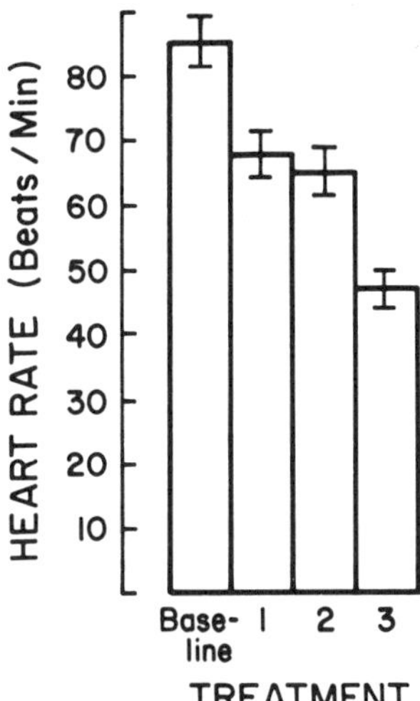

Figure 8.11. Changes in resting heart rates of obese patients participating in a 9-month program of diet and exercise. Treatment periods 1, 2, and 3 correspond to measurements taken at 3-month intervals. (From Lampman RM, Schteingart DE, Foss ML: Exercise as a partial therapy for the extremely obese. *Med Sci Sports Exerc* 18:19–24, 1985.)

Following 3 months of diet and exercise, heart rates declined significantly ($p<0.01$) to 68 ± 3.6 beats·min^{-1}. By the end of 9 months (period 3), resting heart rates had declined further to 47 ± 3.1 beats·min^{-1}. It is not clear why marked bradycardia occurred in these obese patients, but similar results have previously been reported (35, 70). In contrast, maximum heart rates recorded during exercise testing remained unchanged, ranging from 156 to 167 beats·min^{-1}.

Exercise training resulted in enhanced fitness levels as assessed by improvements in $\dot{V}O_2$max (Fig. 8.12). From an initial mean ± SEM of 15.7 ± 0.9 ml·kg^{-1}·min^{-1}, $\dot{V}O_2$max significantly ($p<0.01$) improved at period 1 (3 months) to 20.9 ± 1.2 ml·kg^{-1}·min^{-1}. By 9 months, $\dot{V}O_2$max had continued to improve ($p<0.01$) to 31.3 ± 3.7 ml·kg^{-1}·min^{-1}.

Our previous study did not separate improvements due to increased cardiovascular fitness from those due to loss of body weight. For example, obese patients showed rather rapid improvement in work performance. Prior to treatment, 11 obese patients weighing 150.3 ± 20.8 kg ($\bar{x}$ ± SD) required an average of 20.6 ± 2.6 minutes ($\bar{x}$ ± SD) to walk 1 mile as briskly as possible (64). After a 3-month period of training and a 16.8 ± 3.4-kg loss in body weight, they significantly ($p<0.05$) decreased the mile walk time by 10% (18.3 ± 2.2 minutes). Following another 3-month treatment period, these patients had lost a total of 32.9 ± 17.0 kg and were able to walk 1 mile in 15.8 ± 3.5 minutes. This change in performance represented an additional 23% improvement.

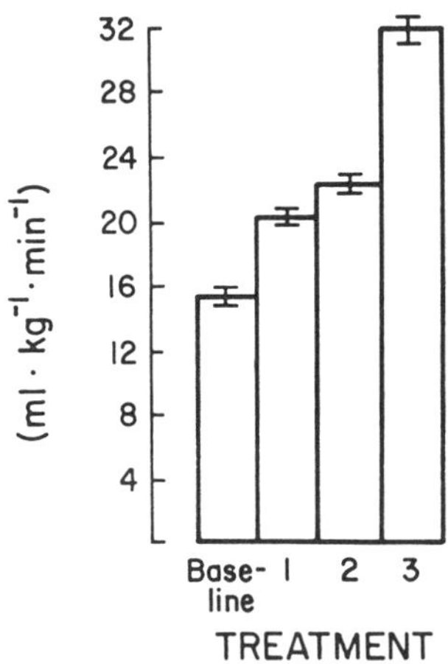

Figure 8.12. Improvements in $\dot{V}O_2$max with diet and exercise training observed in moderately and severely obese patients during treatment over a 9-month period. Treatment periods 1, 2, and 3 correspond to measurements taken at 3-month intervals. (From Lampman RM, Schteingart DE, Foss ML: Exercise as a partial therapy for the extremely obese. *Med Sci Sports Exerc* 18:19-24, 1985.)

The improvement in physical fitness with weight loss occurred in spite of the fact that these patients were eating a severely hypocaloric diet. The hormonal and metabolic changes associated with starvation did not impair their ability to participate successfully in a physical training program, and to show the expected physiological response to exercise training.

Since dietary restriction is by itself an effective way of inducing weight loss and improving the metabolic and psychological consequences of severe obesity, it is not clear what physical training contributes when diet and exercise are combined. We studied the role of physical training in combination with a 600-kcal diet in the treatment of patients with severe obesity to determine if exercise: a) accelerates the rate of weight loss, b) enhances the loss of fat and minimizes the loss of fat-free weight, c) further decreases insulin and glucose levels by improving insulin sensitivity, and d) has beneficial psychological effects. Ten men and 25 women participated in the study. They ranged in age from 20–60 years and were 150–300% of ideal body weight. Fifteen of these patients had either impaired glucose tolerance or noninsulin-dependent diabetes mellitus (NIDDM).

During the 6-month study, patients resided at the University of Michigan Medical Center under supervision by a multidisciplinary team. After initial baseline studies, they were randomly assigned to one of two treatment groups. One group received physical training; the other group received occupational therapy and served as a control. Both groups received a 600-kcal ketogenic, mixed diet and psychosocial interventions consisting of group psychotherapy, individual counseling, and behavior modification.

The exercise sessions consisted of progressive physical training based on fast walking and slow jogging around an indoor track for periods of 45 minutes, three times per week. The metabolic demands of the exercise session were designed to elicit an increase in heart rate equal to 75% of maximal heart rate response as determined by periodic exercise testing on a treadmill. The caloric cost of this exercise was estimated at 200–300 kcal per session. Occupational therapy sessions for the control group were designed to develop manual skills and explore vocational interests. The duration and frequency of these sessions were comparable with the physical training sessions of the experimental group. Studies included: a) measurement of total body weight; b) estimation of total body fat by the hydrostatic weighing technique described by Wilmore using a walk-in densitometric pool (71–73); c) measurements of basal and glucose-stimulated glucose (74) and insulin (75) levels following the oral administration of 75 gm of glucose; d) total body, in vivo measurement of insulin sensitivity by the hyperinsulinemic euglycemic insulin clamp technique (76); and e) measurement of physical work capacity by a continuous, progressive intensity, exercise treadmill test.

Aerobic capacity was determined by measurement of $\dot{V}O_2max$ by open circuit calorimetry and expressed as $ml \cdot kg^{-1} \cdot min^{-1}$ after it was found that a strong positive correlation existed between these units and alternative expressions such as $ml \cdot m^{2-1} \cdot min^{-1}$ and $ml \cdot kg\ fat\text{-}free^{-1} \cdot min^{-1}$. In addition, measurement of the psychological profile was accomplished by means of the SCL-90 test, a self-report clinical rating scale oriented towards symptomatic behavior of psychiatric outpatients (77).

As expected, patients who exercised regularly increased their $\dot{V}O_2max$ by at least 30%. In contrast, there were no significant differences between the patients who exercised and those who received occupational therapy in rate of weight loss, composition of tissue lost, and changes in glucose tolerance. Both groups experienced significant improvement in their measurements of insulin resistance as the result of weight loss and the hypocaloric diet. Results of this study indicated that exercise added to a hypocaloric diet produces a) a further improvement in insulin sensitivity, and b) a greater improvement in psychological status, especially in the areas of anxiety and depression.

It is possible that higher intensity physical exercise would have resulted in more significant differences between patients who received diet plus exercise and those who received diet alone. However, moderately or severely obese people are limited in their ability to exercise strenuously and may not benefit from exercise as readily as less obese individuals. The improvement in insulin sensitivity found in this study may benefit patients with impaired glucose tolerance or NIDDM, and the psychological improvement may better enable them to adhere to a weight reduction program. Others (78) have reported on the importance of physical training in the treatment of obesity for elevating mood, reducing hunger, and improving the possibility of a successful outcome.

CONCLUSION

This chapter has emphasized the many benefits of adding physical training to weight reduction regimens for effectively treating moderately and severely obese people. Exercise testing is a safe procedure; however, standard exercise testing methodology should be modified to overcome the special problems and handicaps of this population.

Individualized exercise prescriptions can be designed from information obtained from the graded exercise test. Such an approach optimizes exercise training, improves safety, enhances motivation, and helps support the patient's effort to lose excess weight. With the approach described in this chapter, people with moderate and severe obesity can achieve a body weight that will enable them to lead a more normal and productive life.

REFERENCES

1. Van Itallie TB: Health implications of overweight and obesity in the United States. *Ann Intern Med* 103:983–988, 1985.
2. National Institutes of Health: Consensus Development Conference Statement. Health implications of obesity, February 11–13, 1985. *Ann Intern Med* 103:981–1077, 1985.

3. Burton BT, Foster WR: Health implications of obesity: An NIH Consensus Development Conference. *J Am Diet Assoc* 85:1117–1121, 1985.
4. Van Itallie TB: Obesity: Prevalence and pathogenesis. In: *Diet Related to Killer Disease*, II. Hearings before Select Committee on Nutrition and Human Needs, United States Senate. Washington, DC: U.S. Government Printing Office, 1977, pp 47–64.
5. Garfinkel L: Overweight and cancer. *Ann Intern Med* 103:1034–1036, 1985.
6. Hubert HB, Feinleib M, McNamara PM, et al.: Obesity as an independent risk factor for cardiovascular disease: A 26-year follow-up of participants in the Framingham Heart Study. *Circulation* 67:968–977, 1983.
7. Kannel WB, Gordon T: Obesity and cardiovascular disease: The Framingham Study. In Burland W, Samuel PD, Yudkin J (eds): *Obesity*. London, Churchill Livingstone, 1974, p 24.
8. Kannel WB, Gordon T: The Framingham Study: An epidemological investigation of cardiovascular disease, Section 30. *Some Characteristics Related to the Incidence of Cardiovascular Disease and Death: Framingham Study, 18-year Follow-up*. Washington, DC: U.S. Department of Health, Education and Welfare, Public Health Service, National Institutes of Health, DHEW Publication No. (NIH) 74–599, February, 1974, p 1.
9. Kannel WB, LeBauer EJ, Dawber TR, et al.: Relation of body weight to development of coronary heart disease: The Framingham study. *Circulation* 35:734–744, 1967.
10. Keys A: Coronary heart disease—the global picture. *Atherosclerosis* 22:149–192, 1975.
11. Keys A, Aravanis C, Blackburn H, et al.: Coronary heart disease: Overweight and obesity as risk factors. *Ann Intern Med* 77(1):15–27, 1972.
12. Mann GV: The influence of obesity on health. *N Engl J Med* 291:178–185, 1974.
13. Rimm AA, Werner LH, Bernstein R, et al.: Disease and obesity in 73,532 women. *Obesity/Bariatric Med* 1:77–82, 1972.
14. U.S. Public Health Service, Division of Chronic Diseases. *Obesity and Health: A Source Book of Current Information for Professional Health Personnel*. Washington, DC: U.S. Government Printing Office, 1986.
15. Van Itallie TB: Obesity: Adverse effects on health and longevity. *Am J Clin Nutr* 32:2723–2733, 1979.
16. Krotkiewski M, Bjorntorp P, Sjostrom L, et al.: Impact of obesity on metabolism in men and women. *J Clin Invest* 72:1150–1162, 1983.
17. Lapidus L, Bengtsson C, Larsson B, et al.: Distribution of adipose tissue and risk of cardiovascular disease and death: A 12-year follow up of participants in the population of women in Gothenburg, Sweden. *Br Med J* 289:1257–1261, 1984.
18. Bjorntorp P: Regional patterns of fat distribution. *Ann Intern Med* 103:994–995, 1985.
19. Ohlson LO, Larsson B, Svardsudd K, et al.: The influence of body fat distribution on the incidence of diabetes mellitus. *Diabetes* 34:1055–1058, 1985.
20. Rabinowitz D: Some endocrine and metabolic aspects of obesity. *Ann Rev Med* 21:241–258, 1970.
21. Seltzer CD: Genetics and obesity in physiopathology of adipose tissue. In, Vague J (ed): Excerpta Medica Monograph, Amsterdam, *Excerpta Med Intl Foundation*, 1969, p 325.
22. Bray GA: The energetics of obesity. *Med Sci Sports Exerc* 15(1):32–40, 1983.
23. Braunstein JJ: Management of the obese patient. *Med Clin North Am* 55:391–401, 1971.
24. Bullen BA, Reed RB, Mayer J: Physical activity of obese and nonobese adolescent girls appraised by motion picture sampling. *Am J Clin Nutr* 14:211–223, 1964.
25. Chirico A, Stunkard AJ: Physical activity and human obesity. *N Engl J Med* 263:935–940, 1960.
26. Johnson ML, Burke BS, Mayer J: Relative importance of inactivity and overeating in the energy balance of obese high school girls. *Am J Clin Nutr* 4:37–44, 1956.
27. Mayer J, Stare F: Exercise and weight control. *J Am Diet Assoc* 29:340–343, 1953.
28. Hirsch J, Leibl RL: What constitutes a sufficient psychobiological explanation for obesity. In Stunkard AJ, Steller E (eds): *Eating and Its Disorders*. New York, Raven Press, 1984, p 121.
29. Schteingart DE, Foss ML, Lampman RM, et al.: Obesity—a multidisciplinary approach to therapy. In Howard A (ed): *Recent Advances in Obesity Research: I. Proceedings from the 1st International Congress on Obesity*. London, Newman Publishers, 1975, p 304.
30. Lampman RM, Schteingart DE, Foss ML: Exercise as a partial therapy for the extremely obese. *Med Sci Sports Exerc* 18:19–24, 1985.
31. Bjorntorp P, Berchtold P, Grimby G, et al.: Effects of physical training on glucose tolerance, plasma insulin and lipids and on body composition in men after myocardial infarction. *Acta Med Scand* 192:439–443, 1972.
32. Barnard J, Lattimore L, Holly RG, et al.: Response of non-insulin-dependent diabetic patients to an intensive program of diet and exercise. *Diabetes Care* 5:370–374, 1982.
33. Bogardus C, Ravussin E, Robbins DC, et al.: Effects of physical training and diet therapy on carbohydrate metabolism in patients with glucose intolerance and non-insulin-dependent diabetes mellitus. *Diabetes* 33:311–318, 1984.
34. Warwick PM, Garrow JS: The effect of addition of exercise to a regime of dietary restriction on weight loss, nitrogen balance, resting metabolic

rate and spontaneous physical activity in three obese women in a metabolic ward. *Int J Obes* 5:25–32, 1981.

35. Krotkiewski M, Sjostrom L, Bjorntorp P: Physical training in hyperplastic obesity. V. Effects of atropine on plasma insulin. *Int J Obes* 4:49–56, 1980.
36. DeFronzo RA: Insulin secretion, insulin resistance and obesity. *Int J Obes* 6 (Suppl): 73–82, 1982.
37. Krotkiewski M, Toss L, Bjorntorp P, et al.: The effect of a very-low-calorie diet with and without chronic exercise on thyroid and sex hormones, plasma proteins, oxygen uptake, insulin and C-peptide concentrations in obese women. *Int J Obes* 5:287–293, 1981.
38. Bjorntorp P, DeJounge K, Krotkiewski M, et al.: Physical training in human obesity. III. Effects of long-term physical training on body composition. *Metabolism* 22:1467–1474, 1973.
39. Lohmann D, Liebold F, Heilmann W, et al.: Diminished insulin response in highly trained athletes. *Metabolism* 27:521–524,1978.
40. Wolf LM, Courtois H, Javet H, et al.: Physical training associated with semistarvation in the treatment of obesity. In Howard A (ed): *Recent Advances in Obesity Research: I. Proceedings of the First International Congress on Obesity*. London, Newman Publishing Ltd., 1975, p 281.
41. Reaven GM: Insulin-dependent diabetes mellitus: Metabolic characteristics. *Metabolism* 29:445–454, 1980.
42. Kahn CR, Neville DM, Roth J: Insulin receptor interaction in the obese-hyperglycemic mouse; a model of insulin resistance. *J Biol Chem* 248:244–250, 1973.
43. Harrison LC, Martin FIR, Melick RA: Correlation between insulin receptor binding in isolated fat cells and insulin sensitivity in obese human subjects. *J Clin Invest* 58:1435–1441, 1976.
44. Kolterman OG, Insel J, Saekow M, et al.: Mechanisms of insulin resistance in human obesity—Evidence of receptor and post-receptor defects. *J Clin Invest* 65:1272–1284, 1980.
45. Esther D, Pruett R, Oseid S: Effect of exercise on glucose and insulin response to glucose infusion. *Scand J Clin Lab Invest* 26:277–285, 1970.
46. Bjorntorp P, Fahlen M, Grimby G, et al.: Carbohydrate and lipid metabolism in middle-aged physically well-trained men. *Metabolism* 21:1037–1044, 1972.
47. Pedersen O, Back-Nielsen H, Heding L: Increased insulin receptors after exercise in patients with insulin-dependent diabetes mellitus. *N Engl J Med* 302:886–892, 1980.
48. Lampman RM, Santinga JT, Savage PJ, et al.: Effect of exercise training on glucose tolerance, in vivo insulin sensitivity, lipid and lipoprotein concentrations in middle-aged men with mild hypertriglyceridemia. *Metabolism* 34:205–211, 1985.
49. LeBlanc J, Nadeau A, Boulay M, et al.: Effects of physical training and adiposity on glucose metabolism and ^{125}I-insulin binding. *J Appl Physiol* 46:235–239, 1979.
50. Fahlen M, Stenberg J, Bjorntorp P: Insulin secretion in obesity after exercise. *Diabetologia* 8:141–144, 1972.
51. Koivisto VA, Soman V, Conrad P, et al.: Insulin binding to monocytes in trained athletes—Changes in the resting state and after exercise. *J Clin Invest* 64:1011–1015, 1979.
52. Sinyor D, Schwartz SG, Peronnet F, et al.: Aerobic fitness level and reactivity to psychosocial stress: Physiological, biochemical and subjective measures. *Psychosom Med* 45:205–217, 1983.
53. Rindskopf KD, Gratch SE: The synergy of running and psychotherapy. Presented at the 133rd Annual Meeting of the American Psychiatric Association, May 6, 1980, San Francisco, California.
54. Pauly JT, Palmer JA, Wright CC, et al.: The effect of a 14–week employee fitness program on selected physiological and psychological parameters. *J Occup Med* 24:457–463, 1982.
55. Lampman RM, Schteingart DE, Henry GC, et al.: Medical management of severe obesity: Graded exercise testing. *J Cardiopul Rehabil* 7:358–364, 1987.
56. Ellestad MH: *Stress Testing Principles and Practice*. Philadelphia, FA Davis Co., 1975, p 9.
57. American College of Sports Medicine: *Guidelines for Graded Exercise Testing and Exercise Prescription*. Philadelphia, Lea & Febiger, 1976, p 11.
58. Montoye HJ, Cunningham DA, Welch HG, et al.: Laboratory methods of assessing metabolic capacity in a large epidemiologic study. *Am J Epidemiol* 91:38–47, 1970.
59. Consolazio CF, Johnson RE, Pecora LJ: *Physiological Measurements of Metabolic Functions in Man*. New York, McGraw-Hill Book Co., Inc, 1963, p 5.
60. Foss ML: Exercise concerns and precautions for the obese. In Storlie J, Jordan HA (eds): *Nutrition and Exercise In Obesity Management*. New York, Spectrum Publications, Inc., 1984, p 123.
61. Schteingart DE, Lampman RM, Savage PJ, et al.: The role of physical training in weight reduction in obesity. In Hansen BC (ed): *Controversies in Obesity*. Endocrinology and Metabolism Series. Vol 5. New York, Praeger Publishers, 1983, p 234.
62. Foss ML, Lampman RM, Watt E, et al.: Initial work tolerance of extremely obese patients. *Arch Phys Med Rehabil* 56:63–67, 1975.
63. Foss ML, Lampman RM, Schteingart DE: Physical training program for rehabilitating extremely obese patients. *Arch Phys Med Rehabil* 57:425–429, 1976.
64. Foss ML, Lampman RM, Schteingart DE: Ex-

tremely obese patients: Improvements in exercise tolerance with physical training and weight loss. *Arch Phys Med Rehabil* 61:119–124, 1980.

65. Foss ML, Strehle DA: Exercise testing and training for the obese. In Storlie J, Jordan HA (eds): *Nutrition and Exercise in Obesity Management.* New York, Spectrum Publications, Inc., 1984, p 93.
66. Alexander JK: Obesity and cardiac performance. *Am J Cardiol* 14:860–865, 1964.
67. Kenrick MM, Ball MF, Canary JJ: Exercise and weight reduction in obesity. *Arch Phys Med Rehabil* 53:323–327,340, 1972.
68. Goodman C, Kenrick M: Physical fitness in relation to obesity. *Obesity/Bariatric Med* 4:12–15, 1975.
69. Harris MB, Hallbauer ES: Self-directed weight control through eating and exercise. *Behav Res Ther* 11:523–529, 1973.
70. Krotkiewski M, Mandroukas K, Sjostrom L, et al.: Effects of long-term physical training on body fat, metabolism, and blood pressure in obesity. *Metabolism* 28:650–658, 1979.
71. Wilmore JH: The use of actual, predicted and constant residual volumes in the assessment of body composition by underwater weighing. *Med Sci Sports* 1:87–90, 1969.
72. Wilmore JH: A simplified method for determination of residual lung volume. *J Appl Physiol* 27:96–100, 1969.
73. Behnke AR, Wilmore JH: *Evaluation and Regulation of Body Build and Composition.* Englewood Cliffs, Prentice Hall, 1974, p 21.
74. Lowry OH, Passoneau JV: *A Flexible System of Enzymatic Analysis.* New York, Academic Press Inc, 1972, p 174.
75. Morgan CR, Lazarow A: Immunoassay of insulin. Two antibody systems. *Diabetes* 12:115–126, 1963.
76. DeFronzo RA, Tobin JD, Andres R: Glucose clamp technique: A method for quantifying insulin secretion and resistance. *Am J Physiol* 237:E214–E223, 1979.
77. Derogatis LR, Rickels K, Rock AF: The SCL-90 and the MMPI: A step in the validation of a new self-report scale. *Br J Psychol* 128:280–289, 1976.
78. Stuart RB: Exercise prescription in weight management: Advantages, techniques and obstacles. *Obesity/Bariatric Med* 4:16–24, 1975.

CHAPTER 9

Exercise in Chronic Obstructive Pulmonary Disease

Michael J. Belman, M.D.

INTRODUCTION

Chronic obstructive pulmonary disease (COPD) pursues a gradual but relentless downhill course over many years. The dyspnea of patients with COPD worsens concomitantly with the progression of the underlying disease. Dyspnea limits patients' activity, leading to a vicious cycle of increasing inactivity, which aggravates the debilitating effects of the disease. Later in the course of the illness, other complications, such as hypoxemia, polycythemia, cor pulmonale, and congestive heart failure, develop. Experience has shown that in chronic progressive diseases, greater success is achieved through comprehensive care programs that utilize multifaceted treatment approaches and a team of trained personnel to deal with the various aspects of the disease.

COPD is no exception, and several groups now recommend comprehensive care programs (1–8). The scope and complexity of these programs may vary, but they are based on the premise that this approach is more likely to be successful than intermittent and occasional patient-physician contact. There are tempting suggestions in the literature that comprehensive programs may reduce mortality (4, 5, 8), but definitive proof is still lacking. On the other hand, ample evidence has been provided that patients participating in such programs experience improved well-being and a reduction in the number of subsequent hospitalizations (3, 5, 8).

While the management of these patients covers many areas, comprehensive care programs need not necessarily be complex in character. *The major ingredient of successful programs is interested and dedicated personnel with appropriate training.* Together with a relatively small investment in equipment, they can achieve satisfying results. The key components of comprehensive programs have been described by several authors (2–8). These are:

1. Patient and family education.
2. Treatment of bronchospasm by means of bronchodilators.
3. Treatment of bronchial infections.
4. Treatment of congestive heart failure.
5. Oxygen therapy.
6. Chest physical therapy, including breathing technique training and, possibly, ventilatory muscle training.
7. Exercise reconditioning.
8. Psychosocial management, including vocational rehabilitation.

On the basis of experimental evidence to date, it is not clear which of these factors are most important. In view of the many components of these programs plus the problems inherent in performing long-term controlled studies, it will be difficult to provide experimental proof in the near future.

The goals of pulmonary rehabilitation have been succinctly stated by the American College of Chest Physicians Committee on Pulmonary Rehabilitation:

> Pulmonary rehabilitation may be defined as an art of medical practice wherein an individually tailored, multi-disciplinary program is formulated which through accurate diagnosis, therapy, emotional support, and

education stabilizes or reverses both the physio- and psychopathology of pulmonary disease and attempts to return the patient to the highest possible functional capacity allowed by the pulmonary handicap and overall life situation.

In the majority of patients in pulmonary rehabilitation programs, the disease has progressed to the point at which there is considerable reduction in the expiratory flow rates. This reduction is relatively fixed, with only minor responses to bronchodilators; therefore, these patients are unlikely to return to normal function. The emphasis should be on setting realistic goals based on knowledge of the effect of impaired pulmonary function on exercise performance. This information provides reasonable expectations for peak or symptom-limited exercise capacity. Accurate assessment of the patients' capacity to improve is important both for the patient and members of the rehabilitation team. In this way, one avoids disappointment when patients fail to meet unrealistic goals.

Several recent reviews have dealt in detail with the multiple aspects of pulmonary rehabilitation. Dudley et al. (9). have reviewed the problem of psychological difficulties and their management in the patient with COPD. Exercise training has been emphasized as an important component in pulmonary rehabilitation, but there is as yet no consensus as to the best methods of exercise or the mechanisms whereby improvements are obtained. This chapter will review the subject of exercise testing and training in COPD.

Pattern of Exercise Response in COPD

At peak exercise levels the maximal exercise ventilation ($\dot{V}$Emax) is close to or exceeds the measured maximum voluntary ventilation (MVV) (10) (Fig. 9.1). In association with the reduced breathing capacity this results in a small breathing reserve (MVV-$\dot{V}$Emax) at maximal work rates (11). Because of the decreased efficiency of gas exchange as evidenced by an increase in the physiologic dead space to tidal volume

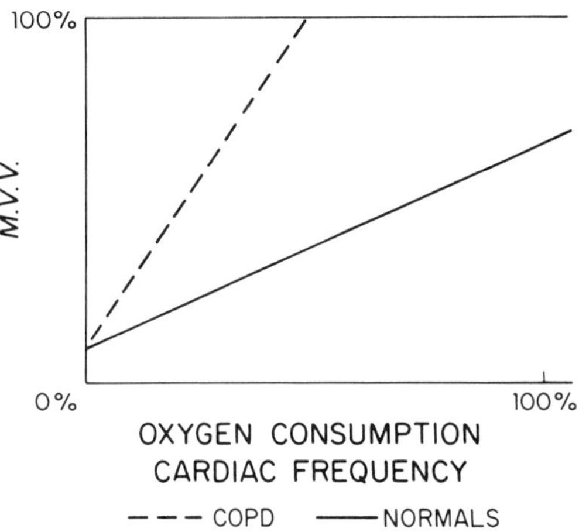

Figure 9.1. This illustrates the major differences between the exercise response in normals versus patients with chronic obstructive pulmonary disease. Normals are illustrated by the *unbroken line* and COPD patients by the *dashed line*. COPD patients reach their maximal power output at a ventilatory level close to the MVV while their cardiac frequency is relatively low. In normals the converse is true. The maximal ventilatory level is well below the MVV while the cardiac frequency achieved is close to the maximum. MVV—maximal voluntary ventilation. (Reproduced with permission from Belman MJ: Exercise in chronic obstructive pulmonary disease. *Clin Chest Med* 7:585–597, 1986.)

ratio (VD/VT ratio), there is an abnormally high ventilatory requirement for the work rate. Breathing frequency rises more rapidly, resulting in a smaller than normal increase in tidal volume. At a minute ventilation of 40 $l \cdot min^{-1}$, breathing frequency is approximately twice as high in COPD patients as in normals (10–12). Cardiac output rises normally with exercise as does the oxygen pulse (O_2P), although absolute values of O_2P tend to be at the lower limits of normal (11). Exercise ceases at relatively low heart rates because of the ventilatory limitation (Fig. 9.1). The absolute heart rate is higher at the same oxygen consumption because of a smaller than normal increase in stroke volume with increasing levels of exercise (11). The VD/VT ratio, which is often abnormally large at rest, fails to decrease at progressively higher work rates (13, 14). Arterial desaturation may occur, particularly in patients with reduced diffusing capacity (15); in more severely limited patients, exercise may produce hypercapnia and respiratory acidosis.

Exercise testing, in general, is used to:

1. Evaluate exercise capacity and the response to exercise training programs;
2. Monitor the electrocardiogram (ECG) during exercise to detect the presence of ischemic heart disease or significant arrhythmias; and
3. Assess the need for supplemental oxygen.

There is considerable controversy as to the best way to assess exercise capacity in COPD patients. An ideal test for assessing exercise capacity would be free of motivational effects and would not require maximal levels of exercise.

EXERCISE TESTS

The following variables and/or exercise tests may be assessed or employed:

1. Maximal oxygen consumption ($\dot{V}O_2max$);
2. Ventilatory or anaerobic threshold (AT);
3. Single-stage tests;
4. Timed maximal walk distances; and,
5. Psychophysical tests.

Maximal Oxygen Consumption ($\dot{V}O_2max$)

The $\dot{V}O_2max$, a reliable index of aerobic capacity in normal subjects, is of limited usefulness in patients with COPD because peak exercise levels are symptom-limited at a level below the plateau of the true $\dot{V}O_2max$. This occurs because of the well-known ventilatory limitation to exercise performance in COPD (10, 11). A "true" $\dot{V}O_2max$ is verified by the attainment of a plateau in $\dot{V}O_2$ despite an increase in work rate. Patients with COPD do not reach this plateau because they stop exercising at a point along the ascending limb; therefore, it is not possible to determine an objective end point. Improvement in this or symptom-limited $\dot{V}O_2$ in COPD patients may result from increased exercise performance or increased motivation (Fig. 9.2).

Ventilatory or Anaerobic Threshold (AT)

The anaerobic threshold (AT), defined as the highest oxygen consumption during exercise above which a sustained lactic acidosis occurs (13, 14), is a useful test in exercise physiology. It can be used as a measure of peak submaximal exercise capacity and to test responses to an endurance training program. After training, normal individuals show a higher AT in absolute terms and as a percentage of the $\dot{V}O_2max$ ($AT/\dot{V}O_2max$). This test, however, is of limited value in moderate to severe COPD because peak exercise levels are often below the AT (11, 14) (Fig. 9.2).

Single-Stage Tests

Single-stage exercise tests can be used to measure submaximal exercise capacity in terms of endurance at a single workload. The test is obviously subject to motivational influences and as with the symptom-limited $\dot{V}O_2$, it is difficult to separate these from true physiologic improvement.

Timed Maximal Walk Distances

In an attempt to simplify exercise testing in COPD patients, maximal walking distance during arbitrarily defined times has been measured. The 12-minute walk is an adaptation of the 12-minute run first described by Cooper (16). In the original description Cooper measured the distance covered during a 12-minute run and showed that it correlated with the laboratory-determined $\dot{V}O_2max$ as measured on a treadmill in normal subjects. Subsequently McGavin and coworkers (17) showed a significant correlation between the distance covered in the 12-minute walk and $\dot{V}O_2max$ during treadmill testing in patients with COPD. This test has now been used in numerous studies of exercise training in COPD, and several modifications have been introduced.

A decision to use 12 minutes was ob-

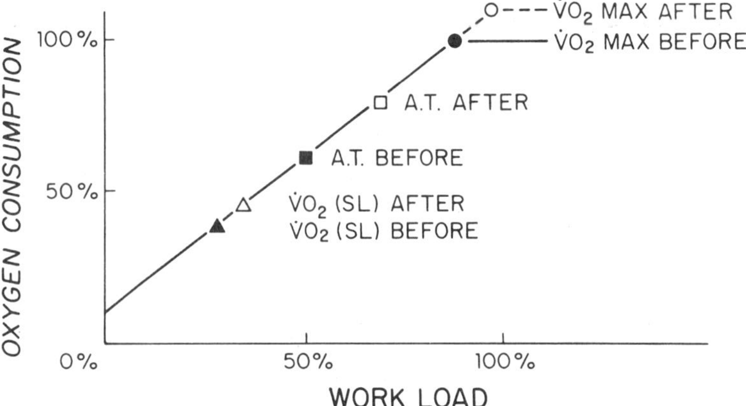

Figure 9.2. Comparison of the $\dot{V}O_2$max and the anaerobic threshold (AT) in exercise testing in normal subjects and in patients with COPD. In normal subjects, the $\dot{V}O_2$max reaches a plateau that provides an objective end point to the test. In addition, the anaerobic threshold is a valuable marker that can be detected at submaximal loads. In the normal subjects, the AT increases both in terms of the absolute value and in terms of the percentage of the $\dot{V}O_2$max after training. In patients with COPD, the peak oxygen consumption is symptom-limited ($\dot{V}O_2$ SL), and if it increases after training this may be ascribed to a motivational effect. In the diagram, which is representative of most symptomatic COPD patients, the $\dot{V}O_2$ SL occurs below the level at which the AT occurs, thus limiting the value of the AT. (Reproduced with permission from Belman MJ: Exercise in chronic obstructive pulmonary disease. *Clin Chest Med* 7:585–597, 1986.)

viously arbitrary and, more recently, other investigators have used 3- and 6-minute walks and shown them to be as useful as the 12-minute walk (18–20). Correlations between static pulmonary function tests such as the FEV_1 and FVC and the 12-minute walk, however, are generally low and therefore walking distance cannot be predicted from these tests (17, 21). The 12-minute walk was shown to have the least variance in studies that compared static pulmonary function tests and other exercise tests in patients with COPD (22, 23).

This finding was also confirmed by Swinburn et al. (21) who compared a variation of the 12-minute walk distance, a step test, and cycle ergometry. These studies emphasized that there is significant improvement after each test; however, there is disagreement as to how many baseline tests should be done before a plateau is reached. These vary from 1 to 3 tests (18, 21). Furthermore, there appears to be a significant effect of encouragement on the performance of a 6-minute walk (19). In this study, the investigators showed that verbal encouragement of the subjects clearly improved performance. This test is as subject to motivational influence as other exercise tests in COPD patients; however, its distinct advantage includes simplicity of performance and a minimum of measuring devices. The test employs a familiar activity and is relatively reproducible after the initial practice attempts. Moreover, patients can perform it alone, thereby facilitating self-monitoring of their progress.

Psychophysical Tests

Because of the lack of objective end points to exercise endurance, clinical scales and psychophysical methods have been used in the measurement of breathlessness. A four-point clinical scale developed by the Medical Research Council of Great Britain has been widely used in epidemiological studies and clinical trials (24). Disadvantages of this scale include the fact that the demarcation between grades may be too coarse to show subtle changes, and substantial improvements or declines in exertional capacity may occur because of differences in the effort with which tasks are performed. A more complex rating system has recently been described by Mahler and coworkers (24), which, in addition to grading dyspnea by means of a clinical scale, considers the effect of magnitude of the task and magnitude of effort during the overall assessment.

Psychophysical methods use continuous scales such as the visual analog scale (VAS). This is a line usually 100 mm in length along which daily activities are ranked according to their associated oxygen cost or severity of a symptom, ranging from 0 for no symptoms to 10 when symptoms are maximal or very severe. This latter method has been used in several recent studies to evaluate the efficacy of therapeutic interventions in COPD, such as the use of O_2 in normoxemic patients or dihydrocodeine, valium, and promethazine as a means of reducing breathlessness (25). In this incremental test the patient walks on the treadmill; at the end of each minute he or she is asked to indicate on a VAS the severity of the breathlessness.

Despite the subjectivity involved in the use of VAS, it appears to have a satisfactory level of reproducibility (20, 25, 26). Further testing is required to assess the validity and reproducibility of these measures of breathlessness, but early results indicate that they are valuable. This is particularly the case in patients with COPD for whom there is a lack of objective end points during exercise testing.

Prediction of Maximal Exercise Ventilation

Static pulmonary function tests including spirometry lung volumes have been used to predict maximal exercise performance in COPD. Prediction equations (Table 9.1) have been developed to estimate the $\dot{V}_{Emax}$ based on the FEV_1 (27). This is suggested as a helpful method of deciding whether a particular patient has performed maximally during an incremental exercise test (28). Failure to reach the predicted $\dot{V}_{Emax}$ may reflect poor motivation.

The recommended prediction formula for $\dot{V}_{Emax}$ in COPD is listed as equation #3 in the Table—a formula that utilizes both inspiratory and expiratory function variables (29). The relationship between the predicted and actual $\dot{V}_{Emax}$ was highly significant with an r value of 0.967. However the 95% confidence interval around the mean was wide ($\pm 18\ l \cdot min^{-1}$). When the formula was calculated using the FEV_1 alone, the 95% confidence interval was even larger ($\pm 27\ l \cdot min^{-1}$). In this study the patients exhibited a wide range of airway obstruction (mean $FEV_1 = 1.75$ liters $\pm$ 0.96 liters). In those with only mild obstruction, impaired ventilatory mechanics may not have played a role in their exercise limitation. However, even studies (10,27) in which patients had moderate to marked impairment showed a wide range of predicted $\dot{V}_{Emax}$ (10). Thus, while the relatively high correlation coefficients suggest that use of these equations is valuable, it is difficult to see how they can be useful when the range of predicted values is so wide.

Evaluating the Need for Oxygen

With the advent of standard oximetry it is now possible to measure oxygen saturations simply and reliably, thereby obviating the need for arterial cannulation and blood gas measurements. However, controversy still exists as to the indications for oxygen therapy in patients who are normoxemic at rest. Multicenter studies (22, 30) have shown that the administration of oxygen was beneficial to patients with chronic hypoxemia at rest in whom the PO_2 was less that 55 mm Hg. Thus, these patients will obviously require oxygen during exercise. However, there are a large number of patients whose oxygenation at rest is satisfactory but who exhibit hypoxemia at low levels of exercise. Whether these patients require supplemental oxygen during exercise is as yet unclear. Suggested levels of PO_2 that indicate a need for oxygen therapy range between 50 and 55 mm Hg (3, 31). It is often difficult to predict which patients will develop oxygen desaturation during exercise, but the availability of ear oximeters makes it practical to screen patients during incremental exercise testing. The practice of examining arterial blood gases after walking is not helpful because even in the presence of hypoxemia during exercise, there may be a rapid return of

Table 9.1
Prediction of $\dot{V}$Emax in COPD [a]

	r	CI	Reference
1. $\dot{V}$Emax $l \cdot min^{-1}$ = $FEV_1 \times 18.9 + 19.7$	0.82	NA	(10)
2. $\dot{V}$Emax $l \cdot min^{-1}$ = $(28.09 \times FEV_1) + 18.4$	0.92	$\pm 27\ l \cdot min^{-1}$	(29)
3. $\dot{V}$Emax $l \cdot min^{-1}$ = $(21.34 \times FEV_1)$ + $(6.28 \times$ PIFR $l \cdot sec^{-1}) + 3.94$	0.97	$\pm 18\ l \cdot min^{-1}$	(29)

[a] Abbreviations: NA = not available; CI = 95% confidence interval; FEV_1 = volume exhaled in first second of maximal forced vital capacity maneuver; PIFR = peak inspiratory flow rate; r = correlation coefficient.

oxygen saturation to a satisfactory level shortly after the cessation of exercise (32).

PRACTICAL APPLICATIONS OF EXERCISE TESTING

Exercise testing is appropriate when the degree of dyspnea is proportional to the pulmonary function test result and when it is unclear whether the underlying disease is cardiac or pulmonary. The equipment needed and the interpretation of these tests have been discussed extensively in several reviews (13, 14, 27, 33). In most patients referred to pulmonary rehabilitation programs, significant obstructive ventilatory defects have already been found by means of spirometry. In this group of patients the main goals are to evaluate exercise capacity and assess the safety of exercise. As described above, exercise capacity evaluation is limited by the lack of objective end points. It is just as useful, therefore, to use the more simple exercise tests, which save both time and money. Such tests include either the 12-minute walk distance or an incremental treadmill test, which allows measurement of O_2 saturation, ECG, and perceived exertion.

Prior to the exercise test arterial blood gas analysis is performed. If the resting PaO_2 is less than 55 or saturation less than 85%, the patient receives supplemental oxygen as per standard recommendations (30). If during the exercise the saturation drops below 50 mm Hg (85%) at walk speeds that are commonly used by the patient (1.5 to 2 $mi \cdot h^{-1}$), oxygen is prescribed for exercise only (Fig. 9.3). As a means of monitoring progress during an exercise training program, one can use the 6- or 12-minute walk. Alternatively, dyspnea may be measured by VAS during standard incremental exercise tests. While both these tests are clearly subject to motivational influences, previous studies have shown a reasonable level of reproducibility (25, 26). Furthermore, they are simple to perform and only minimal equipment is required. These tests do not necessitate progression to maximal levels of exercise and therefore save the patients the discomfort of performing high-level exercise. The use of protocols as described above places exercise testing within the capabilities of all those interested in training programs and obviates the need

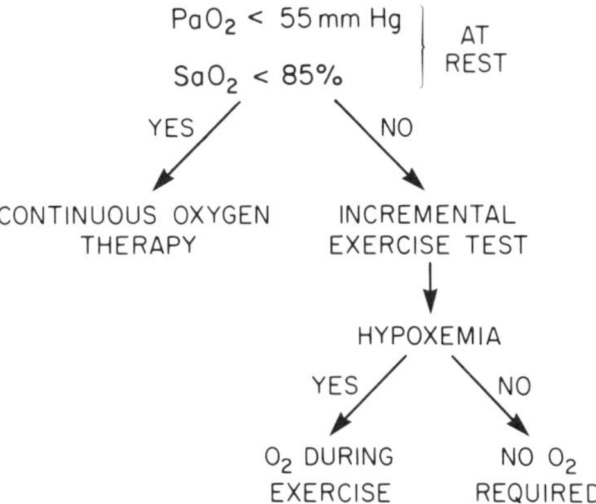

Figure 9.3. This is an illustration of the exercise testing protocol for use of supplementary O_2. (See text for explanation.) (Reproduced with permission from Belman MJ: Exercise in chronic obstructive pulmonary disease. *Clin Chest Med* 7:585–597, 1986.)

for complicated and expensive equipment. It extends the availability of testing to a wide group of interested individuals, not only to expert exercise physiologists.

RESPONSE TO TRAINING IN NORMAL SUBJECTS

Cardiovascular Effects

The hallmark of a training effect in normals is a decreased heart rate at comparable submaximal levels of exercise after training (34, 35). The reduced heart rate or conditioning bradycardia may also be present at rest. The stroke volume at submaximal loads is increased and, together with the decreased heart rate, accounts for similar submaximal levels of cardiac output. It is important to note that oxygen consumption ($\dot{V}O_2$) at submaximal work rates is unchanged. A decrease in $\dot{V}O_2$ at comparable work loads implies improved technique of performance of the task (i.e., mechanical efficiency) rather than a conditioning effect. This point will emerge again in the discussion of effects of training in patients with COPD. Exercise training generally increases the $\dot{V}O_2$max in normal subjects by 5 to 20%; however, the magnitude of increase depends upon the intensity of the training and the initial state of fitness of the subjects. Increased $\dot{V}O_2$max is due to an increase in both cardiac output and arteriovenous oxygen difference (a-v) DO_2. As the maximal heart rate is unchanged after training, the increase in cardiac output is due to an increased stroke volume.

Response of Muscles to Exercise Training

Oxygen transport to mitochondrial enzymes is facilitated after training by an increase in capillary density and myoglobin content in the skeletal muscles. Mitochondrial size and number increase and there are important enzymatic changes. In general, there are substantial increases in enzymes of the citric acid cycle and enzymes responsible for the oxidation of long chain fatty acids. On the other hand, little or no increase is seen in anaerobic glycolytic enzymes. The concentration of glycogen in the trained muscle is increased, and during exercise there is preferential utilization of fat as the carbon source for the citric acid cycle (34–37). This results in a glycogen-sparing effect during prolonged exercise, which may be an important factor in improved endurance after training. Exercise training improves not only the absolute anaerobic threshold (AT) but also improves the AT relative to the $\dot{V}O_2$max (38). This finding is consistent with previous documentation of lower lactate levels at identical submaximal work loads after training.

Response of Ventilation to Exercise Training

Below the AT, the carbon dioxide production ($\dot{V}CO_2$) during exercise is derived from muscle metabolism only. Above the AT the $\dot{V}CO_2$ derives from both muscle metabolism and the buffering of lactic acid by bicarbonate (14).

The fact that lactic acid accumulation and consequently the AT are altered by training causes a delay in the increase in $\dot{V}_E$ necessary to compensate for the metabolic acidosis. Thus, $\dot{V}_E$ is reduced at subanaerobic work loads (39). In general the $\dot{V}_E$max is increased at maximal work loads although the maximal voluntary ventilation (MVV) is unchanged. This implies that a greater percentage of MVV is utilized at maximal effort (39).

Training Threshold

A multiplicity of factors affect the threshold above which the effects of exercise training are seen (38, 40–42). The most important factors include the intensity, duration, and frequency of training and the initial aerobic capacity (i.e., $\dot{V}O_2$max) of the subject. The interaction of these factors is complex but some generalizations are possible. It would appear that an exercise heart rate of 60 to 70% of the maximum or an exercise $\dot{V}O_2$ of 50% of the $\dot{V}O_2$max is an adequate intensity. These exercise intensities should be performed three or four times a week for 30 minutes per session, for a minimum of 4 weeks. This regimen probably represents a threshold exercise dosage (40). After the start of training, a higher steady-state level of fitness is generally reached after 3-4 weeks, and to continue to improve fitness, the intensity needs to be increased proportionately (1).

EXERCISE TRAINING IN COPD

In the past 20 years, multiple studies have examined the progress of COPD patients during exercise training programs. There is little doubt that in general, there is improved exercise tolerance after training (6, 7, 35, 43). Both treadmill and cycle ergometer training showed similar results. An interesting feature of some of the studies is that considerable benefit was seen after relatively short periods of physical conditioning. Studies in which training was performed for as little as 3 to 4 weeks demonstrated beneficial results.

More recently, long-term studies have shown that even though early improvement may be seen, continued training may produce further increases in exercise endurance. In one study (44), maximal improvement occurred at 36 weeks after the start of training. Sinclair and Ingram (45) observed maximal increases only after 8 to 12 months. The supervision provided in a training program is important. The percentage improvement was greater in programs in which the exercise was supervised by experienced personnel. Patients participating in two unsupervised programs (23, 46) showed a 6.3% and 9.2% improvement, whereas those involved in supervised programs (45, 47) showed a 24% improvement in the 12-minute walk. Several recent studies using control groups (23, 45, 48) failed to show an improvement in exercise endurance. In the study by Mungall and Hainsworth (46), a 12-week observation period preceded the training and no change in exercise endurance occurred during this time. In another study (47), a control group that did not improve subsequently underwent supervised training, after which improvement in exercise endurance was noted.

Specificity of Training

In normal subjects, great emphasis has been placed on specificity of training. Thus, it has been recommended that the predominant training of athletes should be in their specific area of competition. This specificity, however, does not seem to apply to exercise training in COPD. Whereas previous studies (12) showed that walking training did not improve cycling performance, more recent studies (23, 46) showed interchangeability of improvement from one form of training to another. One of these demonstrated that a modified Royal Canadian Air Force program improved 12-minute walk distance; another showed that stair climbing and walking improved cycling and the 12-minute walk distance. For logistic reasons, long-term exercise studies are very difficult to perform and there is a paucity of data regarding long-term benefits. However, in studies that followed patients for periods of 6 months to 2 years, maintenance of improvement was shown while training continued (43, 45).

Results of Exercise Training

Pulmonary Function

The striking feature of all the studies to date has been the lack of a significant change in pulmonary function. A wide variety of tests have been employed including spirometry, lung volumes, diffusing capacity, airway resistance, and pulmonary compliance. Occasionally, exceptions have been recorded but even where significant changes have resulted, the magnitude was small and the clinical significance was therefore of dubious value (46). Apart from a study in which a small increase in the resting PaO_2 was noted (49), no change in arterial blood gases has been documented (50–52). In the study in which the resting PO_2 increased, improvement did not persist during exercise. A sensitive measure of gas exchange of the lung is the alveolar-arterial oxygen difference, which apparently remains unchanged during exercise (50).

Hemodynamic Changes

Several recent reviews have commented on the evolution of specific training effects. These include decreases in the exercise heart rate and minute ventilation (1, 3). Confusion exists over the significance of many of these cardiovascular and ventilatory changes; this stems from the fact that cognizance has not always been taken of the $\dot{V}O_2$ at comparable submaximal work loads. As noted in the section on normal exercise physiology, the $\dot{V}O_2$ at comparable submaximal loads remains unchanged after endurance training unless there have been improvements in technique or efficiency of neuromuscular coordination (3). In other words, changes in exercise indices, such as heart rate, $\dot{V}_E$, $(a\text{-}v)DO_2$, and stroke volume, occur despite the fact that the $\dot{V}O_2$ at submaximal loads is unchanged. In several studies of patients with COPD, a decreased $\dot{V}O_2$ occurred despite similar work loads (12, 50, 51, 53, 54). This change reflects improved skill of performance, which itself may be of benefit but confounds comparison of several measurements, such as the submaximal heart rate, $\dot{V}_E$, and blood lactate (44). For these changes to be valid, care must be taken that measurements are made at a similar submaximal $\dot{V}O_2$. When this factor is taken into account, no apparent decreases have been shown for heart rate, stroke volume, cardiac output, $(a\text{-}v)DO_2$, and blood lactate (6, 12, 19, 23, 31, 42, 46, 47, 49, 50, 55, 56). At variance with the majority of studies are the findings of Mohsenifar and coworkers (57) who reported reductions in blood lactate and exercise heart rate after training. However this may have been the result of habituation to the testing procedure.

The abnormally large increase in pulmonary artery pressures at low levels of exercise is well-described in patients with COPD (50). One study (54) showed a decrease in pulmonary artery pressure at rest after training but this and several other studies failed to show reduced pulmonary artery pressure during exercise (52, 53). Cardiac output at submaximal loads is unchanged but this finding is concordant with the physiologic responses in normal subjects. In contrast to normal subjects, COPD patients at maximal exercise showed no increase in the maximal heart rate, cardiac output, stroke volume, or $(a\text{-}v)DO_2$ (49, 52).

Peripheral Changes

In normal persons the postconditioning reduction in heart rate appears to be related to adaptations in peripheral muscles (35, 58). This has been demonstrated in studies involving training one pair of limbs, or in some cases training only one leg. In these situations, muscle enzyme changes are reported to occur in the trained limbs only. The decrease in heart rate is seen when exercise is done with the trained limbs or limb (36). The importance of these peripheral changes has recently been emphasized in a study that showed that after denervation of the heart, a decrease in heart rate was seen after training (59). This evidence points to the importance of peripheral changes rather than central adaptations in the genesis of the posttraining bradycardia.

The fact that posttraining decreases in heart rate have not been shown in patients with COPD may suggest a failure to develop peripheral adaptations in skeletal muscle such as an increase in capillary density and aerobic enzymes. This possibility was evaluated by means of muscle biopsies taken from the arms and legs of patients with COPD (60). One group of patients trained their arms and another trained their legs. Biopsies were taken from the trained arms and legs as well as from the untrained arms and legs, which served as controls. Concentrations of citrate synthetase and 3-β-hydroxyacyl coenzyme A dehydrogenase were measured. Neither of these enzymes increased significantly in the trained or untrained limbs.

The fact that neither the heart rate nor muscle enzyme responses were seen in patients with COPD is consistent with the view that these patients are unable to reach the critical exercise threshold required to induce a training effect (60). In normal subjects it was observed that training intensities of approximately 50% of $\dot{V}O_2max$ are required to elicit beneficial training responses. These coincide with heart rates of approximately 50% of predicted maximum (42). Although patients with COPD are usually able to exercise to heart rates within this range, their heart rates do not necessarily provide a reliable guide to exercise intensity. This stems from the fact that the rise in heart rate with exercise may be more rapid than in normal subjects and probably results from a reduced stroke volume response (10). In addition, there is a greater than normal rise in the oxygen consumption of ventilatory muscles with hyperpnea, and this results in less oxygen availability for the exercising limbs (61). Thus, at a comparable oxygen consumption, the patient with COPD may be exercising at a higher heart rate (Fig. 9.4). Alternatively, at similar heart rates, the work load achieved by a COPD patient will be lower than that of a normal subject.

Generally, training effects occur in normal subjects only when exercise is performed at a higher oxygen consumption than that generally obtainable in the patient

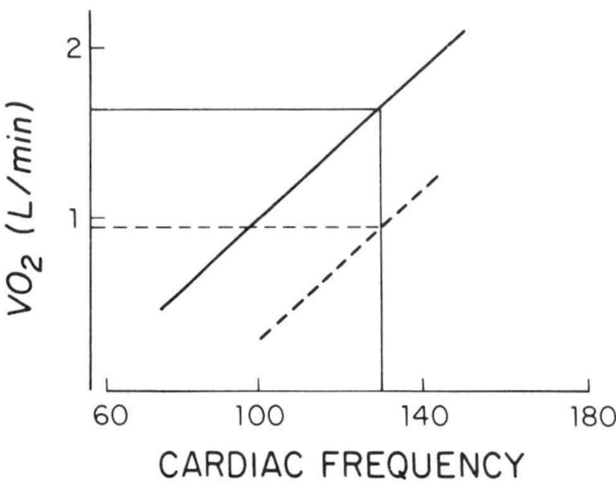

Figure 9.4. Illustration of the problem that arises when target heart rates are used to estimate work loads and training intensity. This figure shows the cardiac frequency/$\dot{V}O_2$ relationship in normal subjects (*unbroken line*) compared with patients with COPD (*dashed line*). The slope of the lines is similar but the absolute values are lower in COPD patients. At a heart rate of 130 beats/min (shown as *vertical line*) the corresponding exercise $\dot{V}O_2$ is less than 1 liter in COPD but almost 1.75 liters in normals. (Data for O_2 pulse derived from reference 50.) (Reproduced with permission from Belman MJ: Exercise in chronic obstructive pulmonary disease. *Clin Chest Med* 7:585–597, 1986.)

with COPD. Davis and coworkers (38) recently showed that normal subjects who trained at a $\dot{V}O_2$ of 1.5 to 2 $l \cdot min^{-1}$ demonstrated a training response. These levels are in excess of those reached by most patients with symptomatic COPD. As will be discussed shortly, the lack of objective training responses in the heart and peripheral muscles has important implications for methods of exercise training in COPD.

Breathing Training

Traditionally, breathing training in COPD involved diaphragmatic breathing and pursed-lip breathing. These have been reviewed extensively and will not be dealt with in detail (1, 2, 8, 55, 62). Although such techniques may help slow breathing, it is not clear whether these methods are used by patients during increased physical effort when they are not being observed. Studies have shown that pursed-lip breathing improves arterial oxygenation with a decrease in breathing frequency and larger tidal volumes (7, 44). Casciari and coworkers (50) have shown that breathing retraining provides additional benefit to exercise conditioning; however, some have criticized this study because it employed estimates of $\dot{V}O_2$max rather than direct measurements. Several investigators have found it useful to use pursed-lip breathing to slow breathing with COPD patients in an attempt to allay anxiety and panic during exercise.

Ventilatory Muscle Training

During the past few years interest has developed in endurance training of the ventilatory muscles (63). The main difference between this and the breathing technique training is the emphasis on improved endurance regardless of the technique. The rationale for this form of training is based on the fact that exercise capacity in patients with symptomatic COPD is often limited by impaired ventilatory mechanics. Two main methods of testing and training ventilatory muscles have emerged: a) resistive methods (Fig. 9.5) and b) hyperpneic methods.

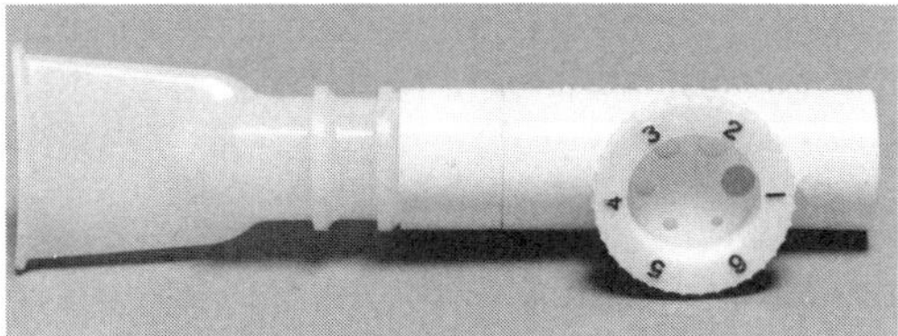

Figure 9.5. This is a typical resistive breathing device. The patient breathes in through the mouthpiece. The inspiratory load can be adjusted by turning the dial on which the orifices are numbered. The orifices are numbered 1 through 6 and range in diameter from 0.54 cm (orifice 1) to 0.17 cm (orifice 6).

In the resistive method, the patient inspires against a resistance so as to generate higher than normal mouth pressures with each breath. Using this method, several investigators have shown that patients are able to breathe against higher resistances after training. However, several of these studies failed to show improved exercise tolerance in patients after such training (7, 27, 58, 63–65). Some of the discrepancies in the results may stem from the fact that in some of the studies, target pressures and pattern of breathing were not monitored during the training (66). It has been shown that by taking long slow inspirations, it is possible to reduce the resistive work of breathing despite breathing through a smaller orifice (67).

In the hyperpneic method, which utilizes a specially constructed rebreathing system, several investigators have shown that it is possible to improve the maximal sustained ventilation (MSV) (Fig. 9.6) (43, 67, 68). The MSV is defined as the maximal ventilation that can be sustained for 15 minutes under isocapnic conditions. This form of training has been used in normal subjects, patients with cystic fibrosis, and patients with COPD. In an earlier study, this method was effective not only in improving the MSV but also overall exercise capacity.

Recently, however, Levine and associates (69) have shown that exercise capacity improved to the same degree in both a ventilatory-trained and control group, thus casting doubt on the role of muscle training in improving exercise tolerance. However, this study also showed that only the trained group improved the MSV during the study.

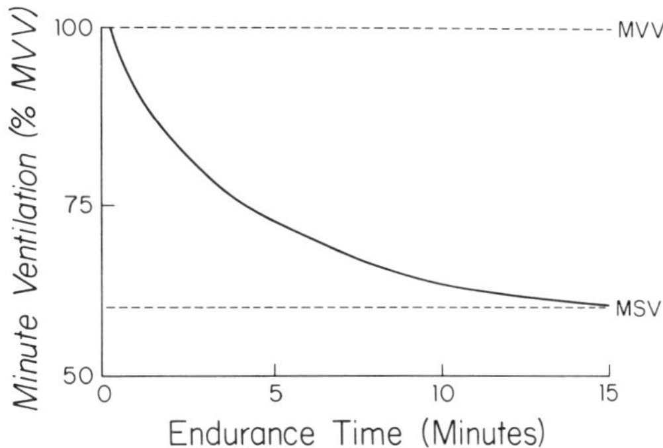

Figure 9.6. This illustrates measurement of the maximal sustained ventilation (*MSV*). The maximum voluntary ventilation (*MVV*) can be maintained for a short time after which there is a gradual decline in the sustained ventilatory level. After 15 minutes this reaches an asymptote and it is this level of ventilation that has been termed the MSV. (Reproduced with permission from Rochester DF, Dudley F, Brown NMT, et al.: The respiratory muscles. *Basics Respir Dis* 6:1–6, 1978.)

Thus, it seems that with the proper use of both methods, it is possible to improve ventilatory muscle endurance capacity.

The clinical importance of an improved ventilatory muscle endurance remains to be defined. The mechanism of this improvement is not yet clear but may be related to changes in aerobic enzyme concentrations of the diaphragm and other inspiratory muscles, as occur in other skeletal muscle. This hypothesis is supported by the fact that animals exposed to high inspiratory resistances developed increases in aerobic enzymes in diaphragms and intercostal muscles (70).

Mechanisms of Improvement

Improvements in exercise tolerance in COPD patients may be ascribed to one or more of the following factors: a) improved aerobic capacity; b) increased motivation; c) desensitization to the sensation of dyspnea; d) improved ventilatory muscle function; and, e) improved technique of performance. Despite the multiplicity of studies, there is as yet no clear consensus as to the predominant mechanism of improvement.

Improved Aerobic Capacity ($\dot{V}O_2max$)

In normal subjects increased $\dot{V}O_2max$ has been ascribed to both central adaptations (i.e., increased maximal stroke volume) and peripheral changes in the trained muscles. These changes occur concomitantly with training-induced decreases in the exercise heart rate and constitute an important component of the aerobic training responses in normal subjects. Similar responses have not been observed in patients with COPD (60) and so it is not possible to ascribe improved exercise endurance to improved aerobic capacity. Furthermore, the $\dot{V}O_2max$, an index of aerobic capacity in normal subjects, is not a reliable measure in patients with COPD. In COPD the increase in $\dot{V}O_2$ is limited by dyspnea secondary to impaired ventilatory mechanics (54) and so in essence is a symptom-limited $\dot{V}O_2$ ($\dot{V}O_2$ SL) (Fig. 9.2).

Increased Motivation

Increased motivation could easily account for the improvement reported in some studies. This could be deduced by noting increases in the maximal $\dot{V}E$ or heart rate. However, neither of these variables has increased consistently in cases that showed an increase in endurance (52, 56). In submaximal steady-state exercise tests, in which exercise endurance time is the measure of improvement, motivation may be a factor.

Desensitization to Dyspnea

Dudley et al. (9) have recently reviewed psychosocial aspects of pulmonary rehabilitation and cited several studies that have found correlations between improved exercise endurance and enhanced well-being. One study (71) found that psychological improvement resulted from pulmonary rehabilitation that included either exercises or psychotherapy alone. Several studies of exercise training have shown improvements in well-being and a reduction in breathlessness (23, 45, 47, 72). Agle and coworkers (72) suggested that these training effects may have, in part, reflected the presence of trained medical personnel who "inadvertently functioned as a desensitizing form of behavior therapy." They felt, therefore, that progressive exercise led to a decrease in the unrealistic fear of activity and dyspnea. This desensitization to dyspnea may be a key component of improved endurance after exercise, but it lacks objective measures of improved exercise endurance. Furthermore it has been shown that there is a better correlation between mood, motivation, and exercise endurance, compared with pulmonary function and exercise endurance (31).

Ventilatory Muscle Training

Ventilatory muscle training has been discussed. Its effect on improving endurance is as yet unclear. Further work will be necessary in order to delineate its true role.

Improved Mechanical Skill

Improved skill in performance among COPD patients has been reported in the literature. For example, early studies by Pierce and colleagues (54) and Paez and coworkers (12) showed that skill in treadmill walking improved with repeated attempts. Clearly, skillful performance of the task decreases the oxygen cost of work and ventilatory requirements, although the work load is unchanged. This constitutes training of technique and can be used to advantage by training COPD patients to perform specific tasks more efficiently. Although the technique of treadmill walking has been shown to improve in some studies, it is not known if this is indeed a component of improvement seen in nontreadmill walking.

From this discussion, it is clear that patients with COPD differ markedly from normal subjects in their response to endurance training. The major mechanism of improved endurance in normal subjects, namely increased aerobic capacity, is not found in these patients. The other factors enumerated here are important, but the relative contribution of each has not been elucidated. Delineation of the key mechanisms is important so that therapeutic efforts can be concentrated to achieve optimal benefits.

Exercise Training Methods

The major factors for consideration here are:

1. Intensity, frequency and duration of exercise;
2. Type of exercise;
3. Use of oxygen;
4. Energy conservation; and,
5. Breathing retraining.

Intensity of Exercise

In order to estimate the appropriate exercise intensity for training, the use of a target heart rate has been advocated (73). This method has achieved its widest application in normal subjects and patients with coronary artery disease. The aim is to provide the patient with an exercise heart rate that is within a safe range but of sufficient intensity to induce a training response. The fact that patients with COPD demonstrate impaired trainability despite the fact that they are able to achieve prescribed heart rates, casts doubt on the usefulness of the target heart rate in this population (60). As noted, an improved aerobic capacity is not essential to enhanced exercise tolerance in COPD. Consequently, there appears to be little justification for advocating this method. One exception might be the use of a target heart rate to ensure that exercise is performed at a level below that at which cardiac arrhythmias are known to occur. However, this would apply only to a minority of COPD patients.

Several studies have used gradually increasing levels of exercise as a means of training. These have been successful and they are simple to implement. In our program we use a progressive walking system, placing the emphasis on duration rather than intensity, and initially aiming to have the patient increase his or her walking time to 45 minutes to 1 hour. Once this has been achieved, an increased intensity is attempted if the patient has adequate ventilatory reserve. It should be emphasized that improvement in walking duration to this level enables these patients to be relatively independent. They are now able to leave their homes or able to walk to stores or cinemas from parking lots. Such achievements are taken for granted by normal persons, but in patients previously housebound or severely limited, these can be major milestones.

As discussed earlier in the section on Exercise Testing, the safety of a walking program can be established by monitoring during preliminary exercise testing to ensure that serious cardiac arrhythmias do not occur. Moreover, the 6- or 12-minute walk described previously can provide a simple means of assessing progress.

Type of Exercise

We recommend regular walking as this is the most natural form of exercise, although treadmill walking has been used in many studies and is certainly effective. Treadmill walking, however, has limitations, which include the fact that it requires a certain skill and many patients require time to develop this. Because of the skill required, there are usually improvements in performance over the first few attempts as patients become familiar with the task. This makes the treadmill generally unsuitable for exercise testing since several practice attempts are needed before a reliable baseline can be obtained. Cycling has also been a popular means of training. However, it is not a familiar task to many older patients, and there is some doubt as to whether the benefits of cycling are transferable to other modalities of exercise, such as walking (53).

Oxygen Administration

Only recently have clear recommendations for supplemental oxygen emerged (9, 30). These apply to patients with COPD at rest. We still do not have sufficient evidence on which to base firm recommendations for oxygen therapy during exercise. Several studies have used supplemental oxygen in training, and the clinical impression is that this has helped patients in initiating their exercise programs. In some cases, supplemental oxygen could later be stopped without adversely affecting exercise tolerance. No systematic study of effective long-term supplemental oxygen in exercising hypoxemic patients is available. In studies that compared supplementary oxygen administration during exercise, decreases were found in breathing frequency and exercise $\dot{V}E/\dot{V}O_2$ (9). A single-blind study failed to find similar changes, although in this case the patients were not hypoxemic (39). As exercise $\dot{V}E$ is reduced by oxygen administration, it has been suggested that supplementary oxygen may be beneficial even in patients who are not hypoxemic at rest. This was substantiated by Woodcock and coworkers (74) who reported that oxygen administration reduced breathlessness in "pink puffers" who were normoxemic. Current recommendations include the use of supplemental oxygen during exercise in patients in whom the PaO_2 is less than 50 to 55 mm Hg (Fig. 9.7) (6).

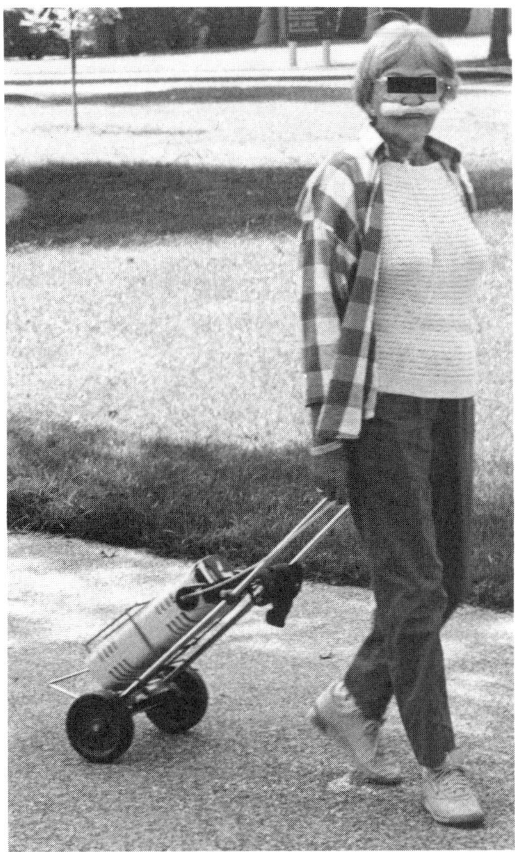

Figure 9.7. A COPD patient is shown walking with the aid of a portable liquid O_2 supply. Indications for O_2 therapy are discussed in the text.

Energy Saving Techniques

In the section on Mechanisms of Improvement, mention is made of improved mechanical skill. With respect to certain tasks of daily living, this can be utilized for the patients' benefit. Many patients perform wasteful movements in the course of daily activities. Occupational therapists are especially attuned to this and considerable reduction in inefficient movement can be achieved through appropriate monitoring and instruction of these patients in the performance of certain tasks (8).

Breathing Retraining

Breathing retraining was discussed previously.

CONCLUSION

Several important differences exist between the training responses in normal persons and in patients with COPD. Important among these are lack of significant cardiovascular and metabolic changes in the latter. Despite this, favorable improvements in functional capacity do occur after exercise training programs. Experience has shown that simple forms of exercise training and testing are effective and safe in patients with COPD. These can be done without the use of complicated and expensive equipment. While elaborate programs may utilize several professionals, including physicians, respiratory nurse specialists, occupational and physical therapists, and dietitians, these are not essential and success can be achieved with a modest number of personnel provided they are well-trained and motivated.

COPD patients who have participated in rehabilitation programs experience substantial benefits, not the least of which is a reduction in the number of hospitalizations (2, 4, 30, 71). This, together with the fact that there is an improved well-being and increased functional capacity, is in our view sufficient justification for third-party reimbursement for comprehensive care programs. While improved prognosis would be an added benefit, this has not been conclusively shown. A future area of research that appears worthwhile is the evaluation of the mechanisms responsible for the improvement so that emphasis can be directed to these.

The fact that both exercise training and testing can be done in a relatively simple fashion should make this modality of treatment more widely available than is currently the case.

REFERENCES

1. Hodgkin JE: Pulmonary rehabilitation. In Simons DH (ed): *Current Pulmonology*. New York, John Wiley & Sons, 1981, p 361.
2. Hodgkin JE, Balchum OJ, Kass S, et al.: Chronic obstructive airways disease. Current concepts in diagnosis and comprehensive care. *JAMA* 232:1243–1260, 1975.
3. Hodgkin JE (ed): Current concepts in diagnosis and comprehensive care. In: *Chronic Pulmonary Disease*: Park Ridge, Illinois, American College of Chest Physicians, 1979, p 34.
4. Hudson LD, Pierson DJ: Comprehensive respiratory care for patients with chronic obstructive pulmonary disease. *Med Clin North Am* 65:629–644, 1981.
5. Lertzman MM, Cherniack RM: Rehabilitation of patients with chronic obstructive pulmonary disease. *Am Rev Respir Dis* 114:1145–1165, 1976.
6. Moser KM, Bokinsky GC, Savage RT, et al.: Results of a comprehensive rehabilitation program. *Arch Intern Med* 140:1596–1601, 1980.
7. Petty TL: Pulmonary rehabilitation. *Basics Respir Dis* 4:1–6, 1975.
8. Petty TL, Nett LM, Fenegan MM, et al.: A comprehensive care program for chronic airway obstruction. Methods and preliminary evaluation of symptomatic and functional improvement. *Ann Intern Med* 70:1109–1131, 1969.
9. Dudley DL, Glaser EM, Jorgenson BM, et al.: Psychosocial concomitants to rehabilitation in chronic obstructive pulmonary disease (Parts 1, 2 and 3). *Chest* 77:413–420, 544–551, 677–684, 1980.
10. Spiro SG, Hahn ML, Edwards RHT, et al.: An analysis of the physiologic strain of submaximal exercise in patients with chronic obstructive bronchitis. *Thorax* 30:415–425, 1975.
11. Nery LE, Wasserman K, French W, et al.: Contrasting cardiovascular and respiratory responses to exercise in mitral valve and chronic obstructive pulmonary diseases. *Chest* 83:446–453, 1983.
12. Paez PN, Phillipson EA, Mosangkay M, et al.: The physiologic basis of training patients with emphysema. *Am Rev Respir Dis* 95:944–953, 1967.
13. Wasserman K: The anaerobic threshold measurement in exercise testing. *Clin Chest Med* 5:77–88, 1984.
14. Wasserman K, Whipp BJ: Exercise physiology in health and disease. *Am Rev Respir Dis* 112:219–249, 1975.
15. Owens GR, Rogers RM, Pennock BE, et al.: The diffusing capacity as a predictor of arterial O_2 desaturation during exercise in patients with COPD. *N Engl J Med* 310:1218–1221, 1984.
16. Cooper KH: A means of assessing maximal oxygen intake. *JAMA* 203:201–204, 1968.
17. McGavin CR, Gupta SP, McHardy GJR: Twelve minute walking tests for assessing disability in chronic bronchitis. *Br Med J* 1:822–823, 1976.
18. Beaumont A, Cockcroft A, Guz A: A self-paced treadmill walking test for breathless patients. *Thorax* 40:459–464, 1985.
19. Guyatt G, Pugsley SO, Sullivan M, et al.: Effect of encouragement on walking test performance. *Thorax* 39:818–822, 1984.
20. Guyatt GH, Thompson PJ, Berman LB, et al.: How should we measure function in patients with chronic heart and lung disease? *J Chronic Dis* 38:517–524, 1985.
21. Swinburn CR, Wakefield JM, Jones PW: Performance, ventilation, and oxygen consumption in three different types of exercise tests in patients with chronic obstructive lung disease. *Thorax* 40:581–586, 1985.
22. Editorial. Oxygen in the home. *Br Med J* 2:1909–1910, 1981.
23. McGavin CR, Gupta SP, Lloyd EL, et al.: Physical rehabilitation for the chronic bronchitic: Results of a controlled trial of exercises in the home. *Thorax* 32:307–311, 1977.
24. Mahler D, Weinberg DH, Wells CK, et al.: The measurement of dyspnea. *Chest* 85:751–758, 1984.
25. Woodcock AA, Gross ER, Gellert A, et al.: Effects of dihydrocodeine, alcohol and caffeine on breathlessness and exercise tolerance in patients with chronic obstructive lung disease and normal blood gases. *N Engl J Med* 305:1611–1616, 1981.
26. Stark RD, Gambles SA, Chattengee SS: An exercise test to assess clinical dyspnea. An estimation of reproducibility and sensitivity. *Br J Dis Chest* 72:269–278, 1982.
27. Spiro SG: Exercise testing in clinical medicine. *Br J Dis Chest* 71:145–172, 1977.
28. Kass I: Evaluation of impairment/disability secondary to respiratory disease. *American Thoracic Society News* 7:2028, 1981.
29. Dillard TA, Piantadosi S, Rajagopal KR: Prediction of ventilation at maximal exercise in chronic airflow obstruction. *Am Rev Respir Dis* 132:230–235, 1985.
30. Nocturnal Oxygen Therapy Trial Group: Continuous or nocturnal oxygen therapy in hypoxemic chronic obstructive lung disease: A clinical trial. *Ann Intern Med* 92:391–398, 1980.

31. Morgan AD, Peck DF, Buchanan DR, et al.: Effect of attitudes and beliefs on exercise tolerance in chronic bronchitis. *Br Med J* 286:171–173, 1983.
32. Reis AL, Fedullo PF, Clausen JL: Rapid changes in arterial blood gas levels after exercise in pulmonary patients. *Chest* 83:454–457, 1983.
33. Jones NL, Campbell EJM: *Clinical Exercise Testing*. Philadelphia, W.B. Saunders, 1982, p 89.
34. Clausen JP: Effect of physical training on cardiovascular adjustments to exercise in man. *Physiol Rev* 57:779–815, 1977.
35. Holloszy JO, Coyle EF: Adaptations of skeletal muscle to endurance exercise and their metabolic consequences. *J Appl Physiol* 56:831–838, 1984.
36. Davies CTM, Sargeant AJ: Effects of training on the physiological responses to one and two legged work. *J Appl Physiol* 38:377–381, 1977.
37. Gollnick PD, Sembrowich WL: Adaptations in human skeletal muscle as a result of training. In Amsterdam EA, Wilmore JH, Demaria AN (eds): *Exercise in Cardiovascular Health and Disease*. New York, Yorke Medical Books, 1977, p 7.
38. Davis JA, Frank MH, Whipp BJ, et al.: Anaerobic threshold alterations caused by endurance training in middle-aged men. *J Appl Physiol* 46:1039–1046, 1979.
39. Longo AN, Moser KM, Luchsinger PC: The role of oxygen therapy in the rehabilitation of patients with chronic obstructive lung disease. *Am Rev Respir Dis* 103:690–697, 1971.
40. American College of Sports Medicine: Recommended Quantity and Quality of Exercise for Developing and Maintaining Fitness in Healthy Adults. *Med Sci Sports Exerc* 10:vii–x, 1978.
41. Åstrand PO, Rodahl K: *Textbook of Work Physiology: Physiological Basis of Exercise*, ed 2, New York, McGraw-Hill Book Company, 1977, p 391.
42. Hellerstein HK: Principles of exercise prescription. In Naughton JP, Hellerstein HK (eds): *Exercise Testing and Exercise Training in Coronary Heart Disease*. New York, Academic Press, 1973, p 120.
43. Leith ED, Bradley M: Ventilatory muscle strength and endurance training. *J Appl Physiol* 41:508–516, 1976.
44. Tydeman DE, Chandler AR, Graveling BM, et al.: An investigation into the effects of exercise tolerance training on patients with chronic airways obstruction. *Physiotherapy* 70:261–264, 1984.
45. Sinclair DJM, Ingram CG: Controlled trial of supervised exercise training in chronic bronchitis. *Br Med J* 1:519–521, 1980.
46. Mungall IPF, Hainsworth R: An objective assessment of the value of exercise training to patients with chronic obstructive airways disease. *Q J Med*, New Series XLIX, 77–85, 1980.
47. Chester EH, Belman MJ, Bahler RC, et al.: Multidiscipline treatment of chronic pulmonary insufficiency. III. The effect of physical training on cardiopulmonary performance in patients with chronic obstructive disease. *Chest* 72:695–702, 1977.
48. Cockcroft AE, Sanders MJ, Berry G: Randomized controlled trial of rehabilitation in chronic respiratory disability. *Thorax* 36:200–203, 1981.
49. Degre S, Sergysels R, Messin R, et al.: Hemodynamic responses to physical training in patients with chronic lung disease. *Am Rev Respir Dis* 110:395–401, 1974.
50. Casciari RJ, Fairshter RD, Harrison A, et al.: Effects of breathing retraining in patients with chronic obstructive pulmonary disease. *Chest* 79:393–398, 1981.
51. Nicholas JJ, Gilbert R, Gabe R, et al.: Evaluation of an exercise therapy program for patients with chronic obstructive pulmonary disease. *Am Rev Respir Dis* 102:1–9, 1978.
52. Woolf CR, Suero JT: Alterations in lung mechanics and gas exchange following training in chronic obstructive lung disease. *Dis Chest* 55:37–44, 1969.
53. Alpert JS, Bass H, Szucs MM, et al.: Effects of physical training on hemodynamics and pulmonary function at rest and during exercise in patients with chronic obstructive pulmonary disease. *Chest* 66:647–651, 1974.
54. Pierce AK, Taylor HF, Archer RK, et al.: Responses to exercise training in patients with emphysema. *Arch Intern Med* 113:28–36, 1964.
55. Mueller RE, Petty TL, Filley GF: Ventilation and arterial blood gas changes induced by pursed-lip breathing. *J Appl Physiol* 28:784–789, 1970.
56. Vyas MN, Banister EW, Morton JW, et al.: Response to exercise in patients with chronic airways obstruction; 1. Effects of exercise training. *Am Rev Respir Dis* 103:390–399, 1975.
57. Mohsenifar Z, Horak D, Brown HV, et al.: Sensitive indices of improvement in a pulmonary rehabilitation program. *Chest* 83:189–192, 1983.
58. Chen H, Dukes R, Martin BJ: Inspiratory muscle training in patients with chronic obstructive pulmonary disease. *Am Rev Respir Dis* 131:251–255, 1985.
59. Ordway GA, Charles JB, Randall SC, et al.: Heart rate adaptation to exercise in cardiac denervated dogs. *J Appl Physiol* 6:1586–1590, 1982.
60. Belman MJ, Kendregan BA: Exercise training fails to increase skeletal muscle enzymes in patients with chronic obstructive pulmonary disease. *Am Rev Respir Dis* 123:256–261, 1981.
61. Rochester DF, Arora NS, Braun NMT, et al.: The respiratory muscles in chronic obstructive pulmonary disease. *Bull Eur Physiopathol Respir* 15:951–975, 1979.
62. Booker HA: Exercise training and breathing control in patients with chronic airflow limitation. Physiotherapy 70:258–260, 1984.
63. Belman MJ, Mittman C: Ventilatory muscle training improves exercise capacity in chronic obstruc-

tive pulmonary disease patients. *Am Rev Respir Dis* 121:273–280, 1980.

64. Andersen JB, Dragsted L, Kann T, et al.: Resistive breathing training in severe chronic obstructive pulmonary disease. *Scand J Respir Dis* 60:151–156, 1979.
65. Bjerre-Jepsen K, Scher NH, Koh-Jensen A: Inspiratory resistance training in severe chronic obstructive pulmonary disease. *Eur J Respir Dis* 62:405–411, 1981.
66. Clanton TL, Dixon G, Drake J, et al.: Inspiratory muscle conditioning using a threshold loading device. *Chest* 87:62–66, 1985.
67. Belman MJ, Thomas SG, Lewis MI: Resistive breathing training in patients with chronic obstructive pulmonary disease. *Chest* 90:662–669, 1986.
68. Keens TG, Krastings IRB, Wannamaker EM, et al.: Ventilatory muscle endurance training in normal subjects and patients with cystic fibrosis. *Am Rev Respir Dis* 116:853–860, 1977.
69. Levine S, Weiser P, Gillen J: Evaluation of a ventilatory muscle endurance training program in the rehabilitation of patients with chronic obstructive pulmonary disease. *Am Rev Respir Dis* 133:400–406, 1986.
70. Keens TB, Chen V, Petel P, et al.: Cellular adaptations of the ventilatory muscles to a chronic increased respiratory load. *J Appl Physiol* 44:905–908, 1978.
71. Lustig FM, Maas A, Castillo R: Clinical and rehabilitation regime in patients with COPD. *Arch Phys Med Rehabil* 53:315–322, 1972.
72. Agle DP, Baum GL, Chester EH, et al.: Multidiscipline treatment of chronic pulmonary insufficiency: Functional status at one year follow-up. In Johnston RF (ed): *Pulmonary Medicine: A Hahnemann Symposium*. New York, Grune and Stratton, 1973, p 355.
73. Adams WC, McHenry MM, Bernauer EM: Longterm physiologic adaptations to exercise with special reference to performance and cardiorespiratory function in health and disease. In Amsterdam EA, Wilmore JH, Demaria AN (eds): *Exercise in Cardiovascular Health and Disease*. New York, Yorke Medical Books, 1977, p 322.
74. Woodcock AA, Gross ER, Geddes DM: Oxygen relieves breathlessness in "pink puffers." *Lancet* 1:907–909, 1981.

CHAPTER 10

Asthmatic Patients and Those With Exercise-Induced Bronchospasm

Bruce G. Nickerson, M.D.

Patients with asthma frequently find that a few minutes of vigorous, physical exercise involving large muscle groups is followed by 30 minutes of misery. They may experience a dry, nonproductive cough, chest tightness, pain, wheezing and dyspnea. This syndrome is called exercise-induced bronchospasm. It can be demonstrated in almost all asthmatic patients.

Asthma is the frequent reason for children to be excluded from physical education. Exercise-induced bronchospasm represents the most common barrier to vigorous physical activity and may afflict 5 to 10% of the population. Because the prevalence of asthma and hyperactive airways is so great, all exercise laboratory personnel should be familiar with this syndrome. They should be familiar with the typical history, physical findings, and effective treatments that are now available.

The purpose of this chapter is to provide a current understanding of the clinical features, mechanisms and pathophysiology, avoidance strategies, and medical treatment of exercise-induced bronchospasm in patients with hyperactive airways. The author believes that nearly every asthmatic person should be able to participate fully in the exercise enjoyed by his or her peers. This requires that the patient and physician have an adequate understanding of the phenomenon of exercise-induced asthma and are willing to treat it vigorously. Thus, the diagnosis of asthma should present virtually no barrier to participation in a program of vigorous physical activity. Recent studies and clinical experience have demonstrated that regular vigorous exercise can be safe and provide good physical conditioning even in severe asthmatics if they are adequately treated.

EXERCISE TESTING

The relationship between exercise and asthma is well described. Observant patients and their physicians (1) have long been aware that several minutes of vigorous physical activity, particularly in cold air, is often followed by coughing, a sensation of tightness, chest pain, or overt wheezing. Kattan et al. (2) found that an exercise challenge test preceded and followed by a flow volume loop demonstrated exercise-induced bronchospasm in 99% of a group of 105 asthmatic children. They also found a close correlation between the results of an exercise challenge test and histamine challenge in children with a history of clinical asthma (3). Comparing exercise challenge to methacholine challenge, other investigators observed a reasonable correlation (4). Children seem to be more vulnerable to exercise-induced bronchospasm than adults (5). Asthmatic patients should be presumed to be subject to exercise-induced bronchospasm. In fact, the absence of exercise-induced bronchospasm should call the diagnosis of asthma into question. History-taking in asthmatic patients should include a careful probe for symptoms following vigorous exercise.

History

The type and intensity of exercise are quite important. Frequently, asthmatic individuals learn to limit the level of physical activity they experience in order to avoid bronchospasm. Some of these patients report no symptoms. Only careful questioning reveals that they have learned to avoid vigorous large-motor exercise lasting more than 3 to 5 minutes.

A history of symptoms immediately following vigorous work involving large muscle groups, which has lasted 5 to 10 minutes, is most consistent with exercise-induced bronchospasm. Shorter periods of heavy work usually do not have this effect. Activities lasting longer than 10 to 15 minutes are generally at a lower intensity so that they also do not elicit exercise-induced bronchospasm. The symptoms of bronchospasm usually do not occur during exercise, but are experienced shortly after the cessation of activity. With intermittent workloads as are found in many team sports, the patient may describe symptoms while still trying to play and need to be taken out of the game.

Exercise-induced bronchospasm can be quite frightening. The patient describes the sudden onset of a dry cough, chest pain or tightness, severe dyspnea, and perhaps wheezing. The phenomenon is more pronounced during cold or dry weather when the subject participates in vigorous activity outdoors. Exercise-induced bronchospasm may be avoided by a warm-up period of increasing intensity of work. Many patients find that after a gradual warm-up period, there is a refractory period when exercise-induced bronchospasm cannot be reinduced, as was documented by Edmunds et al. (6). However, Morton et al. (7) were not able to confirm this observation in their laboratory.

Mechanisms of Exercise-Induced Asthma

Chen and Horton (8) and later McFadden, Ingram and their students (9–15) in the late 1970s proposed the unifying concept of respiratory heat and water loss as the explanation of many clinical observations concerning exercise-induced asthma. They noted that the pulmonary function changes following exercise in susceptible subjects were increased if they were breathing air at −35 °C (9, 10). The investigators were also able to induce bronchospasm without exercise in susceptible subjects by asking them to breathe large volumes of this freezing air (11). However, neither exercise nor hyperpnea while breathing air that was warmed and fully humidified produced bronchospasm (8, 12). Esophageal temperature fell during hyperpnea or exercise sufficient to induce bronchospasm (13).

They proposed that respiratory heat loss was responsible for exercise-induced asthma. They found that exercise-induced bronchospasm represents a continuum of responses that are influenced by the prechallenge state of the airways and, under certain circumstances, can even be demonstrated in normal subjects (15, 16). For example, normal subjects may experience mild exercise-induced bronchospasm for several weeks following a respiratory infection (16).

The theory that exercise-induced asthma was related to respiratory heat loss explained many of the clinical observations. Careful analysis reveals that respiratory heat loss consists of three components: warming the air, warming the water in the air, and vaporizing water from the mucosa.

The equation that describes respiratory heat loss (RH) is composed of minute ventilation $\dot{V}_E$ times three terms:

$$RH = \dot{V}_E\,[\Delta T \cdot H_{DA} + \Delta T \cdot [H_2O]_c \cdot H_{H_2O} + ([H_2O]_B - [H_2O]_c) \cdot H_v]$$

ΔT is the difference between inspiratory and body temperature and H_{DA} (0.304 cal/1 °C) is the specific heat of dry air. Thus, the first term represents the heat required to warm dry air to body temperature. $[H_2O]_c$ is the water content of the inspired air and H_{H_2O} (0.001 cal/gm °C) is the specific heat of water. Therefore, the second term represents the heat required to warm the water present in inspiratory air. $[H_2O]_B$ is the water content of fully saturated air at body temperature (44mg/liter at 37 °C) and H_v (0.58 cal/mg) is the heat of vaporization of water. The third term represents the heat required to vaporize water from the mucosa. For example, for an exercising subject breathing 100 liters/min with a body temperature of 38 °C breathing air at 15 °C and relative humidity of 70%: RH (cal/min) = 100 liters/min [6.99 + 0.21 + 21.63] (cal/liter) = 2883 cal/min.

Thus, in this example, the heat of vaporizing water to humidify the air in the lungs represents 75% of the respiratory heat loss. Warming the inspiratory air and the water it already contains represents the other 25%.

The amount of water fully saturated air carries increases substantially with temperature. Thus, the relative humidity of the ambient air becomes less important as the inspired air has the lower temperature.

During quiet breathing, the nose provides most of the warming and humidification to inspiratory air (17). Both heat and water are supplied to the inspired air as it is inhaled, and are extracted from the expiratory air during exhalation. This countercurrent exchange mechanism decreases heat and water loss from the body (17). Excercise-induced asthma is associated with physical activity that is vigorous enough to produce mouth breathing. When the efficient countercurrent exchange mechanism of the nose is bypassed, cold, dry air enters the airways.

The relative effects of heat and water loss are closely intertwined. As temperature falls, the water bearing capacity of air decreases dramatically. Fully saturated air at 4 °C contains only 6.4 mg/liter of water or only 15% of the water content of alveolar air at body temperature (18). Thus, cold air is dry air as far as the airways are concerned.

Recently, Hahn et al. (19) proposed that drying of the airway rather than cooling was the mechanism responsible for exercise-induced bronchospasm. This was consistent with the observation that osmotic changes in the respiratory mucosa can result in bronchospasm (20). Hahn's studies were confirmed by Aitken and Marini (21). However, Eschenbacher and Sheppard (22) felt that both heat loss and water loss were independently important stimuli provoking bronchospasm. This question is difficult to resolve because cold air even at 100% relative humidity is quite dry when warmed to body temperature. Conversely, breathing warm dry air still entails considerable heat loss due to the heat of vaporization. Thus the effects of water and heat loss are closely intertwined.

Demonstration of Exercise-Induced Bronchospasm

Many satisfactory exercise protocols have been used for testing for exercise-induced bronchospasm. A protocol should be safe, achieve adequate minute ventilation for significant respiratory heat loss and drying, and produce reliable, objective documentation of bronchoconstriction. Protocols may be adapted to the equipment available and the specific purpose of the study. Prior to any exercise test, a thorough history and physical examination should be performed to establish the presence or absence of significant cardiovascular, neuromuscular, or pulmonary disease, and to determine the general level of the patient's fitness. The physician should understand the exact nature of the patient's symptoms, their relation to exercise, and response to previous therapy. The specific goals of the test should be clearly understood and the exact protocol planned accordingly. For example, the type of exercise may need to be adjusted to fit the needs and abilities of the patient.

Tests may be individualized for patients with specific problems or to answer specific questions. A precise understanding of the patient's symptoms and concerns is most important. One of the goals of the test should be to duplicate the patient's clinical symptoms and demonstrate whether they are accompanied by objective changes in pulmonary function. This is particularly important in persons who fear they are suffering from chest pain due to coronary artery disease, or who do not believe they have bronchial hyperactivity. Sometimes a repeat challenge after administration of a suitable bronchodilator can be very convincing to the patient who finds the distressing symptoms are prevented.

Pulmonary Function Measurements

The patient's pulmonary function can be monitored using a number of different devices. The simplest system suitable for field work would include a watch with a second hand and an inexpensive, portable peak flowmeter. The examiner should measure the heart rate during exercise for documentation of the adequacy of the stimulus, and measure the peak expiratory flow rates before and after exercise to document the response. Using a 12.5% fall in peak expiratory flow following exercise as a significant change, Kattan et al. (2) were able to detect approximately 80% of asthmatic children.

A more elaborate system, which the author uses in a well-equipped pulmonary function laboratory, includes a wedge spirometer suitable for generating a flow volume loop before and after exercise. This allows measurement of the forced expiratory volume in 1 second (FEV_1), and forced expiratory flow between 25 and 75% of vital capacity (FEF_{25-75}) and peak expiratory flow rate. In Kattan's study, 99% of asthmatic children had either a 10% fall in FEV_1, a 26% fall in FEF_{25-75}, or a 12.5% fall in peak expiratory flow following exercise.

A still more sophisticated test would also include measurements of airways resistance and lung volumes so that specific conductance could be calculated. Cropp (23) found that specific conductance changed by large percentages, and suggested that this was the most sensitive test for detecting exercise-induced bronchospasm. In addition to sensitivity, reproducibility must be evaluated. Nickerson et al. (24) found that FEV_1 was the most reproducible test of airway obstruction. They also found that persons with clinically significant lung disease had pulmonary function that was substantially less reproducible than that in those without lung disease. Thus, there is a trade-off between more sensitive tests of pulmonary function and a greater number of false-positive results.

Ambient Air Measurements

In view of the importance of inspired air in the induction of exercise-induced bronchospasm, a careful recording of the air temperature and relative humidity should be made at the time of the test. Although exercise-induced bronchospasm can usually be demonstrated under laboratory conditions with a room temperature of around 23 °C and a relative humidity of 75%, a negative study at a time when the air in the laboratory is particularly warm and humid would not be sufficient to rule out exercise-induced bronchospasm.

Physiologic Measurements

Several systems are now available for the measurement of minute ventilation, oxygen consumption, carbon dioxide production, respiratory quotient, anaerobic threshold, and oxygen saturation, and for the transcutaneous measurement of oxygen and carbon dioxide during exercise. Physicians and technicians should be cognizant of all the potential pitfalls and inaccuracies involved before using such a system. In particular, attention must be paid to the use of low dead space valves to separate inspiratory air from the warm, humid expiratory air. Systems designed for adults are frequently not satisfactory for children because the dead space is too large. Systems that calculate oxygen consumption and carbon dioxide production based on breath-by-breath measurements must have a very rapid sample rate. For accurate calculations, extreme precision must be used in matching the response time of the gas analyzers and measurements of flow. Before the calculated values can be relied upon and reported, these systems should be calibrated against the oxygen consumption measured using a collection system such as a Tissot or Douglas bag.

Noninvasive measurements of oxygen saturation are now available in many pulmonary function laboratories and can be very helpful in recognizing patients with severe obstructive lung disease who may have a fall in oxygen saturation level during exercise. The finding of oxygen saturation falling below 90% during exercise should raise suspicion of lung disease other than asthma, although, occasionally, severe asthmatics may also desaturate at high workloads (25). Measurement of transcutaneous oxygen levels during exercise has been found to be useful by Schonfeld and his colleagues (26). Transcutaneous carbon dioxide measurements can also be valuable under special circumstances (27). Familiarity with appropriate corrections and response time of the instruments used is always necessary (27, 28). These sophisticated measurements of pulmonary physiology are helpful in sorting out complex clinical problems or in documenting the physiological response, but are not necessary for screening most patients with exercise-induced bronchospasm if that is the only goal of the test.

The cardiovascular response to exercise can be monitored and recorded by taking the pulse and blood pressure every minute during the test. These measurements are especially important in demonstrating that a sufficient level of work has been achieved. Usually, one should document that the heart rate exceeds 70% of the maximal predicted value in order to establish that an adequate level of exercise has occurred. In suspected cardiac disease a multi-lead ECG should be recorded before, during, and after the test.

Type of Exercise

A number of different types of exercise involving large-muscle groups can be used to induce bronchospasm in susceptible patients (29). The most easily available form of exercise is free running, but it precludes precise measurement of the work obtained and the cardiovascular response (30). However, free running obviates the problems of selecting an appropriate workload because the intensity of exercise is determined by the patient. The actual running should be directly observed by the examiner, and the subject should be encouraged by all bystanders to perform a high level of work.

In most laboratories bronchospasm is induced using exercise on a cycle ergometer or a treadmill, which allows the subject to remain stationary for measurement of physiologic parameters. Because larger muscles are used, treadmill exercise generally evokes a greater minute ventilation and a higher heart rate (31). Anderson et al. (32) found that treadmill exercise was more likely to provoke bronchospasm than cycle ergometry. However, the expense and necessity for close supervision are relative disadvantages of the treadmill.

The author prefers the cycle ergometer (33) because it is relatively stationary and provides more accurate physiologic measurements. The workload can easily be determined by the physician and varied for the specific patient. Also, most subjects are more familiar and comfortable with the stationary cycle ergometer than the treadmill. Cycle ergometers with precise calibration of workloads are available but are more expensive than uncalibrated stationary bicycles. The proper workload must be selected with some care. Experience with patients of different ages, sizes, and degree of physical fitness is necessary to gain this judgment, although tables are available (34) and corrections can quickly be made if the level of exercise is found to be too high or low for that individual.

Cold Air Sources

The stimulus for provoking bronchospasm can be enhanced by the use of cold, dry air. A widely available environmental chamber is a large food freezer or meat locker. For several years, the author performed exercise tests in the hospital freezer, which provided a readily available source of cold air. Bronchospasm could easily be provoked in patients riding the cycle ergometer in the food freezer. Disadvantages of this system were the necessity of making arrangements with the food services department and the need for the technician and physician to dress warmly for adequate supervision of the test. Also, since the freezer was located some distance from the pulmonary function laboratory, subjects and technicians had to hurry back to the laboratory for the measurements of pulmonary function.

Recently, we have used a Hilsch tube (Fig. 10.1) connected to a compressed air tank as a convenient source of cold, dry air

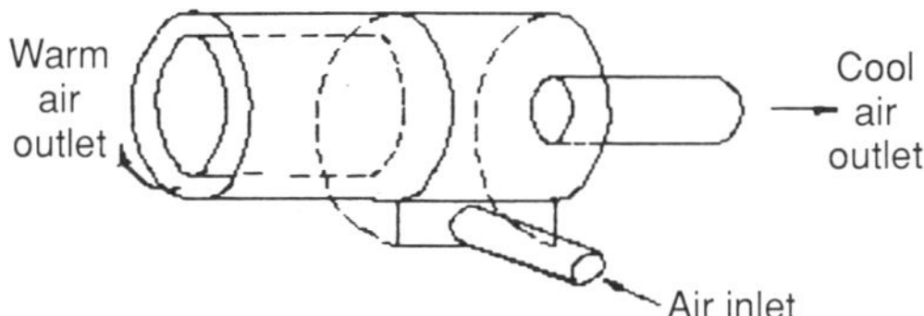

Figure 10.1. A Hilsch tube used to generate cold, dry air in the laboratory for exercise-induced bronchospasm challenge testing. Compressed air is released through the air inlet, forming a vortex. Warm air stays near the circumference and exits to the left. Cold air spirals to the center and leaves via the outlet on the right where it is breathed by the patient.

in the laboratory. Air from the tank is already quite dry so that a low water content is obtained. The Hilsch tube is a device that separates molecules with different kinetic energies so that a stream of cold air emanates from one end, and hot air from the other. This is accomplished by releasing pressurized air through a nozzle tangential to the cylindrical tube. The air then rotates rapidly around the cylinder. The Hilsch tube has two avenues for the air to escape, one near the circumference at one end, the other at the axis of the opposite end. The higher kinetic energy of warm molecules causes them to stay in the circumference of the cylinder and exit through the port at the circumferential end. Cold air spirals to the center of the cylinder and exits out the axial port. Under practical situations, cold air at 4 °C with very low water content is produced and is quite effective in provoking bronchospasm in susceptible subjects but does not produce bronchospasm in healthy persons. Hilsch tubes may be bought commercially or fabricated by a good machinist.

Clinical Evaluation

In addition to physiologic measurements, the subject should be questioned about symptoms experienced following exercise, and careful auscultation of the chest to detect wheezing should be performed. The physician's presence at this time is frequently crucial for confirming or ruling out exercise-induced asthma and explaining the presence or absence of symptoms to the patient. It is the author's practice and that of most other clinical laboratories to reverse exercise-induced bronchospasm with a suitable bronchodilator. Following administration of the bronchodilator, pulmonary function may be repeated to document the fact that bronchospasm has been fully reversed.

EXERCISE PRESCRIPTION

There are two approaches to exercise prescription in the asthmatic patient. The approach chosen depends on the philosophy and desires of the patient. One may choose strategies to avoid provocation of exercise-induced bronchospasm. This frequently requires limiting the patient's activities. The approach favored by the author is to use safe medications to control the asthma sufficiently well to allow participation without symptoms in whatever form of exercise the patient desires.

Strategies to Avoid Exercise-Induced Bronchospasm

Some patients desire to avoid taking medications at all cost. This may be due to side effects, expense, aversion to medications, inconvenience, or fear. In these cases, symptoms can be avoided by limiting exercise to activities unlikely to induce bronchospasm. Alternatively, the inspiratory air during exercise can be prewarmed and humidified.

The type of physical activity most likely to provoke bronchospasm has been studied by several groups. Fitch and Morton (35) found that treadmill and cycle ergometer exercise were more likely to provoke bronchospasm than kayaking or swimming. Anderson, Connolly, and Godfrey (32) found that free running resulted in even more severe reduction in pulmonary function than did treadmill exercise or the cycle ergometer.

Intermittent work of short duration with high intensity, such as weight lifting or baseball, does not usually produce exercise-induced bronchospasm because the patient's volume of ventilation is not sufficient to produce cooling or drying of the airway mucosa. Alternatively, a gradual warm-up period and prolonged exercise of relatively low intensity, such as walking, hiking, or aerobic dancing, can be selected. As long as the intensity is low enough and the patient can breathe through the nostrils, bronchospasm is unlikely to be provoked.

Exercise can be performed with warmed, humidified inspiratory air, but is uncomfortable because it is difficult to obtain enough heat loss to maintain a normal body temperature. However, swimming allows for adequate heat loss and does not provoke bronchospasm because the swimmer breathes air that is already warmed and humidified by the water. An alternative strategy is to exercise while wearing a face mask or bandana tied over the mouth. Rebreathing some of the air helps to prewarm and humidify the inspiratory air, thus preventing symptoms.

Few are able to breathe solely through their noses during intense exercise to take advantage of the efficient countercurrent exchange mechanism of the nose. This is especially true for patients with nasal allergies or upper respiratory infections.

Treatment of Exercise-Induced Asthma with Medications

For most patients with significant bronchospasm, the strategy of avoiding exercises likely to induce bronchospasm entails losing many opportunities for vigorous activities and foregoing the many physiologic and social benefits. Therefore, the author favors treatment so that patients with asthma can indulge in vigorous exercise with impunity.

Several classes of medications are effective and safe in the treatment of exercise-induced asthma. Thus, treatment can be individualized to the patient's preference and life-style. Choices among safe treatments for each person are based on acceptability to the individual, effectiveness, and cost. The goal in chronic therapy should be to control the asthma so that the patient can participate in the same forms of exercise as his or her peers without experiencing adverse symptoms. This goal can be achieved in nearly all asthmatic patients.

The three safe classes of drugs useful for treating exercise-induced asthma are the β-adrenergic aerosols, aerosolized sodium cromolyn, and oral methylxanthines. All these medications have been used for many years for a wide variety of patients. They have generally proven safe and effective; side effects are minor when properly used.

β-adrenergics

Often the simplest, most convenient, and inexpensive treatment for the patient with occasional symptoms of exercise-induced asthma is the β-adrenergic metered-dose inhaler taken prior to exercise. Before indulging in vigorous exercise, the patient inhales two deep breaths of the prescribed agent. Since the onset of action is almost immediate, the patient can promptly begin vigorous exercise.

Use of a metered-dose inhaler requires the medication to be released during inhalation through a properly held mouthpiece. Careful instruction and observation of the patient's technique are needed to ensure that this method is effective. For patients unable to coordinate inhalation and spraying simultaneously, use of an additional spacer device may provide some advantage. The medication is sprayed into the chamber and then inhaled with the next breath.

Used correctly, metered-dose β-adrenergic inhalers are quite safe. Common side effects are tremor, palpitations, and occasionally a significant rise in blood pressure. Also, some patients, particularly adolescents, on finding that the metered-dose inhaler gives rapid relief from bronchospasm, may overdose themselves by taking repeated dosages during a severe attack when additional agents may be indicated. The physician should discuss the potential dangers of overdosage of sympathomimetics with the patient and family, and avoid providing excessive refills of prescriptions for metered-dose inhalers.

Although physicians recommend taking inhaled sympathomimetics prior to exercise, many patients wait until they experience symptoms and then use the metered-dose inhaler to reverse the bronchospasm. During bronchospasm, less medication is delivered to the lungs so this strategy may not always be as effective as taking the inhalations before exercise.

Portable electric pumps for aerosolization of sympathomimetics provide a more potent and consistent effect than metered-dose inhalers. For the patient with more severe asthma who requires an aerosol machine to avoid frequent emergency room visits and hospitalizations, these pumps can also be used to deliver sympathomimetics prior to exercise. However, the expense and inconvenience of using these devices make them less practical for those who have only occasional symptoms following exercise. Oral sympathomimetics may be used, but in the author's experience, they are seldom potent enough to adequately block exercise-induced bronchospasm.

There are many β-adrenergic agents currently available (36). In the author's experience and as documented by numerous studies, all of them are quite effective if used in appropriate dosage. Some patients find that the unpleasant side effects, particularly tremor or a sensation of cardiac pounding, govern the choice of agents. Often the tremulousness, which can be very distressing on the first trial, diminishes after a few days so that it becomes unnoticeable to the patient.

Sodium Cromolyn

Sodium cromoglycate or cromolyn is also effective in preventing exercise-induced asthma. It is available as an aerosol solution or a metered-dose inhaler. It is effective in blocking symptoms of exercise-induced asthma (37–39), but must be used on a regular basis for consistent effect. If the patient has a home aerosol machine, cromolyn can also be given as a liquid aerosol solution and even mixed with a β-adrenergic agent. A major advantage of cromolyn is that patients seldom experience troublesome side effects and it is quite safe without the risk of overdosage as encountered with the β-adrenergics. Cromolyn currently is more costly that β-adrenergic agents.

Methylxanthines

Methylxanthines, such as theophylline, are effective agents for blocking exercise-induced asthma (40–42). However, the dosage needs to be adjusted for the desired effect since each patient absorbs and metabolizes these agents at different rates. Thus, they are more practical for patients who require chronic asthma therapy than for those who require intermittent, symptomatic relief. However, some patients find that theophylline alone controls their asthma and exercise-induced bronchospasm symptoms quite well.

The availability of long-acting theophylline preparations makes it possible to take two or three doses per day to achieve an adequate therapeutic effect. Some patients cannot tolerate methylxanthines because of nausea, vomiting, stomach discomfort, or headache. Others find the convenience of taking oral capsules the most acceptable form of therapy.

Glucocorticosteroids

Konig et al. (43) studied the effect of glucocorticosteroids on exercise-induced asthma. They found that neither oral prednisone nor aerosolized beclomethasone blocked exercise-induced bronchospasm in more than one-third of asthmatic patients. Henriksen and Dahl (44) found only a small improvement in exercise-induced bronchospasm after 4 weeks of inhaled steroids. Thus, steroids are not likely to be effective treatment of this condition. The potential side effects of chronic glucocorticosteroids also limit their use for this indication.

Some patients with asthma who require chronic glucocorticosteroids may require special consideration in exercise testing and prescription. Patients on chronic steroids are more prone to pathological fractures, particularly compression fractures of the vertebral bodies, so that forms of exercise that put extra compression stress on the vertebral bodies might not be appropriate. Some clinicians try to ameliorate this by treatment with supplemental calcium or vitamin D. However, appropriately controlled studies have not been done to demonstrate the efficacy of such supplements. Also, patients on chronic steroids may have decreased strength of the ventilatory muscles, which might limit their exercise capacity (45) although this has not been established.

Other Agents

Parasympatholytics, such as atropine (46) or ipatropium bromide (47), have been found to prevent exercise-induced asthma. However, the frequency of side effects such as dry mouth, urinary retention, and, until recently, the lack of a convenient commercial preparation for aerosol use, has prevented widespread use of parasympatholytics. It is quite likely that these agents will be introduced and promoted in the near future. Calcium channel blockers such as nifedipine (48) may soon also have a place in the therapeutic armamentarium.

Some patients with asthma may have other special considerations. For example, milk allergy may cause them to limit their intake of dairy products. They may suffer from hypocalcemia and be at greater risk for compression fracture or symptoms of hypocalcemia with hyperventilation. Thus, a careful dietary history should be taken. Patients who believe they have a large number of food allergies should receive very careful dietary counseling to ensure that they consume sufficient quantities of essential nutrients.

Patients with asthma may take other medications, such as troleandoic acid (TAO), other antibiotics, antihistamines, decongestants, eye drops, and supplemental vitamins. Since asthma is a chronic disease that waxes and wanes, patients are particularly susceptible to advertisements of foods or dietary supplements alleged, but not proven, to be effective. Thus, a very careful history should be taken regarding over-the-counter medications, dietary supplements, and other unconventional treatments.

In summary, selection of medical treatment to prevent exercise-induced bronchospasm is a choice between intermittent aerosolized sympathomimetics, chronic aerosolized sodium cromolyn, or oral theophylline. The choice should be based on patient preference, the severity of symptoms, and cost. Steroids should not be used for prevention of exercise-induced asthma because of their poor efficacy and the significantly greater risk of side effects.

Patients may adopt a variety of strategies for avoiding exercise-induced bronchospasm, such as choosing activities that are unlikely to provoke symptoms or breathing warm, humid air during exercise. This should be an informed choice, with the patient understanding that safe medications are now available so that he or she may participate in virtually any form of exercise.

CHRONIC ADAPTATIONS TO TRAINING

Since exercise-induced bronchospasm limits vigorous activities in many asthmatic patients, one might presume that they are poorly conditioned. The long-term consequences of this phenomenon represent a major portion of their disability. Nickerson et al. (49) studied the safety of a vigorous exercise program likely to achieve conditioning. The program was designed to repeatedly precipitate exercise-induced bronchospasm in 15 children with asthma and chronic airway obstruction despite multiple daily medications.

Following a 6-week control period, the subjects ran 3.2 kilometers around a grassy park, 4 days a week for 6 weeks. They developed symptoms and were treated with additional β-2 sympathomimetic inhalations. Their fitness improved significantly as assessed by their performance in a 12-minute run. There was no change in their daily symptoms, peak flow rate, resting pulmonary function, or propensity to develop exercise-induced asthma when studied in the laboratory. Thus, these children with severe asthma were able to participate in very vigorous physical activity that provoked exercise-induced asthma and experience the benefits of increased fitness.

Unfortunately, the psychological benefits of this program were not measured. Many of the subjects experienced an obvious and dramatic change in their self-image and self-esteem when they found they could exercise as well as their peers. In a long-term study, Szentagothai et al. (50) found that a vigorous exercise program for 121 children with asthma was accompanied by a decrease in symptoms, need for medication, and hospitalization.

Orenstein et al. (51) studied a 4-month running program for asthmatics. The subjects ran after inhalation of β-2 adrenergic agents. The investigators also found a significant increase in fitness with no change in the severity of asthma. They concluded: "We urge physicians caring for young asthmatics to encourage them to take advantage of exercise opportunities and not let the fear of exercise-induced asthma prevent them from leading a full, active life."

Ventilatory Muscle Function

The muscles of respiration are of particular importance with lung disease. One view of hypercarbic respiratory failure is that it is failure of the muscles of respiration to perform the work of breathing to eliminate enough carbon dioxide. Thus, ventilatory muscle conditioning might be a protective mechanism for asthmatics.

Nickerson and Keens (52) designed a valve suitable for measuring ventilatory muscle endurance as the sustainable inspiratory pressure in patients with chronic lung disease. This device requires a subject to generate a preset inspiratory pressure with each breath in order to open the valve and sustain respiration. Sustainable inspiratory pressure is defined as the highest pressure a subject can generate with each breath for 10 minutes, and is a measure of ventilatory muscle endurance.

We found that in asthmatic subjects, both ventilatory muscle endurance measured by sustainable inspiratory pressure and strength expressed as maximum inspiratory pressure far exceeded the values found in healthy subjects (49). This indicates that patients with chronic asthma have ventilatory muscles that are conditioned by their lung disease. In these asthmatic subjects, distance running did not further improve the sustainable inspiratory pressure or maximal inspiratory pressure, which were already elevated. We concluded that intermittent episodes of airway obstruction, which increased the work of breathing, led to conditioning of the ventilatory muscles.

SPECIAL EXERCISE PRECAUTIONS, LIMITATIONS, AND PROBLEMS

This chapter has emphasized the safety of exercise for asthmatic subjects. This is because historically, physicians have proscribed vigorous activities for fear of provoking episodes of exercise-induced asthma. The author's enthusiasm for vigorous exercise in asthmatic patients is in the context of a program of excellent medical control, a thorough understanding of the condition by the patient and physician, and a willingness to recognize and aggressively treat airway obstruction.

The strategies outlined to avoid exercise-induced bronchospasm should be used in situations in which such strict medical control is not feasible (53). The patient should be fully informed that vigorous exercise is practical and safe with an aggressive medical treatment program. The patient's choice to forego the benefits of vigorous exercise should be an informed one. Exercise-induced bronchospasm should be avoided in asthmatics who are unstable or chronically ill until adequate control of their disease is achieved.

SUMMARY AND CONCLUSIONS

Exercise-induced bronchospasm is a nearly universal manifestation of asthma. Its absence makes the diagnosis of asthma questionable. Exercise-induced bronchospasm may manifest as a dry cough, chest tightness, or wheezing following a period of 5 minutes of vigorous large-motor exercise performed in cool or dry air. The stimulus for exercise-induced asthma is related to either cooling, drying, or the osmotic changes in the airway provoked by breathing large volumes of relatively cool, dry air through the mouth.

A variety of protocols may be used to test for exercise-induced bronchospasm. They are adequate if they consist of several minutes of vigorous exercise involving large-muscle groups while patients breathe relatively cool, dry air. Objective assessment of the patient's level of exercise, symptoms, physical findings, and documentation of pulmonary function before and after exercise is needed to establish the presence or absence of exercise-induced bronchospasm.

The choice of protocols depends on the question being asked, equipment available, and experience of the physician. Free running, cycle ergometry, and treadmill exercise are most commonly used. Bronchospasm can be assessed with a simple peak flowmeter, spirometer, flow volume loop, or body plethysmograph before and after exercise. Bronchospasm should be reversed following a positive test.

Exercise-induced bronchospasm can be avoided by warming and humidifying the air by breathing through the nose or a mask. Alternatively, exercise of high intensity and moderate duration can be avoided. A preferable alternative is vigorous medical treatment so that the patient can indulge in vigorous exercise in any form. Exercise-induced asthma is eminently treatable with inhaled β-adrenergic agents, sodium cromolyn, or oral methylxanthines. The condition is seldom responsive to steroids and the risks of side effects do not justify their use for exercise-induced bronchospasm.

Even patients with severe asthma can safely embark on vigorous physical activity programs if their exercise-induced bronchospasm is adequately treated. The author feels that the goal of therapy is to control the asthma sufficiently well to allow vigorous exercise without the development of exercise-induced bronchospasm.

REFERENCES

1. Green MA: Exercise-induced asthma. *N Engl J Med* 302:522, 1980.
2. Kattan M, Keens TG, Mellis CM, et al.: The response to exercise in normal and asthmatic children. *J Pediatr* 92:718–721, 1978.
3. Mellis CM, Kattan M, Keens TG, et al.: Comparative study of histamine and exercise challenges in asthmatic children. *Am Rev Respir Dis* 117:911–915, 1978.
4. Chatham M, Bleecker ER, Smith PL, et al.: A comparison of histamine, methacholine, and exercise airway reactivity in normal and asthmatic subjects. *Am Rev Respir Dis* 126:235–240, 1982.
5. Weiss ST, Tager IB, Weiss JW et al.: Airways responsiveness in a population sample of adults and children. *Am Rev Respir Dis* 129:898–902, 1984.
6. Edmunds AT, Tooley M, Godfrey S: The refractory period after exercise-induced asthma: Its duration and relation to the severity of exercise. *Am Rev Respir Dis* 117:247–253, 1978.
7. Morton AR, Fitch KD, Davis T: The effect of warm up on exercise-induced asthma. *Ann Allergy* 44:257–260, 1979.
8. Chen WY, Horton DJ: Heat and water loss from the airways and exercise-induced asthma. *Respiration* 34:305–313, 1977.
9. Strauss RH, McFadden ER, Ingram RH, et al.: Enhancement of exercise-induced asthma by cold air. *N Engl J Med* 297:743–747, 1977.
10. Strauss RH, McFadden ER, Ingram RH, et al.: Influence of heat and humidity on the airway obstruction induced by exercise in asthma. *J Clin Invest* 61:433–440, 1978.
11. Deal EC, McFadden ER, Ingram RH, et al.: Hyperpnea and heat flux: Initial reaction sequence in exercise-induced asthma. *J Appl Physiol* 46:476–483, 1979.
12. Deal EC, McFadden ER, Ingram RH, et al.: Role of respiratory heat exchange in production of exercise-induced asthma. *J Appl Physiol* 46:467–475, 1979.
13. Deal EC, McFadden ER, Ingram RH, et al.: Esophageal temperature during exercise in asthmatic and nonasthmatic subjects. *J Appl Physiol* 46:484–490, 1979.
14. Haynes RL, Ingram RH, McFadden ER: An assessment of the pulmonary response to exercise in asthma and an analysis of the factors influencing it. *Am Rev Respir Dis* 114:739–752, 1976.
15. O'Cain CF, Dowling NB, Slutsky AS, et al.: Airway effects of respiratory heat loss in normal subjects. *J Appl Physiol* 49:875–880, 1980.
16. Aquilina AT, Hall WJ, Douglas RG, et al.: Airway reactivity in subjects with viral upper respiratory tract infections: The effects of exercise and cold air. *Am Rev Respir Dis* 122:3–10, 1980.
17. Schmidt-Nelson K: Countercurrent systems in animals. *Sci Am* 244: 118–128, 1981.
18. Weast RC (ed): *Handbook of Chemistry and Physics*, ed 50, Cleveland, The Chemical Rubber Co., 1969, p E 35.
19. Hahn A, Anderson SD, Morton AR, et al.: A reinterpretation of the effect of temperature and water content of the inspired air in exercise-induced asthma. *Am Rev Respir Dis* 130:575–579, 1984.
20. Eschenbacher WL, Boushey HA, Sheppard D: Alteration in osmolarity of inhaled aerosols cause bronchoconstriction and cough, but absence of a permeant anion causes cough alone. *Am Rev Respir Dis* 129:211–215, 1984.
21. Aitken ML, Marini JJ: Effect of heat delivery and

extraction on airway conductance in normal and in asthmatic subjects. *Am Rev Respir Dis* 131:357–361, 1985.
22. Eschenbacher WL, Sheppard D: Respiratory heat loss is not the sole stimulus for bronchoconstriction induced by isocapnic hyperpnea with dry air. *Am Rev Respir Dis* 131:894–901, 1985.
23. Cropp GA: Relative sensitivity of different pulmonary function tests in the evaluation of exercise-induced asthma. *Pediatrics* 56:860–867, 1975.
24. Nickerson BG, Lemen RJ, Gerdes CG, et al.: Within subject variability and percent change for significance of spirometry in normal subjects or cystic fibrosis patients. *Am Rev Respir Dis* 122:859–866, 1980.
25. Young IH, Corte P, Schoeffel RE: Pattern and time course of ventilation-perfusion inequality in exercise-induced asthma. *Am Rev Respir Dis* 125:304–311, 1982.
26. Schonfeld T, Sargent CW, Bautista D, et al.: Transcutaneous oxygen monitoring during exercise stress testing. *Am Rev Respir Dis* 121:457–462, 1980.
27. Nickerson BG, Patterson C, McCrea R, et al.: In vivo response times for a heated skin surface CO_2 electrode during rest and exercise. *Pediatr Pulmonol* 2:135–140, 1986.
28. Monaco F, McQuitty JC, Nickerson BG: Calibration of a heated transcutaneous CO_2 electrode to reflect arterial CO_2. *Am Rev Respir Dis* 127:322–324, 1983.
29. Fitch KD: Comparative aspects of available exercise systems. *Pediatrics* 56(Suppl):904–907, 1975.
30. Pierson WE, Bierman CW: Free running test for exercise-induced bronchospasm. *Pediatrics* 56(Suppl):890–892, 1975.
31. Godfrey S, Silverman M, Anderson SD: The use of the treadmill for assessing exercise-induced asthma and the effect of varying the severity and duration of exercise. *Pediatrics* 56(Suppl):893–898, 1975.
32. Anderson SD, Connolly NM, Godfrey S: Comparison of bronchoconstriction induced by cycling and running. *Thorax* 26:396–401, 1971.
33. Eggleston PA: The cycloergometer as a system for studying exercise-induced asthma. *Pediatrics* 56(Suppl):899–903, 1975.
34. Godfrey S: *Exercise Testing in Children: Applications in Health and Disease*. London, WB Saunders, 1974, p 68.
35. Fitch KD, Morton AR: Specificity of exercise in exercise-induced asthma. *Br Med J* 4:577–581, 1971.
36. Sly RM: Effects of beta adrenoreceptor stimulants on exercise-induced asthma. *Pediatrics* 56(Suppl):910–915, 1975.
37. Silverman M, Andrea T: Time course of effect of disodium cromoglycate on exercise-induced asthma. *Arch Dis Child* 47:419–422, 1972.
38. Shapiro GG, Pierson WE, Bierman CW: The effect of cromolyn sodium on exercise induced bronchospasm using a free running system. *Pediatrics* 56(Suppl):923–926, 1975.
39. Corkery C, Mindorff C, Levison H, et al.: Comparison of three different preparations of disodium cromoglycate in the prevention of exercise-induced bronchospasm. *Am Rev Respir Dis* 125:623–625, 1982.
40. Godfrey S, Konig P: Suppression of exercise induced asthma by salbutomol, theophylline, atropine, cromolyn and placebo in a group of asthmatic children. *Pediatrics* 56(Suppl):930–934, 1975.
41. Pollock J, Kiechel F, Cooper D, et al.: Relationship of serum theophylline concentration to inhibition of exercise-induced bronchospasm and comparison with cromolyn. *Pediatrics* 60:840–844, 1977.
42. Bierman CW, Shapiro GG, Pierson WE, et al.: Acute and chronic theophylline therapy in exercise-induced bronchospasm. *Pediatrics* 60:845–849, 1977.
43. Konig P, Jaffe P, Godfrey S: Effect of corticosteroids on exercise induced asthma. *J Allergy Clin Immunol* 54:14–19, 1974.
44. Henriksen JM, Dahl R: Effects of inhaled budesonide alone and in combination with low-dose terbutaline in children with exercise induced asthma. *Am Rev Respir Dis* 128:993–997, 1983.
45. Melzer E, Souhrada JF: Decrease of respiratory muscle strength and static lung volumes in obese asthmatics. *Am Rev Respir Dis* 121:17–22, 1980.
46. Deal EC, McFadden ER, Ingram RH, et al.: Effects of atropine on potentiation of exercise induced bronchospasm by cold air. *J Appl Physiol* 45:238–243, 1978.
47. Chan-Yeung M: The effect of SCH 1000 and disodium cromoglycate on exercise-induced asthma. *Chest* 71:320–323, 1977.
48. Corris PA, Nariman S, Gibson GJ: Nifedipine in the prevention of asthma induced by exercise and histamine. *Am Rev Respir Dis* 128:991–992, 1983.
49. Nickerson BG, Bautista DB, Namey MA, et al.: Distance running improves fitness in asthmatic children without pulmonary complications or changes in exercise-induced bronchospasm. *Pediatrics* 71:147–152, 1983.
50. Szentagothai K, Gyene I, Szocska M, et al.: Physical exercise program for children with bronchial asthma. *Pediatr Pulmonol* 3:166–172, 1987.
51. Orenstein DM, Reed ME, Grogan FD, et al.: Exercise conditioning in children with asthma. *J Pediatrics* 106:556–560, 1985.
52. Nickerson BG, Keens TG: Measuring ventilatory muscle endurance in humans as sustainable inspiratory pressure. *J Appl Physiol* 52:768–772, 1982.
53. Plaut TF: *Children with Asthma—a Manual for Parents*. Amherst, Pedipress, 1983, p 1.

CHAPTER 11

Patients with Cystic Fibrosis

David M. Orenstein, M.D.
Patricia A. Nixon, Ph.D.

INTRODUCTION

Cystic fibrosis (CF) is the most common life-shortening inherited disease in white populations, occurring in approximately 1 in 2000 live births (1). To date, there is no cure for the disease. However, recent advances in treatment have increased median survival age from 10.6 years in 1966 to 20.0 years in 1981 (2). The disease is characterized by noticeably salty sweat and the production of abnormally thick mucus that clogs ducts, tubules, and bronchioles. Although the mucus blockage affects almost every organ system, the most important adverse effects are in the pancreas and lungs (1). In the pancreas, the mucus blocks the ducts, preventing digestive enzymes (lipases and proteases) from breaking down dietary fat and protein. In the lungs, the mucus causes bronchiolar obstruction and infection, which leads to bronchiolitis, bronchitis, bronchiectasis, and, eventually, fibrosis and loss of pulmonary function. It is the pulmonary involvement that accounts for more than 90% of the mortality (1).

Treatment is directed at both the digestive and pulmonary problems. The digestion of dietary fats and proteins is enhanced with pancreatic enzyme supplements. Antibiotics are prescribed to fight pulmonary bacterial infection, and various physical means, such as chest clapping, are employed to prevent or relieve bronchiolar obstruction (3).

Exercise intolerance and exertional dyspnea are common complaints of CF patients and worsen as the disease progresses. In general, exercise tolerance is directly related to pulmonary function (4–6). Patients who are mildly affected by CF will have better exercise tolerance than those with severe disease. Although this relationship holds true when patients are grouped by disease severity, it is not possible to predict exercise tolerance for an individual from the results of the pulmonary function tests (7). For example, as shown in Figure 11.1, disease severity (indicated by the ratio of residual volume to total lung capacity (RV/TLC)), is directly related to exercise tolerance (measured by peak oxygen uptake ($\dot{V}O_{2\,peak}$)) for the total group. However, the variability in peak oxygen uptake among individuals for a given RV/TLC ratio is readily apparent.

Exercise intolerance appears to be related to ventilatory rather than cardiac limitations. Cystic fibrosis patients meet the increased oxygen demands of exercise by employing large minute ventilation ($\dot{V}_E$) to compensate for increased dead space (6, 8). In people with normal lungs, peak minute ventilation during exhaustive work usually does not exceed 60–70% of maximal voluntary ventilation (MVV). In CF patients,

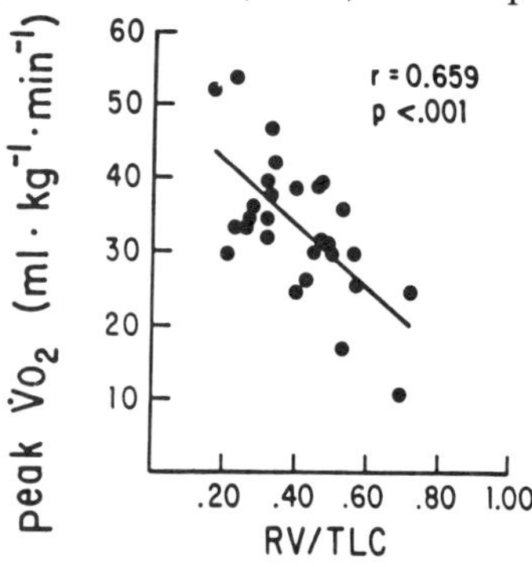

Figure 11.1 Peak oxygen uptake ($\dot{V}O_{2\,peak}$) in ml·kg^{-1}·min^{-1} plotted against residual volume *(RV)*/total lung capacity *(TLC)* for 28 patients.

minute ventilation during maximal exercise often approaches or even exceeds resting maximal voluntary ventilation, suggesting limited ventilatory reserve (9). The exaggerated minute ventilation may further impair exercise performance by requiring oxygen to be shunted away from exercising muscles to ventilatory muscles to meet the increased oxygen cost of breathing.

In most CF patients, proper gas exchange is maintained by increased minute ventilation and improved ventilation/perfusion ratio ($\dot{V}/\dot{Q}$) (6, 10). In patients with severe disease, minute ventilation may be insufficient to maintain adequate alveolar ventilation, resulting in oxyhemoglobin desaturation and carbon dioxide retention (11). Some patients may experience oxyhemoglobin desaturation without carbon dioxide retention, presumably because of altered $\dot{V}/\dot{Q}$ matching. The extent to which oxyhemoglobin desaturation itself limits exercise tolerance is not known.

Cardiovascular factors do not appear to limit exercise capacity in the majority of patients with cystic fibrosis. Most patients are able to reach age-predicted levels of maximal heart rate with normal cardiac output (9). In many of the sicker patients, impaired ventilatory capacity may limit their ability to exercise to a level below that at which the cardiovascular system would be maximally stressed, resulting in a peak heart rate below age-predicted levels (7, 9). Stroke volume may also be reduced in sicker patients (9). In some patients, radionuclide studies show evidence of right ventricular dysfunction, and more rarely, left ventricular dysfunction (12–14). For the most part, these cardiovascular limitations are less important than the ventilatory limitations in impairing exercise performance.

EXERCISE TESTING IN CYSTIC FIBROSIS

The exercise test provides important information about the patient's pulmonary function and reserve that cannot be obtained from standard pulmonary function tests. The specific objectives of exercise testing in CF are to:

1. evaluate disease severity
2. determine aerobic fitness (maximal or peak oxygen uptake) and functional exercise capacity
3. examine cardiorespiratory adaptive responses to exercise
4. provide a basis for prescribing exercise within safe limits
5. assess changes that occur with treatment intervention (e.g., pharmacologic, chest physical therapy, exercise training) or with disease progression

Safety Precautions

Exercise testing may be contraindicated for some patients, particularly those with late-stage disease with cor pulmonale and overt right heart failure. In these patients, discretion should be used to determine if the benefits of the evaluation outweigh the potential risks and discomfort involved with testing.

Exercise testing during an acute pulmonary exacerbation may not be appropriate, depending on the objective of testing. With an acute infection, exercise tolerance will be reduced, and therefore not representative of the patient's "normal" exercise capacity. However, exercise testing during an infection will provide specific information about the patient's exercise tolerance while sick, as well as the patient's response to intervention.

Hundreds of patients with CF, including many with severe pulmonary involvement, have been tested with no untoward effects. Nevertheless, we recommend that standard safety precautions be taken during tests with this population. Testing should be conducted by personnel trained in cardiopulmonary resuscitation and emergency procedures. The laboratory should be equipped with emergency equipment and drugs (15). Furthermore, prior to the test, the test procedures should be explained and written informed consent should be obtained from the patient or a legal guardian if the patient is a minor.

Types of Exercise Tests

The purpose of the test and the information desired will dictate the mode of testing and the protocol that should be used. The two modes of testing most commonly used are the treadmill and the cycle ergometer. Although walking on the treadmill is similar to everyday weight-bearing activities, the cycle ergometer is more widely used for testing CF patients for several reasons. A large proportion of this population includes children and adolescents, for whom bicycle riding is a familiar and easily mastered task. The likelihood of falling off the cycle is minimal compared to the potential for stumbling on the treadmill. The upper body is also more stationary, which enables the breathing apparatus to remain steady. Power output is more easily quantified on the cycle ergometer because it is independent of body weight (15, 16). Furthermore, because of the popularity of the cycle ergometer as the mode for testing in children, more extensive normal standards are available for comparisons with other populations (17–20).

Maximal Incremental Tests

Functional exercise capacity and aerobic fitness are best evaluated by a progressive maximal exercise test, such as the Godfrey protocol (18). This protocol is based on height and is performed on the cycle ergometer. The test starts at "0" resistance and increases by 10, 15, or 20 watts (W) each minute for subjects who are shorter than 125 cm, between 125 and 150 cm tall, or taller than 150 cm, respectively. The test ends when the patient can no longer maintain the prescribed pedaling frequency.

Protocols that adjust work load according to weight may also be used. For instance, Cerny and associates (8) report using a protocol with power increments equivalent to 0.3 $W \cdot kg^{-1}$ every 2 minutes, starting at 0.3 $W \cdot kg^{-1}$ for severely ill patients, and at 0.6 $W \cdot kg^{-1}$ for all other patients. This protocol permits the comparison of responses between individuals for each power output because each work level is adjusted for body weight.

If testing is to be conducted on a treadmill, a progressive maximal testing protocol such as the Balke protocol can be used (21). With this protocol, the speed is held constant at 3.4 $mi \cdot h^{-1}$ and the grade increases by 1% each minute, or by 2% each minute in the modified version. Oxygen consumption at each work level will vary according to the patient's weight and mechanical efficiency of walking (22).

Minute-by-minute incremental tests or the more rapidly increasing "ramp" protocols do not allow the subjects to reach a steady-state at each work load. In most cases, this is not a drawback provided that the same protocol is employed when comparisons are made between individuals or between groups.

Expanding the time at each work load to 2 or 3 minutes may allow more careful examination of cardiorespiratory responses to increasing work loads. If "true" steady-state is the goal, work stages of 5 minutes may be required (23). However, 5-minute stages will significantly prolong the test and may not be a realistic goal for sicker patients.

With the maximal exercise test, it is important to verify that a maximal effort has been made by the patient. This verification can be made by examining the peak heart rate (HR), peak minute ventilation ($\dot{V}E$), and/or peak oxygen consumption ($\dot{V}O_{2\,peak}$) attained at the highest work load. Peak heart rate should reach age-predicted maximal levels ($\pm$ 10 $beats \cdot min^{-1}$) (24), unless it is limited by ventilatory factors as reflected in a peak $\dot{V}E$ that exceeds 70% of MVV. Peak respiratory exchange ratio (RER) should exceed 1.15 (25). A commonly used criterion is that oxygen uptake at maximal levels of work should plateau or not increase with an increase in work rate (26). This plateau, however, is often not observed, particularly in protocols in which the work rate increases each minute. In rare cases, intolerable dyspnea may cause the patient to terminate exercise before other factors can reach maximal levels.

Maximal exercise tests are often very difficult for patients, who may experience hard coughing spells and shortness of breath. Sicker patients may be fatigued for many hours following a maximal test. Discretion should be used to determine if the information to be gained from a maximal effort warrants the fatigue and discomfort endured by the patient.

Submaximal Tests

Although the maximal exercise test is the only method for assessing peak exercise capacity, valuable information about the cardiorespiratory responses to exercise can be obtained with a steady-state submaximal exercise test. The test is often performed with the patient exercising at work loads equivalent to ⅓ or ⅔ of his or her predetermined maximal work level (23). It can also be performed at an arbitrarily selected work load or intensity (e.g., as determined by heart rate). Each stage should be a minimum of 5 minutes to ensure that the responses have stabilized, indicating that a true steady-state has been reached. The cardiorespiratory responses during a steady-state submaximal test will reflect the patient's ability to adapt to submaximal work associated with everyday activities.

Changes in response to treatment may be evaluated by a submaximal progressive test. For example, the effects of exercise training can be assessed by having the patient exercise progressively up to a heart rate of 150 beats·min^{-1} (or approximately 75% of peak heart rate). If a positive training effect has occurred, greater power output will be accomplished before reaching the predetermined heart rate (75% of peak HR) (27). In this manner, the effects of exercise training can be evaluated at more frequent intervals without unduly fatiguing the patient. Similarly, either a submaximal progressive test or a 5- to 6-minute steady-state test can be administered at frequent intervals (e.g., every other day) to provide objective information about the patient's response to treatment (pharmacologic, chest physical therapy) during hospitalization for therapy of an acute exacerbation of pulmonary infection.

Observations to be Made During the Test

During the exercise test, the following measurements are recommended to provide optimal information about the patient's cardiorespiratory responses to exercise: power output, minute ventilation ($\dot{V}E$), oxygen uptake ($\dot{V}O_2$), carbon dioxide production ($\dot{V}CO_2$), end-tidal carbon dioxide tension ($PetCO_2$), oxygen saturation (SaO_2), respiratory exchange ratio (RER), and heart rate (HR). The electrocardiogram (ECG) should be monitored continuously and blood pressure measured periodically throughout the test. Oxygen saturation should be monitored continuously and can be measured noninvasively by an ear or pulse oximeter. End-tidal carbon dioxide tension can be measured breath by breath or averaged over short intervals of time. These noninvasive measurements of oxygen saturation and end-tidal carbon dioxide provide fairly valid estimates of arterial levels of oxygen and carbon dioxide, without the pain involved with obtaining arterial blood. Furthermore, the noninvasive measurements of oxygen saturation and end-tidal carbon dioxide tension are displayed continuously, while actual blood gas results are seldom available before the test has ended.

In the absence of metabolic equipment, the measurements of oxygen saturation, power output, blood pressure, and heart rate (with continuous monitoring of the ECG) can provide sufficient information about the patient's exercise tolerance.

If the CF patient is suspected of suffering from exercise-induced asthma, measurements of forced expiratory flow rate, such as forced expired volume in 1 second (FEV_1), forced expiratory flow for the middle half of forced vital capacity (FEF_{25-75}), and peak expiratory flow rate (PEFR), should be made before and several times after the exercise test (for at least 15 minutes postexercise) (18).

Ratings of perceived exertion (RPE) may also provide additional information about the patient's subjective tolerance of the exercise (28). Furthermore, some estimate of coughing should be made.

Criteria for Terminating the Test

The exercise test should be terminated for any of the following reasons:

1. The patient is unable to maintain the pedaling rate on a cycle ergometer or is unable to "keep up" with the speed of the treadmill;
2. the patient requests that the test be stopped because of extreme discomfort of any kind;
3. the oxygen saturation drops below 80% (This criterion is precautionary; we have never observed any irreversible ill effects from short-term hypoxemia in this setting);
4. the appearance of significant ST-segment depression (i.e., > 2 mm) and/or serious ventricular dysrhythmias;
5. the systolic blood pressure exceeds 250 mm Hg, or decreases, or fails to increase with increased power output;
6. the diastolic blood pressure exceeds 110–120 mm Hg.

More detailed criteria for terminating an exercise test are presented in the American College of Sports Medicine's *Guidelines for Graded Exercise Testing and Exercise Prescription* (15). In our own experience with the CF population, most tests are terminated because a maximal level is reached. Rarely have we been forced to stop a test because of cardiovascular abnormalities.

Interpretation of the Test Results

Exercise tolerance varies greatly among CF patients. When grouped by severity of disease, those with the mildest disease may have normal exercise tolerance. However, as the disease progresses, exercise tolerance decreases significantly.

Specifically, peak work capacity and oxygen uptake may often be normal in mildly affected patients with CF, but these values decrease substantially as the disease progresses (4, 7). The trend for decreasing peak oxygen uptake with progressive pulmonary deterioration is evident in Figure 11.2. Furthermore, as in the normal population, the peak oxygen uptake of female patients is lower than that of male patients.

High minute ventilation ($\dot{V}E$) is commonly observed in patients when compared with normals, with the peak minute ventilation approaching or even exceeding maximal voluntary ventilation (MVV) (4, 8,

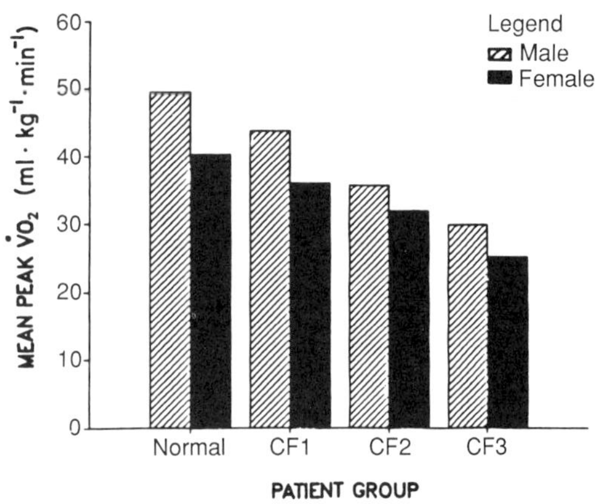

Figure 11.2 Mean peak oxygen uptake ($ml \cdot kg^{-1} \cdot min^{-1}$) for 56 male and 51 female healthy control subjects, and for 57 male and 52 female CF patients categorized into 3 groups by degree of pulmonary obstruction: *CF1*—mild obstruction ($FEV_1 \geq 70\%$ FVC); *CF2*—moderate obstruction ($FEV_1 = 50$ to 69% FVC); and *CF3*—severe obstruction ($FEV_1 < 50\%$ FVC).

9). In normal subjects, minute ventilation during exercise testing generally does not exceed 70% of MVV. Oxygen uptake may be greater at a given submaximal work load due to the added oxygen cost of breathing (29). The ventilatory equivalent for oxygen ($\dot{V}E/\dot{V}O_2$) is often elevated, suggesting that the increased $\dot{V}E$ is primarily to compensate for increased dead space (29).

Peak heart rate may also reach normal levels predicted for age (220 minus age in years) in patients with mild disease, but may be significantly below age-predicted levels in severely affected patients (7–9). Heart rate at a given submaximal work load may often be disproportionately high (8) because of deconditioning, hypoxemia, the increased work of breathing, or any combination of these factors.

As with most normal subjects, patients with CF are able to exercise beyond their anaerobic threshold, i.e., at levels of work where the oxygen supply is insufficient to meet the energy requirements, and aerobic metabolism must be supplemented with anaerobic metabolism to meet these demands. Therefore, the respiratory exchange ratio (RER = $\dot{V}CO_2/\dot{V}O_2$) will reach levels between 1.1 and 1.3 in most patients who exercise to exhaustion (29, 30).

In most CF patients, normal arterial levels of oxygen and carbon dioxide are maintained throughout exercise (11). However, in patients with severely diminished pulmonary function, oxyhemoglobin desaturation, with or without carbon dioxide retention, may occur. It is probably important to identify these patients and the work level and heart rate at which they desaturate. As demonstrated in Figure 11.3, patients with an FEV_1 less than 50% of forced vital capacity (FVC) are more likely to exhibit oxygen desaturation than patients with an FEV_1 greater than 50% of FVC. However, even in these patients with pronounced airway obstruction, it is clear that oxyhemoglobin saturation often stays the same or even increases with exercise.

The results of maximal exercise testing in four CF patients are presented in Table 11.1. In Case 1, the high peak minute ventilation (equivalent to 105% MVV) and the high RER of 1.2 indicate that a maximal effort was put forth despite the low workload achieved (50% of predicted physical work capacity). The high $\dot{V}_E$/MVV and low peak heart rate (75% of predicted) indicate that exercise was limited by ventilatory mechanics before the heart rate could reach its predicted maximum. The decrease in oxyhemoglobin saturation (SaO_2) from 93 to 91% probably did not impair exercise performance because arterial blood is still well-oxygenated at this level.

In Case 2, a better than normal peak work load (110% of predicted) was achieved, with a normal peak heart rate (100% of predicted). These results are very similar to those seen in normal subjects, and would be consistent with the normal cardiac limitation to exercise. And yet, the very high $\dot{V}_E$/MVV ratio is not normal, and indicates that there was no ventilatory reserve.

In Case 3, peak physical work capacity was 50% of predicted, and was achieved aerobically, as indicated by the peak RER of 0.85. The peak heart rate was substan-

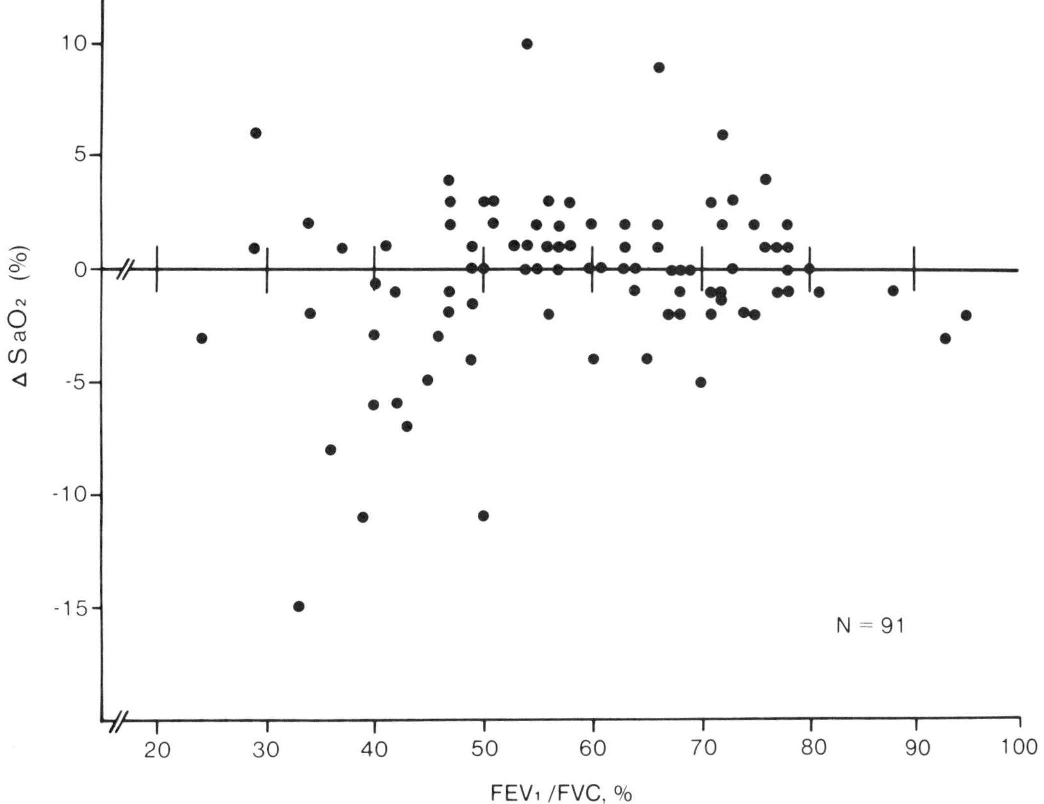

Figure 11.3 Changes in oxyhemoglobin saturation (SaO_2) with exercise plotted against FEV_1/FVC. (From Henke KG, Orenstein DM: Oxygen saturation during exercise in cystic fibrosis. *Am Rev Respir Dis* 129:708–711, 1984.)

Table 11.1
Results From Progressive Exercise Tests In Four Cystic Fibrosis Patients

	Case 1	Case 2	Case 3	Case 4
Pre-test FEV_1 (% FVC)	45%	80%	70%	30%
Physical work capacity (% pred)	50%	110%	50%	40%
Peak heart rate (% pred)	75%	100%	70%	70%
Peak $\dot{V}_E$ (% MVV)	105%	110%	40%	55%
Peak RER	1.20	1.31	0.85	0.98
Initial SaO_2	93%	96%	92%	79%
Peak SaO_2	91%	96%	94%	64%

tially below predicted levels, and was achieved with no impingement on the ventilatory capacity. The increase in SaO_2 from 92 to 94% suggests improved ventilation/perfusion matching. It is likely that this patient did not give a maximal effort.

In Case 4, the peak heart rate and peak work capacity were substantially below predicted levels (70% and 40%, respectively). The peak RER of 0.98 was lower than the normal range of 1.1 to 1.3, and suggests that the work was achieved aerobically. The relatively low $\dot{V}_E$/MVV ratio indicates that ventilatory capacity was not a limiting factor. The oxyhemoglobin saturation (SaO_2) was initially low (79%) and decreased significantly with exercise. In this case, it is likely that low oxyhemoglobin saturation limited the patient's ability to exercise to a level at which the ventilatory and cardiovascular system could reach maximal levels.

BENEFITS OF EXERCISE TRAINING

Few well-controlled experimental studies have directly addressed the effects of exercise training in CF patients. However, the results of several published studies provide evidence to suggest that CF patients may benefit from a variety of exercise training programs in several ways.

Keens and associates (31) reported that 4 weeks of upper body exercise (swimming and canoeing) or daily sessions of ventilatory muscle training (breathing against increased resistance) were each effective in increasing ventilatory muscle endurance. No changes in the standard pulmonary function test results were observed with either type of training.

Similar results were obtained by Asher and associates (32) with 4 weeks of inspiratory muscle training. The patients showed an increase in inspiratory muscle endurance, with no change in pulmonary function. Exercise tolerance was also measured and did not change with the inspiratory muscle training program.

Improvements in ventilatory muscle endurance were also observed in CF patients who participated in 3 months of supervised aerobic exercise conditioning (running and walking) at 70% of peak heart rate, three times per week (7). As shown in Figure 11.4, these patients also responded to training with improvements in exercise tolerance, as reflected in a higher peak oxygen

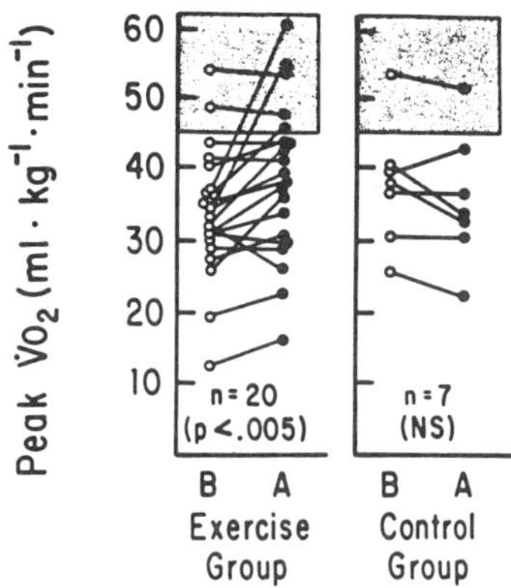

Figure 11.4 Peak oxygen uptake of exercise group and control group before (*B*) and after (*A*) the 3-month exercise conditioning program. The *shaded area* indicates normal range. (From Orenstein DM, Franklin BA, Doershuk CF, et al.: Exercise conditioning and cardiopulmonary fitness in cystic fibrosis. *Chest* 80:392–398, 1981.)

uptake. The nonexercising control subjects exhibited no change in peak oxygen uptake over the same period of time. Heart rate at a given submaximal work level decreased significantly after 3 months of training, while no change in submaximal heart rate was evident in the control subjects (Fig. 11.5). Pulmonary function did not change significantly in either group, except for a deterioration in FEV_1 in the control group.

Similar results were observed in another study with a 12-week swimming program (33). Total exercise test time and estimated peak $\dot{V}O_2$ increased in the exercise group, with no change occurring in the nonexercise control group. Likewise, neither group demonstrated improvement in pulmonary function.

In contrast, Zach and associates (34) reported favorable alterations in pulmonary function following a 17-day exercise program that included vigorous participation in swimming, jogging, and sports for several hours each day. At the end of the program, the patients exhibited significant improvements in FEV_1, FVC, FEF_{25-75}, and PEFR. Follow-up measurements taken 8 weeks later indicated that all pulmonary function tests except PEFR had returned to

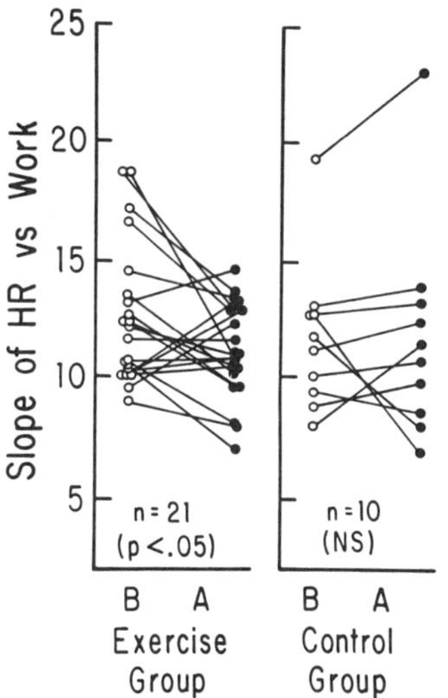

Figure 11.5 Slope of heart rate vs. work curve (beats·min^{-1}·kp·m·min^{-1}) for exercise group and control group before (*B*) and after (*A*) the 3-month conditioning program. (From Orenstein DM, Franklin BA, Doershuk CF, et al.: Exercise conditioning and cardiopulmonary fitness in cystic fibrosis. *Chest* 80:392–398, 1981.)

pretraining baseline levels. Aerobic fitness was not measured.

Furthermore, Zach and associates (35) found that swimming facilitated sputum production and mucus clearance when compared with nonswimming days. There is some evidence to suggest that exercise may be as effective as chest physical therapy (postural drainage and percussion) for clearing mucus (35) and maintaining pulmonary function (36). However, we feel that stronger evidence is needed before chest physical therapy is discontinued or replaced by exercise as the method for enhancing mucus clearance.

Weight training has also been shown in a preliminary and controversial study to affect pulmonary function (37). A 6-month program of variable upper body weight training was associated with a significant improvement in residual volume, suggestive of diminished air trapping, but also a significant decrease in FEF_{25-75}. However, the training program was not associated with any other changes in pulmonary function or ventilatory muscle endurance.

The results of these studies suggest that the CF patient may benefit from a variety of physical conditioning programs. Ventilatory muscle training may improve ventilatory muscle endurance, but the training is tedious. Aerobic exercise conditioning may likewise improve ventilatory muscle endurance, and has the additional benefits of increasing exercise tolerance and perhaps promoting mucus clearance. The increased ability to tolerate exercise and the exertion of everyday activities may in turn improve the patient's sense of well-being and overall quality of life. The effects of exercise training on pulmonary function are equivocal, and better controlled studies are needed to examine the potential benefits of long-term exercise training in maintaining pulmonary function, or perhaps, retarding disease progression.

EXERCISE PRESCRIPTION

The aerobic exercise conditioning program should be prescribed for each individual based on his or her exercise test results. The program should take into account the modality, intensity, duration, and frequency of exercise.

Modality

To promote an increase in exercise tolerance and cardiorespiratory fitness, endurance activities that involve rhythmic contraction of large-muscle groups, such as walking, jogging, cycling, or swimming, should be selected for training. As with any exercise treatment for any group of people, in order to promote compliance, the activity should be one that the patient enjoys.

Intensity

The intensity of exercise should take into consideration the peak exercise tolerance and any maladaptive responses occurring during the exercise test. In the absence of significant clinical signs or symptoms, the exercise intensity may be prescribed at a work level that elicits a heart rate of 70 to 85% of the patient's peak heart rate. Exercise in this heart rate range has been shown to be well-tolerated and effective in increasing cardiorespiratory fitness in CF patients (7).

In patients who demonstrate abnormal exercise responses, such as extreme oxygen desaturation, intolerable dyspnea, or ECG abnormalities, training intensity should be prescribed at a heart rate level at least 10 beats below which these responses occur. In these patients, exercise in a monitored setting under medical supervision may be advisable.

Duration

Initially, the conditioning or stimulus period of each exercise session should be at least 10 minutes. As the patient's functional capacity improves, the stimulus period can be increased gradually to 20 to 30 minutes. We have found an increase of 1 to 2 minutes each session per week is well-tolerated by most CF patients. If the weekly increase is perceived as excessive, it should be emphasized that there is no rush in reaching the goal of 20- to 30-minute sessions, since we are dealing with the establishment of a life-long exercise habit. The extra time should make little difference in reaching the ultimate goal, particularly at the expense of patient compliance. In some individuals with very low functional capacities, exercise may be carried out for shorter durations of 5 to 10 minutes two to three times per day, until longer durations can be tolerated.

Each exercise session should include a 5- to 10-minute warm-up period before, and a 5- to 10-minute cool-down period after the conditioning phase. The warm-up period should consist of stretching exercises to warm the skeletal muscles (38), and low-intensity aerobic exercise (walking or cycling, etc.) at approximately 50% of peak heart rate to increase the heart rate gradually from resting levels to near the target heart rate range (39). The cool-down should also include low-intensity walking to avoid venous pooling (40), and stretching to alleviate muscle tightness (41).

Frequency

In general, exercise sessions should be carried out three to five times per week to accomplish a conditioning response. More frequent training has not been shown to be beneficial in the normal population (42), and may increase the risk of a musculoskeletal injury, particularly with weight-bearing activities (43).

Special Considerations

Oxygen Supplementation

Exercise should be prescribed cautiously for persons who exhibit significant decreases in oxygen saturation during the exercise test. The exercise should be carried out under medical supervision at submaximal levels below which the significant decrease in oxyhemoglobin saturation occurred. An alternative may be to have the patient exercise while breathing supplemental oxygen. Supplemental oxygen has been shown to improve exercise tolerance and oxygenation in adult patients with chronic obstructive pulmonary disease (44, 45). In CF patients, it has been shown to reduce minute ventilation and heart rate during exercise (5). However, the effect of oxygen supplementation on oxygen saturation has not yet been examined in this population.

Exercise in the Heat

In spite of abnormally high concentrations of sodium and chloride in their sweat, CF patients exhibit normal thermoregulation during exercise (46). At work loads equivalent to 50% $\dot{V}O_2$ max in 100 °F, rectal temperatures, heart rates, and rise of serum renin and aldosterone levels of CF patients were shown not to differ significantly from those of normal control subjects; however, the CF patients lost more sodium and chloride in their sweat. The patients also significantly reduced their serum chloride concentration, while normal subjects maintained serum electrolyte balance.

Similar differences in acclimation were observed between CF patients and normal control subjects in response to 70 minutes of cycle exercise in the heat on 8 consecutive days (47). Rectal temperature and heart rate decreased similarly from day 1 to day 8 in both CF and control subjects. However, the sweat chloride concentration of the control group decreased significantly from day 1 to day 8, while that of the CF patients remained high and did not change with each exercise bout. The elevated chloride loss in sweat was again associated with decreased serum chloride concentration in the CF patients. In spite of the daily ion loss during exercise, the serum electrolyte concentrations of the CF patients returned to within normal limits by the start of the next day's exercise session. It should be noted that each exercise bout in the heat was relatively short, and any adverse effects of longer bouts of exercise in the heat have yet to be determined. With regard to the present findings, we encourage ample fluid intake and free use of the salt shaker.

CONCLUSION

Exercise testing provides useful information about the CF patient's exercise tolerance and cardiorespiratory adaptive responses to exercise that cannot be obtained from standard pulmonary function tests and clinical evaluations. It provides an objective method for following disease progression, as well as for assessing changes in exercise tolerance in response to treatment intervention. The results of the exercise test also serve as a basis for prescribing aerobic exercise training as part of the treatment regimen. The CF patient may benefit from aerobic exercise training with improvements in exercise tolerance and ventilatory muscle endurance, and perhaps facilitated mucus clearance. Pulmonary function may not improve, but pulmonary deterioration may be retarded with training. Further research is needed to examine fully the potential benefits of long-term exercise training on pulmonary function, disease progression, and mortality in the CF patient.

REFERENCES

1. Wood RE, Boat TF, Doershuk CF: State of the art: Cystic fibrosis. *Am Rev Respir Dis* 113:833–878, 1976.
2. Wood RE: Prognosis. In Taussig LM (ed): *Cystic Fibrosis*, New York, Thieme-Stratton Inc., 1984, p. 434.
3. Taussig LM, Landau LF, Marks MI: Respiratory system. In Taussig LM (ed): *Cystic Fibrosis*, New York, Thieme-Stratton Inc., 1984, p. 115.
4. Cropp GJ, Pullano TP, Cerny FS, et al.: Exercise tolerance and cardiorespiratory adjustments at peak work capacity in cystic fibrosis. *Am Rev Respir Dis* 126:211–216, 1982.
5. Coates, AL, Boyce P, Muller D, et al.: The role of nutritional status, airway obstruction, hypoxia, and abnormalities in serum lipid composition in limiting exercise tolerance in children with cystic fibrosis. *Acta Paediatr Scand* 69:353–358, 1980.
6. Godfrey S, Mearns M: Pulmonary function and response to exercise in cystic fibrosis. *Arch Dis Child* 46:144–151, 1971.
7. Orenstein DM, Franklin BA, Doershuk CF, et al.: Exercise conditioning and cardiopulmonary fitness in cystic fibrosis. *Chest* 80:392–398, 1981.
8. Cerny FJ, Pullano TP, Cropp GJA: Cardiorespiratory adaptations to exercise in cystic fibrosis. *Am Rev Respir Dis* 126:217–220, 1982.
9. Marcotte JE, Grisdale RK, Levison H, et al.: Multiple factors limit exercise capacity in cystic fibrosis. *Pediatr Pulmonol* 2:274–281, 1986.
10. Dantzker DR, Patten GA, Bower JA: Gas exchange at rest and during exercise in adults with cystic fibrosis. *Am Rev Respir Dis* 125:400–405, 1982.

11. Henke KG, Orenstein DM: Oxygen saturation during exercise in cystic fibrosis. *Am Rev Respir Dis* 129:708–711, 1984.
12. Canny GJ, de Souza ME, Gilday DC, et al.: Radionuclide assessment of cardiac performance in cystic fibrosis. *Am Rev Respir Dis* 130:822–826, 1984.
13. Benson LN, Newth CJD, de Souza M, et al.: Radionuclide assessment of right and left ventricular function during bicycle exercise in young patients with cystic fibrosis. *Am Rev Respir Dis* 130:987–992, 1984.
14. Chipps BD, Alderson PO, Roland JMA, et al.: Noninvasive evaluation of ventricular function in cystic fibrosis. *J Pediatr* 95:379–384, 1979.
15. American College of Sports Medicine: *Guidelines for Graded Exercise Testing and Exercise Prescription,* ed 3, Philadelphia, Lea & Febiger, 1985, p. 13.
16. Fox SM, Naughton JP, Haskell WL: Physical activity and the prevention of coronary heart disease. *Ann Clin Res* 3:404–432, 1971.
17. Wilmore JH, Sigerseth PO: Physical work capacity of young girls, 7-13 years of age. *J Appl Physiol* 22:923–928, 1967.
18. Godfrey S: *Exercise Testing in Children.* Philadelphia, W.B. Saunders Co., 1974, p. 66.
19. Knuttgen HG: Aerobic capacity of adolescents. *J Appl Physiol* 22:655–658, 1967.
20. James FW, Kaplan S, Glueck CJ, et al.: Responses of normal children and young adults to controlled bicycle exercise. *Circulation* 61:902–911, 1980.
21. Balke B, Ware RW: An experimental study of physical fitness of air force personnel. *U.S. Armed Forces Med J* 10:675–688, 1959.
22. Cavagna GA, Saibene FP, Margaria R: External work in walking. *J Appl Physiol* 18:1–9, 1963.
23. Sjostrand T: Functional capacity and exercise tolerance in patients with impaired cardiovascular function. In Gordon BL (ed): *Clinical Cardiopulmonary Physiology,* New York, Grune & Stratton Inc., 1960, p. 201.
24. Davies C, Barnes C, Godfrey S: Body composition and maximal exercise performance in children. *Hum Biol* 44:195–214, 1972.
25. Issekutz R Jr., Birkhead NC, Rodahl K: The use of respiratory quotients in assessment of aerobic work capacity. *J Appl Physiol* 17:47–50, 1962.
26. Mitchell JH, Sproule BJ, Chapman CB: The physiological meaning of the maximal oxygen intake test. *J Clin Invest* 37:538–547, 1958.
27. Raab W: Metabolic protection and reconditioning of the heart muscle through habitual physical exercise. *Ann Intern Med* 53:87–105, 1960.
28. Borg G: Perceived exertion as an indicator of somatic stress. *Scand J Rehabil Med* 2:92–98, 1970.
29. Hjeltnes N, Stanghelle JK, Skyberg D: Pulmonary function and oxygen uptake during exercise in 16 year old boys with cystic fibrosis. *Acta Paediatr Scand* 73:548–553, 1984.
30. Orenstein DM, Henke KG, Cerny FJ: Exercise and cystic fibrosis. *Phys Sportsmed* 11:57–62, 1983.
31. Keens TG, Krastins JRB, Wannamaker EM, et al.: Ventilatory muscle endurance training in normal subjects and patients with cystic fibrosis. *Am Rev Respir Dis* 116:853–860, 1977.
32. Asher MI, Pardy RL, Coates AL, et al.: The effects of inspiratory muscle training in patients with cystic fibrosis. *Am Rev Respir Dis* 126:855–859, 1982.
33. Edlund LD, French RW, Herbst JJ, et al.: Effects of a swimming program on children with cystic fibrosis. *Am J Dis Child* 140:80–83, 1986.
34. Zach M, Oberwaldner B, Hausler F: Cystic fibrosis: Physical exercise versus chest physiotherapy. *Arch Dis Child* 57:587–589, 1982.
35. Zach MS, Purrer B, Oberwaldner B: Effect of swimming on forced expiration and sputum clearance in cystic fibrosis. *Lancet* 2:1201–1203, 1981.
36. Cerny F, Cropp GJA: Effects of regular prescribed home exercise with no chest physical therapy on lung function in patients with cystic fibrosis. (Abst) Proceedings of Cystic Fibrosis Club, Anaheim, Cystic Fibrosis Foundation, 1985.
37. Keens TG, Stabile MW, Gold C-I, et al.: Variable weight training reduces hyperinflation and increases body weight in cystic fibrosis. *Am Rev Respir Dis* 131:A239, 1985.
38. Asmussen E, Boje O: Body temperature and capacity for work. *Acta Physiol Scand* 10:1–22, 1945.
39. Barnard RJ, Gardner GW, Diaco NV, et al.: Cardiovascular responses to sudden strenuous exercise—heart rate, blood pressure, and ECG. *J Appl Physiol* 34:833–837, 1973.
40. Astrand PO, Rodahl K: Physiological bases of exercise. In: *Textbook of Work Physiology,* ed 2. New York, McGraw-Hill, 1977, p. 168.
41. deVries, HA: *Physiology of Exercise,* ed 4. Dubuque, Wm C Brown Co, 1977, p. 303.
42. Gettman LR, Pollock ML, Durstine JL, et al.: Physiological responses of men to 1, 3, and 5 day per week training programs. *Res Q* 47:638–646, 1976.
43. Pollock ML, Gettman LR, Milesis CA, et al.: Effect of frequency and duration of training on attrition and incidence of injury. *Med Sci Sports* 9:31–36, 1977.
44. Bradley BL, Garner A, Billiu D, et al.: Oxygen-assisted exercise in chronic obstructive lung disease. *Am Rev Respir Dis* 118:239–243, 1978.
45. Bye BTP, Esau SA, Levy RD, et al.: Ventilatory muscle function during exercise in air and oxygen in patients with chronic airflow limitation. *Am Rev Respir Dis* 132:236–240, 1985.
46. Orenstein DM, Henke KG, Costill DL, et al.: Exercise and heat stress in cystic fibrosis patients. *Pediatr Res* 17:267–269, 1983.
47. Orenstein DM, Henke KG, Green CG: Heat acclimation in cystic fibrosis. *J Appl Physiol* 57:408–412, 1984.

CHAPTER 12

Healthy Elderly Patients

Herbert A. deVries, Ph.D.

Exercise testing and prescription for individuals with various disease states are well-covered in the other chapters of this book. This review highlights the special requirements of the healthy elderly individual (age 60 and over). Furthermore, emphasis is directed primarily to the fundamentals of exercise prescription. Other excellent texts are available detailing the principles of cardiovascular diagnosis through exercise testing.

As little as 20 years ago, the trainability of the older organism was still in doubt. However, in the past two decades, increasing experimental evidence has accumulated to show that healthy, older individuals improve their functional capacity through physical conditioning programs (1–6). In percentage terms, their improvement is comparable to that in the young, although they start at and progress to lower achievement levels and usually require a lower training stimulus to bring about the desired response. Available evidence also suggests that certain health benefits accompany the improvement in function. In general, the effects of physical conditioning upon older people are opposite to those commonly associated with the aging process.

EXERCISE TESTING

One of the major problems in the exercise testing of the elderly lies in the fact that a large proportion of older people simply do not have the muscular capacity to fully load the cardiorespiratory system. This seems to be especially true when exercise testing is accomplished on the cycle ergometer. For this reason, the commonly used and widely accepted measurement of aerobic power ($\dot{V}O_2max$) as a criterion of physical working capacity (PWC) is not feasible for many sedentary, deconditioned older individuals. Therefore, exercise testing will be discussed at two levels: 1) maximal testing ($\dot{V}O_2max$) for the relatively fit elderly, and 2) submaximal estimation of PWC for the long-term sedentary elderly who cannot satisfactorily perform a maximal test.

Measurement of PWC ($\dot{V}O_2max$)

Preliminary Medical Examination

It is essential that every individual over 60 be examined and have the approval of a physician before entering a physical conditioning program. Guidelines for the conduct of a history and physical examination for this purpose have been established by the American College of Sports Medicine (7). Since measurement of $\dot{V}O_2max$ requires the subject to work to his aerobic capacity and somewhat beyond, the availability of a physician is required during testing, and emergency equipment, including a defibrillator, oxygen, and appropriate drugs, must be organized and readily available.

In a pilot study in the author's laboratory, 31 asymptomatic men (mean age 69 years) who had medical clearance, including a normal 12-lead resting ECG, were tested to define $\dot{V}O_2max$. Of the 31, 14 had premature ventricular contractions (PVCs); in nine instances the tests were prematurely terminated—five due to multifocal PVCs, two because of ischemic ST-segment depression over 0.3 mV, and one due to severe angina. One subject developed ventricular tachycardia, which reverted to normal rhythm upon cessation of exercise (8).

Exercise Modality

Both the cycle ergometer and the treadmill are widely used in exercise testing, and each has its advantages and disadvantages. The treadmill uses a skill with which everyone is familiar (walking or running), and it elicits a slightly better involvement of large-muscle masses than the cycle ergometer since the muscles of the upper body become involved. However, it has three major disadvantages. First, the subject's movement during exercise makes it difficult to record electrocardiographic and blood pressure data. Second, the units of achieved work and power must be expressed in an arbitrary fashion—as running at 7 mi·h^{-1} on a 10% incline—because much of the work is done in a horizontal direction and this does not allow evaluation in standard units of kilogram-meters of work or watts of power. Most importantly, for this age group, an accidental fall, although unlikely, can occur; and the potential anxiety in some subjects regarding this possibility may adversely affect the results.

The cycle ergometer has several advantages. First, it is comparatively inexpensive. Second, the subject's upper body is relatively motionless, facilitating the measurement of quality ECG recordings, blood pressure determinations, and metabolic gas analysis. Third, the exercise load is expressed in standard units of work or power and, perhaps most importantly, there is no potential hazard of accidental falls. The major disadvantage lies in the fact that for persons unaccustomed to bicycle riding, local muscle fatigue may preclude fully loading the cardiovascular system to produce a valid $\dot{V}O_2$max.

Exercise Protocol

For the clinical situation the "continuous step incremental loading" protocol, which can be applied to either the cycle ergometer or the treadmill, is recommended as the simplest and least time-consuming method of testing. This procedure is typified on the cycle ergometer by the Luft protocol in which the power output required for the first 3 minutes is 50 watts (W). Each minute thereafter, the load is increased by 12.5 W (approximately 75 kg·m·min^{-1}) until the subject is unable to continue. The protocol can generally be completed in less than 20 min, and may be modified to use step increments such as 10 W·min^{-1}, 20 W·2 min^{-1}, 25 W·2 min^{-1} or 30 W·3 min^{-1} without substantial differences in result.

The Balke treadmill protocol is commonly used in testing elderly persons and requires the subject to walk at 3.3 mi·h^{-1} for the first 2 minutes on the horizontal. Every minute thereafter the incline is increased by 1% until volitional fatigue.

Parameters To Be Measured

Ideally the following primary parameters, from which many secondary data can be derived, should be recorded at each exercise load:

A. Primary data
  1. % O_2 in expired gas
  2. % CO_2 in expired gas
  3. Minute ventilation ($\dot{V}_E$)

  (items 1–3) —For calculation of $\dot{V}O_2$ max

  4. Heart rate (HR)
  5. Systolic and diastolic blood pressure (BP), i.e., SBP/DBP
  6. ECG—lead CM_5 if only one-lead can be taken

B. Derived data
  1. R = $\dot{V}CO_2/\dot{V}O_2$
  2. O_2 pulse = $\dot{V}O_2$ per heart beat
  3. Double product = [(HR × SBP)/100]
  4. Ventilatory equivalent for O_2 = $\dot{V}_E/\dot{V}O_2$
  5. Lactate threshold

Of the derived data, the respiratory exchange ratio (R) is often employed to define the point when anaerobic metabolism becomes prominent. As such, it is also useful as one criterion that $\dot{V}O_2$max has indeed been achieved. Various authorities use different criteria, but until $R > 1.05$, it is unlikely that a true $\dot{V}O_2$max had been attained.

O_2 pulse directly reflects the stroke volume and/or arteriovenous O_2 difference responses.

The double product or rate-pressure product, defined as the heart rate (HR) times systolic blood pressure (SBP) [(HR × SBP)/100], has been found to be well correlated ($r = 0.92$) with myocardial O_2 consumption and, therefore, reflects the work of the heart at each exercise level. The ventilatory equivalent for O_2 defines how many liters of lung ventilation are required for 1 liter of O_2 uptake by the tissues. Thus, this is an important reflection of the efficiency of O_2 transport mechanisms.

Lactate threshold, or its noninvasive analogue, ventilatory threshold, appears to be a very important determinant of the level of endurance performance that can be sustained.

Indications for Terminating an Exercise Test

Criteria for terminating an exercise test include: 1) anginal symptoms, 2) > 2 mm horizontal or downsloping ST-segment depression or elevation, 3) sustained supraventricular tachycardia, 4) ventricular tachycardia, 5) fall in systolic blood pressure with increase in exercise load, 6) dizziness or signs of peripheral circulatory insufficiency, 7) excessive blood pressure rise (SBP >250 mm Hg, DBP >120 mm Hg), 8) onset of second- or third-degree heart block, and 9) volitional fatigue (i.e., subject requests to stop).

Estimation of PWC from Submaximal Tests

Many tests have been devised for estimation of PWC (or $\dot{V}O_2max$) from submaximal data. In general, use of submaximal tests represents a trade-off of the precision of maximal testing in favor of increased safety and decreased demands upon both subject and laboratory. The loss of precision in evaluation of the subject with respect to his peers may be considerable, and, for this reason, submaximal tests have been justly criticized. However, for purposes of evaluating a training effect within one individual over a period of time, the error is no greater than that in the actual measurement of $\dot{V}O_2max$ (9). In the interest of space limitations, only three submaximal test procedures will be presented here. The first two tests, O_2 pulse at a specified submaximal heart rate and the Åstrand-Ryhming nomogram, have proven very satisfactory in our laboratory for use with the elderly (2); the third, PWC_{FT}, was developed by the author and his colleagues (10) specifically for testing unfit elderly subjects.

O_2 Pulse

It was shown more than two decades ago that for any level of submaximal exercise the individual with the highest oxygen (O_2) pulse is the most fit (11). More recent studies have confirmed this finding, reporting rank-order correlations of 0.854 (cycle ergometer) and 0.873 (treadmill) between submaximal O_2 pulse and measured $\dot{V}O_2max$ (12). Furthermore, this parameter was found to be a better predictor of $\dot{V}O_2max$ than either submaximal oxygen consumption or heart rate.

Two groups of investigators have demonstrated the feasibility and sensitivity of the O_2 pulse to assess exercise training effects in older individuals. The author reported a 29% improvement in O_2 pulse at a heart rate of 145 beats·min^{-1} among elderly men (mean age 69.5) who underwent aerobic conditioning for 42 weeks (2). A subgroup that underwent low-intensity exercise training (i.e., walking alone) showed a 14% improvement in O_2 pulse at a heart rate of 120 beats·min^{-1}. A more recent exercise training study among retirees also reported a 14.7% increase in O_2 pulse at a heart rate of 125 beats·min^{-1} (1). Thus, if metabolic instrumentation is available, O_2 pulse at submaximal workloads that elicit a heart rate of 120 beats·min^{-1} appears to be the method of choice. It should be emphasized that this method requires working the average 70-year-old to only approximately 60-70% of his or her capacity. Moreover, the exercise protocols previously described for measurement of $\dot{V}O_2max$ may be used.

The Åstrand-Ryhming Nomogram

Åstrand and Ryhming (13) reported that heart rate responses for healthy male and female subjects averaged 128 and 138 beats·min^{-1} after 6 minutes of work at a load that required 50% of the $\dot{V}O_2max$. When their subjects exercised at a greater workload, demanding an oxygen consumption equal to 70% of their aerobic capacity, the mean heart rate was 154 for men and 164 for women; however, the standard deviation was considerable, eight to nine beats·min^{-1}.

Åstrand and Ryhming used these data to develop nomograms (see Tables 12.1 and 12.2) to predict maximal oxygen uptake from the heart rate response to one 6-minute submaximal workload. The accuracy of prediction varied with the level of the workload selected. For example, on the cycle ergometer at 900 kg·m·min^{-1}, the standard error of prediction for men was ± 10.4%, and at 1200 kg·m·min^{-1} it was ± 6.7%. The author found a correlation of 0.74 between predicted maximal oxygen uptake by the Åstrand-Ryhming method and $\dot{V}O_2$max as measured directly in his laboratory. These data yielded an error of prediction of ± 9.3%, in agreement with the aforementioned figures.

For the elderly a correction factor must be applied to the data in Tables 12.1 and 12.2 (14). The estimated $\dot{V}O_2$max data provided for young men and women must be multiplied by 0.70 for persons aged 60 and above. Norms for maximal oxygen con-

Table 12.1
Calculation of Maximal Oxygen Uptake from Pulse Rate and Exercise Load on a Cycle Ergometer (Men) [a]

Working Pulse	Maximal Oxygen Uptake (l·min^{-1})					Working Pulse	Maximal Oxygen Uptake (l·min^{-1})				
	300	600	900	1200	1500		300	600	900	1200	1500
	kg·m·min^{-1}						kg·m·min^{-1}				
120	2.2	3.5	4.8			148		2.4	3.2	4.3	5.4
121	2.2	3.4	4.7			149		2.3	3.2	4.3	5.4
122	2.2	3.4	4.6			150		2.3	3.2	4.2	5.3
123	2.1	3.4	4.6			151		2.3	3.1	4.2	5.2
124	2.1	3.3	4.5	6.0		152		2.3	3.1	4.1	5.2
125	2.0	3.2	4.4	5.9		153		2.2	3.0	4.1	5.1
126	2.0	3.2	4.4	5.8		154		2.2	3.0	4.0	5.1
127	2.0	3.1	4.3	5.7		155		2.2	3.0	4.0	5.0
128	2.0	3.1	4.2	5.6		156		2.2	2.9	4.0	5.0
129	1.9	3.0	4.2	5.6		157		2.1	2.9	3.9	4.9
130	1.9	3.0	4.1	5.5		158		2.1	2.9	3.9	4.9
131	1.9	2.9	4.0	5.4		159		2.1	2.8	3.8	4.8
132	1.8	2.9	4.0	5.3		160		2.1	2.8	3.8	4.8
133	1.8	2.8	3.9	5.3		161		2.0	2.8	3.7	4.7
134	1.8	2.8	3.9	5.2		162		2.0	2.8	3.7	4.6
135	1.7	2.8	3.8	5.1		163		2.0	2.8	3.7	4.6
136	1.7	2.7	3.8	5.0		164		2.0	2.7	3.6	4.5
137	1.7	2.7	3.7	5.0		165		2.0	2.7	3.6	4.5
138	1.6	2.7	3.7	4.9		166		1.9	2.7	3.6	4.5
139	1.6	2.6	3.6	4.8		167		1.9	2.6	3.5	4.4
140	1.6	2.6	3.6	4.8	6.0	168		1.9	2.6	3.5	4.4
141		2.6	3.5	4.7	5.9	169		1.9	2.6	3.5	4.3
142		2.5	3.5	4.6	5.8	170		1.8	2.6	3.4	4.3
143		2.5	3.4	4.6	5.7						
144		2.5	3.4	4.5	5.7						
145		2.4	3.4	4.5	5.6						
146		2.4	3.3	4.4	5.6						
147		2.4	3.3	4.4	5.5						

[a] **Modified from Åstrand I: *Acta Physiol Scand* 49 (Suppl 169), 1960 by P-O. Åstrand in *Work Test with the Bicycle Ergometer.* Varberg, Sweden: Monark, 1965.**

Table 12.2
Calculation of Maximal Oxygen Uptake from Pulse Rate and Exercise Load on a Cycle Ergometer (Women) [a]

Working Pulse	Maximal Oxygen Uptake ($l \cdot min^{-1}$)					Working Pulse	Maximal Oxygen Uptake ($l \cdot min^{-1}$)				
	300	450	600	750	900		300	450	600	750	900
	$kg \cdot m \cdot min^{-1}$						$kg \cdot m \cdot min^{-1}$				
120	2.6	3.4	4.1	4.8		148	1.6	2.1	2.6	3.1	3.6
121	2.5	3.3	4.0	4.8		149		2.1	2.6	3.0	3.5
122	2.5	3.2	3.9	4.7		150		2.0	2.5	3.0	3.5
123	2.4	3.1	3.9	4.6		151		2.0	2.5	3.0	3.4
124	2.4	3.1	3.8	4.5		152		2.0	2.5	2.9	3.4
125	2.3	3.0	3.7	4.4		153		2.0	2.4	2.9	3.3
126	2.3	3.0	3.6	4.3		154		2.0	2.4	2.8	3.3
127	2.2	2.9	3.5	4.2		155		1.9	2.4	2.8	3.2
128	2.2	2.8	3.5	4.2	4.8	156		1.9	2.3	2.8	3.2
129	2.2	2.8	3.4	4.1	4.8	157		1.9	2.3	2.7	3.2
130	2.1	2.7	3.4	4.0	4.7	158		1.8	2.3	2.7	3.1
131	2.1	2.7	3.4	4.0	4.6	159		1.8	2.2	2.7	3.1
132	2.0	2.7	3.3	3.9	4.5	160		1.8	2.2	2.6	3.0
133	2.0	2.6	3.2	3.8	4.4	161		1.8	2.2	2.6	3.0
134	2.0	2.6	3.2	3.8	4.4	162		1.8	2.2	2.6	3.0
135	2.0	2.6	3.1	3.7	4.3	163		1.7	2.2	2.6	2.9
136	1.9	2.5	3.1	3.6	4.2	164		1.7	2.1	2.5	2.9
137	1.9	2.5	3.0	3.6	4.2	165		1.7	2.1	2.5	2.9
138	1.8	2.4	3.0	3.5	4.1	166		1.7	2.1	2.5	2.8
139	1.8	2.4	2.9	3.5	4.0	167		1.6	2.1	2.4	2.8
140	1.8	2.4	2.8	3.4	4.0	168		1.6	2.0	2.4	2.8
141	1.8	2.3	2.8	3.4	3.9	169		1.6	2.0	2.4	2.8
142	1.7	2.3	2.8	3.3	3.9	170		1.6	2.0	2.4	2.7
143	1.7	2.2	2.7	3.3	3.8						
144	1.7	2.2	2.7	3.2	3.8						
145	1.6	2.2	2.7	3.2	3.7						
146	1.6	2.2	2.6	3.2	3.7						
147	1.6	2.1	2.6	3.1	3.6						

[a] **Modified from Åstrand, I:** ***Acta Physiol Scand*** **49 (Suppl 169), 1960 by P-O. Åstrand in** ***Work Test with the Bicycle Ergometer.*** **Varberg, Sweden: Monark, 1965.**

sumption, expressed as $l \cdot min^{-1}$ or $ml \cdot kg^{-1} \cdot min^{-1}$, are provided in Table 12.3.

PWC_{FT} Estimation of PWC at Onset of Muscle Fatigue Instead of at Total Exhaustion—A Method Designed for Elderly or Unfit Populations

The PWC_{FT} test is an objective noninvasive test of physical working capacity, which has been shown to be valid and highly reproducible. Its salient advantage lies in requiring only a submaximal effort to an objectively determined criterion consisting of the onset of muscular fatigue as measured by a noninvasive electromyographic (EMG) technique. Thus, the method is ideally suited to evaluate PWC and to monitor progress in physical conditioning programs for geriatric populations. The authors' data also suggest that the identification of PWC_{FT} is not seriously influenced by differences in the protocol leading to the fatigue threshold.

Figure 12.1 illustrates the method used to individually establish the rate of work at which the fatigue threshold or PWC_{FT} oc-

Table 12.3
Norms for Absolute ($l \cdot min^{-1}$) and Relative Maximal O_2 Consumption[a]

Women

Age	Low	Fair	Average	Good	High
20–29	1.69	1.70–1.99	2.00–2.49	2.50–2.79	2.80+
	28	29–34	35–43	44–48	49+
30–39	1.59	1.60–1.89	1.90–2.39	2.40–2.69	2.70+
	27	28–33	34–41	42–47	48+
40–49	1.49	1.50–1.79	1.80–2.29	2.30–2.59	2.60+
	25	26–31	32–40	41–45	46+
50–65	1.29	1.30–1.59	1.60–2.09	2.10–2.39	2.40+
	21	22–28	29–36	37–41	42+

Men

Age	Low	Fair	Average	Good	High
20–29	2.79	2.80–3.09	3.10–3.69	3.70–3.99	4.00+
	38	39–43	44–51	52–56	57+
30–39	2.49	2.50–2.79	2.80–3.39	3.40–3.69	3.70+
	34	35–39	40–47	48–51	52+
40–49	2.19	2.20–2.49	2.50–3.09	3.10–3.39	3.40+
	30	31–35	36–43	44–47	48+
50–59	1.89	1.90–2.19	2.20–2.79	2.80–3.09	3.10+
	25	26–31	32–39	40–43	44+
60–69	1.59	1.60–1.89	1.90–2.49	2.50–2.79	2.80+
	21	22–26	27–35	36–39	40+

[a] Lower figure = $ml \cdot kg^{-1} \cdot min^{-1}$. From Åstrand I: *Acta Physiol Scand* 49 (Suppl. 169), 1960.

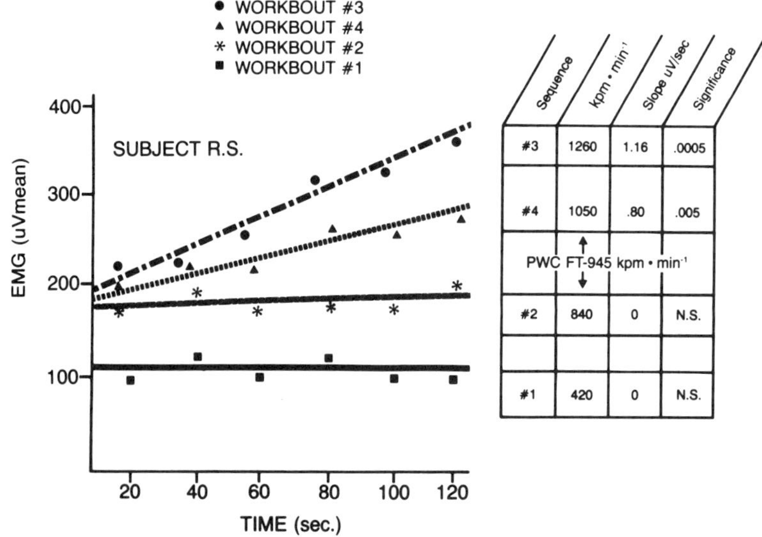

Figure 12.1. Illustration of the PWC_{FT} method and protocol.

curs. Discontinuous work bouts on the cycle ergometer are employed. For subject R.S., the first work bout of 420 kpm·min^{-1} produced a relatively constant electrical output from the quadriceps muscle of about 110 μV with zero slope. After a rest period sufficient to return the heart rate to within 10 beats·min^{-1} of its previous resting value, the second bout at 840 kpm·min^{-1} resulted in a constant electrical output of about 180 μV, also with zero slope. However, the third work bout at 1260 kpm·min^{-1} required an ever-increasing level of electrical activation for its maintenance (slope of 1.16 μV·sec^{-1}, which is significantly different from zero at $P < .0005$, and thus indicates the occurrence of neuromuscular fatigue). Therefore, the fatigue threshold occurred between 840 and 1260 kpm·min^{-1}.

To increase the precision for estimation of PWC_{FT}, the subsequent work bout was determined by selecting the midpoint (1050 kpm·min^{-1}) between the highest nonsignificant work load (840 kpm·min^{-1}) and the first (lowest) significant work load (1260 kpm·min^{-1}). Figure 12.1 carries this procedure only through one interpolation in the interest of clarity of exposition, but two interpolations are typical and, on rare occasions, a third. The fourth work bout (Fig. 12.1) was set at 1050 kpm·min^{-1}, $(840 + 1260)/2 = 1050$, resulting in a slope of 0.80 μV·sec^{-1}, which was still significantly different from zero at $p < .005$. A second interpolation (not shown) was then made at 945 kpm·min^{-1}, $(840 + 1050)/2$, with a resulting slope of 0.61 μV·sec^{-1}, which was still significantly different from zero at $P < .01$. Therefore, we may estimate the PWC_{FT} as $(840 + 945)/2$, or 892.5 kpm·min^{-1}, with a probable error of no more than ± 6%.

Relatively inexpensive EMG instrumentation has been developed for administering this test (National Medical Sales, 23881 Via Fabricante, #512, Mission Viejo, CA 92691), and the method correlates ($r = 0.84$) with other physiological measurements of PWC (Lactate threshold, HR − work load relationship, and percent of HR range utilized at PWC_{FT}). Its reproducibility in test-retests 1 week apart was $r = 0.95$ (10).

To summarize this section, the author considers submaximal testing to be the most satisfactory for the older population for reasons of : (a) increased safety, (b) greater simplicity, (c) decreased time and expense for both laboratory and subject, and (d) the reduced demand upon the subject.

It should also be noted that the most commonly accepted approach to the measurement of PWC, that is, the measurement of aerobic capacity itself, has several serious limitations. Although this measure, $\dot{V}O_2max$, has become recognized as the criterion against which all other PWC test procedures are evaluated, it can be criticized on at least four grounds: (a) the subject must be taken to a state of exhaustion, (b) the results of the test may vary considerably with test method and protocol, (c) the data are expressed in physiologic terms while the physician or technician deals with the physical parameters of work and power, and (d) the test requires sophisticated laboratory equipment, trained staff, and considerable testing time.

$\dot{V}O_2max$ tests would be the methods of choice for the elderly athlete, and can be justified for evaluation of highly-trained persons in Masters competitions, Senior Olympics, or marathon running. Such competitive individuals find the test challenging and are at low risk because of their training history.

For the untrained sedentary older individual, the simplest procedure is the Åstrand test. In a laboratory appropriately instrumented, both the O_2 pulse test and the new PWC_{FT} method provide more comprehensive physiologic data with no greater demands upon the individual's reserve capacity.

EXERCISE PRESCRIPTION

Principles Involved in Scientific Prescription of Exercise

The following aspects of a proposed exercise program must be considered and, where possible, defined on the basis of scientifically derived data.

Objective of the Exercise Program

There is good evidence that we can elicit desirable adaptations in human functional capacities and health-related parameters such as (a) muscular strength, (b) muscular endurance, (c) cardiorespiratory endurance, (d) muscular efficiency, (e) speed of movement, and (f) flexibility. However, each of these physical attributes requires a different and specific exercise program.

Exercise Modality

For strength gains one would recommend progressive resistance exercise, whereas for enhancement of cardiorespiratory function, one would prescribe one of many endurance-type exercise programs, such as walking or jogging.

Exercise Intensity

Here we are concerned with the dose-response relationship, or the level of exercise (e.g., power output) that is required to bring about favorable adaptation and improvement in the human organism.

Exercise Duration

How long must the exercise be continued to elicit the desired result? Is more always better, or is there a practical limit or desirable duration that optimizes the gain for time spent?

Exercise Frequency

How many times a week should one workout for optimal training effects?

Intensity Threshold for Training Effect

Is there a minimal exercise training intensity below which no training adaptations occur?

Rate of Training Adaptation as a Function of Pretraining Fitness Level

Do all individuals progress at the same rate in a conditioning program, or is progress dictated by the level of fitness at entry into the program?

Objective of the Exercise Program

Our discussion in this section will emphasize the development of cardiorespiratory fitness. However, strength and flexibility are also important to normal function in the elderly, and these fitness components will be described in the design of the "cool-down" phase of the daily workout. We can consider cardiorespiratory fitness of three-fold importance to optimal health status because the type of exercise program (endurance exercise) used for its development also contributes significantly to weight control and to relief from neuromuscular tension. Thus, we achieve three important health benefits for the price of one workout.

Exercise Modality

It should be recognized that many different exercise modalities (types of exercise) can be used to enhance cardiorespiratory fitness. The chosen exercise modality should:

1. involve a large proportion of total muscle mass.
2. maximize the use of large muscles.
3. minimize the use of small muscles.
4. maximize dynamic muscle contraction.
5. minimize static muscle contraction.
6. be rhythmic, allowing relaxation phases alternating with contraction phases.
7. minimize the work of the heart per unit training effect.
8. be quantifiable with respect to intensity.

The types of exercise commonly used among healthy elderly individuals include jogging, walking, swimming, and cycling. Many other activities of an endurance nature can be used. Recent evidence shows that singles tennis (15) and vigorous rowing (16) can also provide an aerobic training effect. Even dancing, when developed as an aerobic endurance exercise through control of rhythm and cadence, can elicit a $\dot{V}O_2$ as high as 40 $ml \cdot kg^{-1} \cdot min^{-1}$ (17). Among the modalities commonly used—jogging, walking, swimming, and cycling—there is probably little difference in training effect if equal levels of total work are achieved (18—20). The inclusion of walking may be surprising, but Pollock and associates (18) found large and very significant improvement in $\dot{V}O_2$max in healthy, middle-aged, sedentary men from walking. This corroborates the author's earlier work (2) with the elderly, and more recent work also supports this notion (4).

Of the eight criteria listed above for choice

of exercise modality, seven relate to the importance of getting the most exercise for the least cardiac work. The author (21) has provided data that show clearly the differing effects of walking, cycling, and a crawling type of exercise on the relationship between myocardial and total body work in older men (mean age 69). At all levels of total body work, crawling required greater cardiac demands than cycling, and the work of the heart rose with increasing total work more rapidly in both crawling and cycling than in walking. Obviously, when working with sedentary, middle-aged, and older people, it is desirable to minimize the ratio of cardiac effort to total body effort to achieve maximum conditioning at minimum risk. The most important determinants of cardiac work are the heart rate and systolic blood pressure. The latter is moderately elevated when large muscles are used rhythmically in dynamic contractions (22). In contrast, systolic blood pressure is disproportionately increased when small muscles are used at high fractions of their capacity or when muscles are held in static contraction. Thus, the previously described crawling exercise imposed considerable cardiac demands because it relies heavily on the small muscles in the shoulder girdle and upper limbs; moreover, it involves static contractions of the trunk muscles to maintain the crawling posture. Cycling also caused greater blood pressure changes than walking because, as we showed by EMG techniques (22), there is considerable static contraction in the upper limb muscles. Similarly, recent studies in young men showed greater blood pressure responses to the cycle ergometer than to the treadmill at equal, heavy exercise loads (23).

We may conclude that for all but the highly trained elderly, walking is the conditioning method of choice. We shall also consider the needs of the better conditioned elderly, for whom jogging is one of the more attractive choices of exercise modality.

Duration

The dose-response data for the elderly presently available do not yet allow a precise graphic presentation of the relationship between exercise duration and per cent improvement in $\dot{V}O_2max$, but Figure 12.2 shows the author's conceptualization based on a review of the literature on middle-aged men with particular reference to the work of Hartung and associates (24) and of Pollock (25), both of whose data points are shown. In general, it appears that a minimum duration of 15 minutes is required at an optimal training intensity before significant physiologic adaptation and improvement are brought about (24). However, best results probably require 30 to 60 minutes (25).

It should be emphasized, however, that with previously sedentary or deconditioned elderly subjects, one may not initially achieve even the minimum 15-minute duration of continuous exercise. Consequently, progression to even that duration may be required.

There is also some reason to believe that there is an interaction between exercise intensity and duration. Pollock (25) has shown that for middle-aged men (40 to 57), walking for 40 minutes per day, 4 days a week, produced a training effect equal to that obtained from jogging 30 minutes a day, 3 days a week, when the weekly energy cost of the two programs was equal. We have seen similar results in our work with older men (2).

In a well-controlled walk-jog study of prison inmates, Pollock and associates (26) showed that the injury rate was more than double in inmates who trained for 45 minutes as compared with those who trained for 30 minutes (54% and 24%, respectively). The injuries were largely shin splints and knee problems. In our experience the incidence of shin splints can be reduced and virtually eliminated by use of static stretching (discussed below). In any event, the data suggest that to hold injury rates to a minimum, the duration should be limited to 30 minutes or less for beginning joggers. As aerobic capacity and general fitness improve, duration can be increased.

Although this chapter is directed to cardiorespiratory fitness, note that the endurance exercise prescribed here is also one of the best means of weight control, and of course, all other things being equal, the

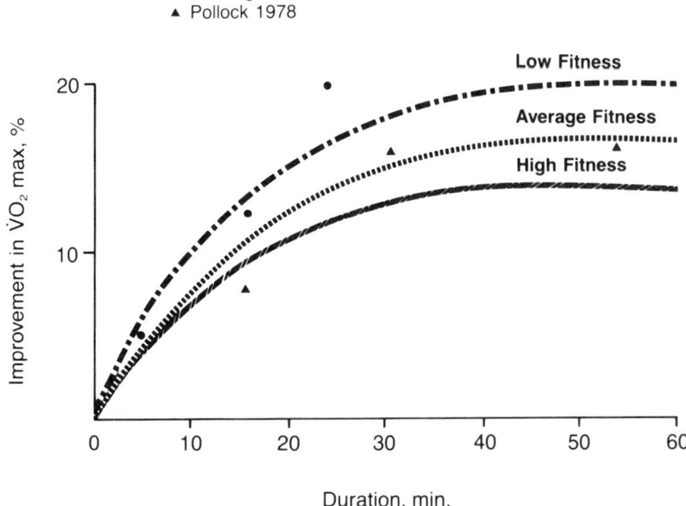

Figure 12.2. Hypothetical relationship between per cent improvement in $\dot{V}O_2$max and the duration of exercise training and baseline fitness. (Curves based on data of Hartung GH, Smolensky MH, Harrist RB, et al.: Effects of varied durations of training on improvement in cardiorespiratory endurance. *J Human Ergol* 6:61–68, 1977 (●), and Pollock, ML: How much exercise is enough? *Phys Sports med* 6:50–64, 1978 (▲); Hartung data at intensity of 65% (HRR), Pollock data at intensity of 85%–90% HRR.) Relative improvement in $\dot{V}O_2$max is inversely related to the baseline fitness level, i.e., at a given exercise intensity and duration, highly fit subjects demonstrate the lowest percentage improvement in $\dot{V}O_2$max.

caloric expenditure is directly proportional to the duration.

Frequency

Figure 12.3 shows the dose-response curve for exercise frequency and corresponding improvement in $\dot{V}O_2$max as conceptualized from selected training studies on young and middle-aged adults (20, 27–29). In general, the available data suggest little if any improvement from one workout per week. Improvement in $\dot{V}O_2$max accelerates rapidly when workouts are increased to four or five per week, with a levelling off thereafter. Moreover, high frequency training regimens (i.e., exercising six or seven times per week) are associated with a disproportionate incidence of injury (26).

It appears that optimal physiologic improvement occurs with three to five workouts per week. What effect does the spacing of the workouts have? There appears to be no difference in training effect in young men when the exercise program is conducted on Monday, Tuesday, and Wednesday as compared with Monday, Wednesday, and Friday. Furthermore, a conditioning effect once accomplished can be maintained with as little as two exercise sessions per week if intensity and duration are maintained (30). It is likely these findings apply to the elderly as well.

For the novice jogger the injury rate is three times greater for five workouts per week than it is for three workouts per week (26). But there are significant advantages in longer and more frequent workouts for weight reduction. Thus, on the basis of available evidence it would seem prudent to initially prescribe no more than three workouts of 30 minutes' duration per week of walking or jogging; subsequently, the

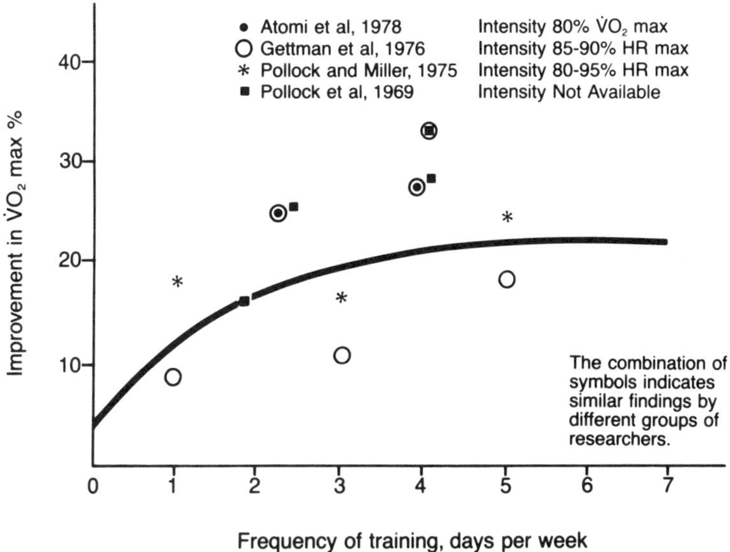

Figure12.3. Relationship of per cent improvement in $\dot{V}O_2$max to frequency of workout (Curves based on data from references as in Fig. 12.2.)

dosage could be increased, if desired, for weight reduction purposes to five workouts of 45 to 60 minutes each. As the exercise sessions become longer and more frequent, intensity would need to be reduced commensurately to prevent overtraining (staleness).

Intensity

Now that we have considered the questions regarding choice of exercise type and the desirable duration and frequency of workout, the most important question remains—that of intensity, which is the greatest single determinant of physiologic response and, therefore, of greatest concern for safety in exercise prescription for the elderly.

Nomenclature

First we need to clarify terminology on the basis of dose or response. We can define the intensity of the exercise in the case of jogging, for example, by spelling out the distance to be accomplished and the rate of running (time for each mile). This is prescription by dose. On the other hand, we can also describe the intensity of the exercise in terms of physiologic responses such as the heart rate achieved. Obviously, the latter is the safer and more effective method because the physiologic strain or challenge of any given workout, defined as distance and rate, can vary greatly with such factors as weather, changing physical fitness, or incipient illness. However, to use response as the prescription basis requires that we train our participants to take their own heart rates quickly and accurately. Our discussion will be based on the heart rate-response concept.

In using heart rate response, we are again faced with two choices. We can express heart rate (HR) as a straight percentage of maximum HR or as a percentage of heart rate range (HRR). Because we start with a resting HR, which is a large fraction of the maximum HR, there is not a very good proportionality between per cent maximum HR and the per cent $\dot{V}O_2$max, which is really the measurement with which we are concerned. Figure 12.4 shows the clear advantage in expressing the exercise target HR in per cent HRR. It is apparent that per cent HRR relates quite accurately to the actual per cent $\dot{V}O_2$max. That is to say, 50% HRR approximates 50% of $\dot{V}O_2$max, but it would require about 68% of maximum HR in a young subject to produce an actual $\dot{V}O_2$ of 50%, and in the elderly the per cent maximum HR would be about 75 to produce the 50% $\dot{V}O_2$max.

Intensity Threshold

Since the classic study of Karvonen and colleagues (31) in 1957, we have been aware that some threshold or certain minimal level of exercise intensity must be attained before measurable training effects are achieved. Karvonen showed that to achieve a training effect required 60% of HRR. However, his findings were based on only six young male subjects, and no considerations were given to the possible effects of age, sex, and physical fitness differences. In general, later work has supported the threshold concept, and the 60% HRR seems to be valid for young subjects of *average* fitness. However, the author (32) has found considerable difference with respect to age and fitness. *The average threshold value for men in their 60s and 70s is only 40% HRR, and there is a well-defined effect of level of fitness at the beginning of the training program.* On the basis of the available evidence, Figure 12.5 seems to provide the best conceptualization of the dose-response relationship. The important points to be noted are: (a) there is a point in the HRR below which no training effect is achieved (intensity threshold); (b) the intensity threshold increases with higher levels of fitness; (c) once the threshold is reached, the response is relatively proportional to the dose but with somewhat less response per unit dose as fitness improves; and (d) the percentage improvement potential grows smaller with increasing fitness at the beginning of training.

The Exercise Prescription

As we have discussed above, there are four elements to the exercise prescription that must be defined. For purposes of our

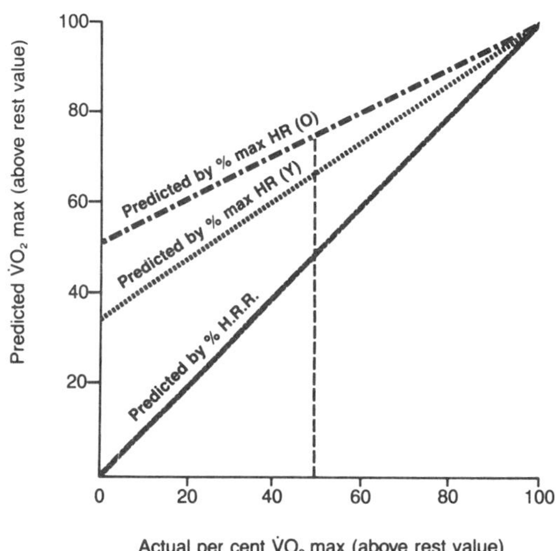

Figure 12.4. Illustration of the errors in using per cent maximum heart rate for exercise prescription compared with the use of per cent heart rate range. *Y* = college ages, *O* = 80-year-old.

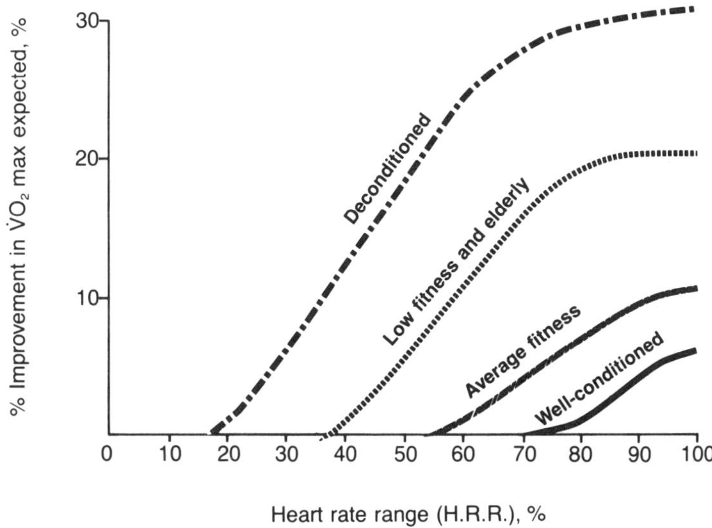

Figure 12.5. Family of curves showing exercise intensity threshold, dose-response relationship, and probable maximum results as related to pretraining $\dot{V}O_2$max (Conceptualization based on data of deVries HA: Exercise intensity threshold for improvement of cardiovascular—respiratory function in older men. Geriatrics 26:94–101, 1971, and Saltin B, et al.; AHA Monograph #23, 1968).

discussion, we will define the exercise modality as walking or jogging, or a combination thereof. We shall recommend an exercise training frequency of three to five sessions per week (Fig. 12.3) and a duration of 20 to 30 minutes per session (Fig. 12.2). However, previously sedentary individuals may require from 6 to 10 weeks to achieve this exercise duration. The remainder of our discussion will be directed to the most important factor of intensity, for which we will need the following definitions:

RHR = resting HR
EHR = exercise HR
MHR = maximum RH
HRR = HR range = MHR − RHR

$$\%HRR = \frac{EHR - RHR}{MHR - RHR} \times 100$$

Using these definitions, we now need to define three HRs for the participant:

Minimum HR—the intensity threshold value of HR, below which improvement is unlikely.

Target HR—the HR to which the participant should work to assure optimal training progress with minimal hazard.

Do-not-exceed HR—the HR above which intensity may be unnecessarily high for optimal results and that may be counterproductive for some.

Although the intensity threshold is approximately 40% HRR on the average for the elderly, the threshold is higher for the relatively fit and lower for the unfit (32). This finding is fortuitous in providing greater safety for the unfit elderly.

Figure 12.6 shows that the threshold for a training effect in older people requires that they exercise above that percentage of their heart rate range (HRR) represented by their measured $\dot{V}O_2$max or Åstrand prescore for estimated $\dot{V}O_2$max, expressed as milliliters of oxygen per kilogram per min-

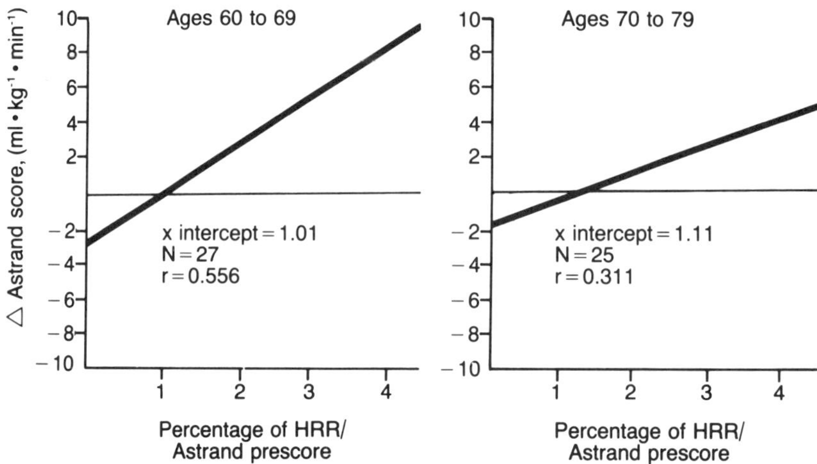

Figure 12.6. Change in Åstrand test score (ml·kg^{-1}·min^{-1}) after 6 weeks of training as a function of percentage of heart rate range divided by the Åstrand prescore. The Åstrand prescore is essentially the preconditioning $\dot{V}O_2$max, expressed as ml·kg^{-1}·min^{-1}. It should be noted that in both age groups (60 to 69 and 70 to 79), the *x intercept* is 1 or more, indicating that the selected training intensity, expressed as % HRR, should equal or exceed the preconditioning $\dot{V}O_2$max, expressed as ml·kg^{-1}·min^{-1}. (From deVries, HA: Exercise intensity threshold for improvement of cardiovascular-respiratory function in older men. *Geriatrics* 26:94–101, 1971.)

ute. For example, an estimated $\dot{V}O_2$max of 30 ml·kg^{-1}·min^{-1} would require exercising at levels that bring HR at least 30% of the way from resting toward maximal (33). Thus, a sedentary man or woman 70 years old with a resting heart rate of 80 and a maximal rate of 150 (220-age) would need to work at an HR above:

$$80 + .30\,(150 - 80) = 80 + 21$$
$$= 101 \text{ beats·min}^{-1}$$

Since 101 beats·min^{-1} represents the calculated "threshold" for a training effect, one might raise that value by 15%–20% and estimate the desirable target HR as approximately 115 to 120, which would be a safe load for the healthy normotensive older individual. Indeed, Sidney and Shephard (5) have reported exercise training HRs as high as 130-140 beats·min^{-1} among elderly subjects. Thus, we have the *minimum HR* in this example established at about 100 beats·min^{-1}. For the *target HR* we add 20% to minimum HR for approximately 120 beats·min^{-1}. Adding another 20% gives us a *do-not-exceed HR* of 140 beats·min^{-1}.

Now using those figures as a target HR, we may use the nomogram of Figure 12.7 to find what combination of jog-walk would furnish the appropriate exercise challenge. For a $\dot{V}O_2$max of 30 ml·kg^{-1}·min^{-1}, the 50 steps run-50 steps walk would seem appropriate, as it would raise the HR to 118 beats·min^{-1} after five sets of 50–50.

If we confine our discussion to the use of walking or jogging as our exercise modality, we must decide at what fitness level it is necessary to use jogging in order to get optimal results from the training program. In the author's opinion, there is now sufficient evidence to suggest prescribing progressive walking exercise for the elderly unless they are habitually active and have a high level of fitness, defined here as a measured or estimated $\dot{V}O_2$max of 40 ml·kg^{-1}·min^{-1}. This offers the greatest possible safety and yet seems to provide something close to the optimal challenge for elderly men and women. More recent studies also support the choice of walking for the elderly (34).

Physiological Monitoring. Subjects should be taught to take their own heart rate, usually at the radial artery. They should find the artery quickly (in 5 to 10 seconds) and count pulse beats accurately over a 15-second period immediately following exercise. While such a count immediately after exercise in the young may involve considerable error because of the

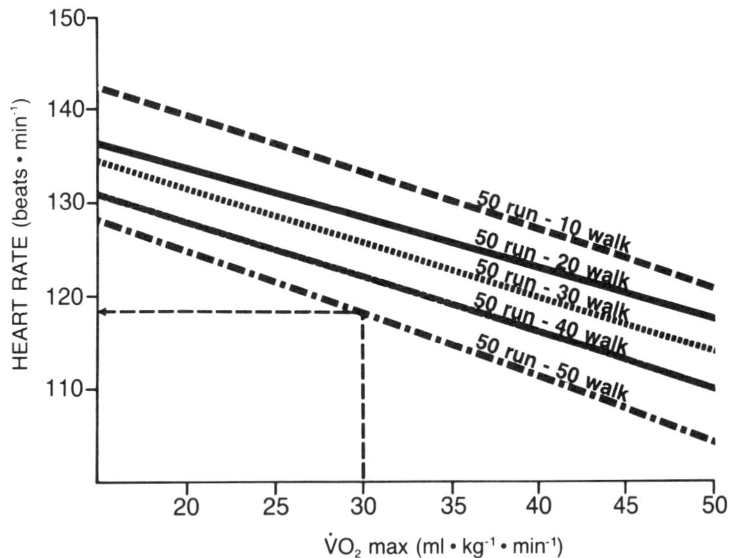

Figure 12.7. Nomogram for the estimation of heart rate response to a given dose of jogging for men 60 to 79. Example: For a man in this age bracket with a measured (or estimated from Åstrand test) $\dot{V}O_2$max of 30 $ml{\cdot}kg^{-1}{\cdot}min^{-1}$, go vertically from 30 on the horizontal axis to the intersection with the 50 run-50 walk regression line. Now go horizontally to the heart rate axis to read 118 $beat{\cdot}min^{-1}$, which represents the mean response to this dose. The standard error for the five regression lines is 8 to 10 beats (From deVries HA: Exercise intensity threshold for improvement of cardiovascular-respiratory function in older men. *Geriatrics* 26:94–101, 1971.)

very rapid exponential decline in rate, the rate of decline in older people is much slower, and the rate counted is a valuable index of the exercise intensity during any given workout.

Progression. Table 12.4 provides a program for progressive walking, which has proven to be very effective in the author's laboratory experiments (2). The table is self-explanatory. If the first day objective was completed in the recommended time (20 min), then, on the next workout day, the subject will do the second-day workout, that is 1 1/4 miles in 25 min, and so on. If, however, on the first day the subject either could not complete the distance or if HR exceeded the *do-not-exceed HR*, then he or she will continue with the first-day objective in subsequent workouts until it is completed successfully. This applies to each day's objective.

It should be noted that the major method of progression employed here is that of increasing distance by modest amounts. This method is recommended because increasing the distance makes only very small increases in demand on the heart. In contrast, increasing the intensity (speed or rate of walking) necessitates an increase in heart rate and myocardial oxygen demands. The "break" in the table does not occur until the 10th workout day. That is, the intensity (speed of walking) is not increased until completion of 3 miles at 20 minutes per mile. This is called the "double progressive" method, because both duration and intensity are modified.

Progression for Jogging Workout. In general, the "game plan" for the jog-walk program revolves around another "double progressive" training procedure. That is, one starts with only a very modest challenge to the cardiovascular and respiratory systems, initially modifying only distance jogged, and later modifying the intensity by shortening the rest periods (walking). This system has been shown to work very well both in laboratory experiments and in practical experience with older individuals.

Each day, one performs from five to ten sets of jog-walk activity. Each set consists of a given number of steps jogged, and a

Table 12.4
Progressive Walking Objectives

Workout Day	Distance	Time	
1	one mile	20 minutes	
2	1 ¼	25	
3	1 ½	30	
4	1 ¾	35	
5	2	40	20 min per mile
6	2 ¼	45	
7	2 ½	50	
8	2 ¾	55	
9	3	60	
10	2 miles	32 minutes	
11	2 ¼	36	
12	2 ½	40	
13	2 ¾	44	
14	3	48	16 min per mile
15	3 ¼	52	
16	3 ½	56	
17	3 ¾	60	
18	4	64	

given number of steps walked to provide the rest interval. The 1st day one does five sets of 50 steps jogging and 50 steps walking. The 2nd day six sets, the 3rd day seven sets, and so on, until completion of 10 sets of 50 jog, 50 walk.

To this point, progression has been achieved by increasing duration or distance. As emphasized earlier, distance progression is very gentle, in that it makes only a small increase in demands on the heart and lungs.

Having completed 10 sets of 50-50, the subject is ready to progress by increasing the intensity of exercise. This can be done either by moving faster or by decreasing the walk interval. The latter is the safer course, so one now jogs 50 steps but walks only 40. However, one also goes back to doing only five sets. The entire progression is shown in Table 12.5.

Table 12.5
Jog-Walk Program

1) 50 steps jog, 50 steps walk
    a) 5 sets the first day
    b) Each day increase the number of sets by one until 10 sets have been completed
    c) Use the same set procedure for each new series of jog-walk
2) 50 steps jog, 40 steps walk
3) 50 steps jog, 30 steps walk
4) 50 steps jog, 20 steps walk
5) 50 steps jog, 10 steps walk
6) 75 steps jog, 10 steps walk
7) 100 steps jog, 10 steps walk
8) 125 steps jog, 10 steps walk
9) 150 steps jog, 10 steps walk
10) 175 steps jog, 10 steps walk
11) 200 steps jog, 10 steps walk
12) Individual program

The subject should check his heart rate immediately at the end of each 50-step-jog interval. So long as it remains below the *do-not-exceed HR* (limit rate), he or she will stay with the progression outlined in Table 12.5.

If the limit rate is exceeded, the subject may be jogging too fast. If this is not the case, he or she can increase the walk interval by 10 steps and then return to the appropriate point of progression in Table 12.5.

The subject will arrive at "individual program," the final step of Table 12.5, in about 6 months' time if training three times per week at an average rate of progress.

He or she then will take the next step, which is to jog steadily for one-quarter mile, at the end of which he or she will check the heart rate. As long as the subject remains under "limit rate," the jogging distance may be increased by increments of one-eighth mile ad libitum until the ultimate goal of 1 mile continuous jogging without rest is achieved, and without exceeding the limit heart rate.

After completing all the sets of jog-walk or continuous jogging on any given workout day, it is important to walk for an additional 3 minutes or more. This will provide a gradual "cooling-down" from the vigorous exercise to the resting state.

When 1 mile of continuous jogging is achieved, time for this distance will vary between 9 and 12 minutes, depending on age and lifetime history of physical activity. Some older individuals who have pursued marathon running throughout their lifetimes can, of course, do far better than 9 minutes for a mile, but this is not necessary to achieve optimal levels of health and physical fitness.

Table 12.6 gives the estimated heart rate responses to various levels of jog-walk, according to physical fitness level. It is designed specifically to determine the appropriate starting level of jog-walk for those who found the 50 jog-50 walk set too easy on the 1st day, as indicated by a heart rate considerably below 130; and for those who scored "excellent" or "very good" on the $\dot{V}O_2$max test.

It should be noted that similar guidelines can be applied to other exercise modalities of an endurance type. It is also interesting that while age and fitness level at entrance to a conditioning program are important considerations, sex is not. The aforementioned procedures can be applied to elderly women as well as men, and the results are quite similar (35).

Daily Workout Plan. In general, there should be three phases in any well-designed exercise program: (a) the "warm-up", (b) the cardiorespiratory workout, and (c) the "cool-down". In the program proposed here, either walking or jogging is of low enough intensity to serve as its own warm-up medium. This necessitates slow jogging, of course, at the beginning of the workout. The endurance work in either case should result in a rise in deep muscle temperature, which will facilitate the use of strength and flexibility exercises described below for the cool-down phase.

Strength and Flexibility Exercises for Cool-Down. Figure 12.8 shows the exercises recommended for improving muscular fitness. The author has shown by radiotelemetry that none of these exercises raises the heart rate above 100 beats·min^{-1} if performed for 2 minutes at the following cadences: (a) toe touchers, three repetitions per minute, (b) modified sit-ups, seven per

Table 12.6
Maximum Heart Rate in Five Sets [a]

Fitness Category $\dot{V}O_2$max	50 jog 50 walk	50 jog 40 walk	50 jog 30 walk	50 jog 20 walk	50 jog 10 walk
≥40 ml·kg^{-1}·min^{-1}	110	115	119	122	126
Excellent	(102–118)	(107–123)	(111–127)	(114–130)	(118–134)
36–39	113	118	122	124	128
Very Good	(105–121)	(110–126)	(114–130)	(116–132)	(120–136)
27–35	117	122	125	128	133
Average	(109–125)	(114–130)	(117–133)	(120–136)	(125–141)
22–26	122	126	130	132	137
Below Average	(114–130)	(118–134)	(122–138)	(124–140)	(129–145)
≤21	126	128	132	135	140
Poor	(118–134)	(120–136)	(124–140)	(127–143)	(132–148)

[a] **These data were established in the author's laboratory by radiotelemetry methods. The upper figure represents the average heart rate response. The lower figures represent the range for plus or minus 1 standard deviation. (From de Vries HA: Exercise intensity threshold for improvement of cardiovascular-respiratory function in older men. *Geriatrics* 26:94–101, 1971).**

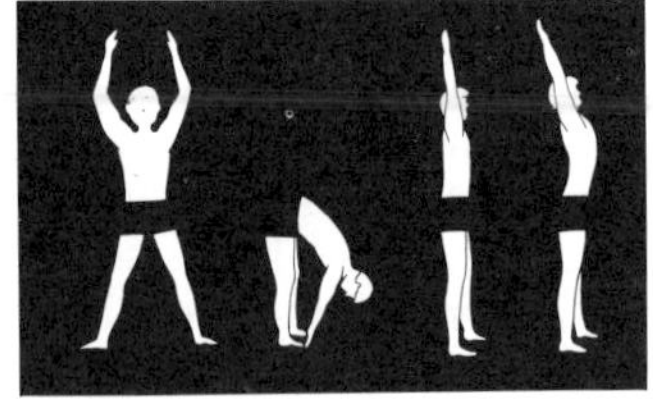

1 TOE TOUCHER

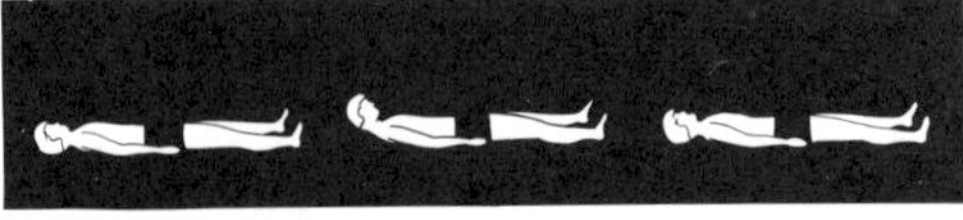

2 MODIFIED SIT·UP

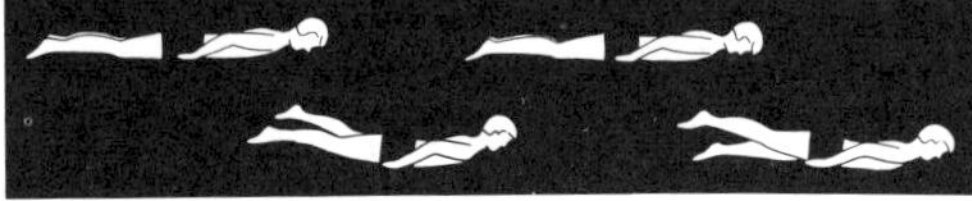

3 ALTERNATE LEG RAISERS

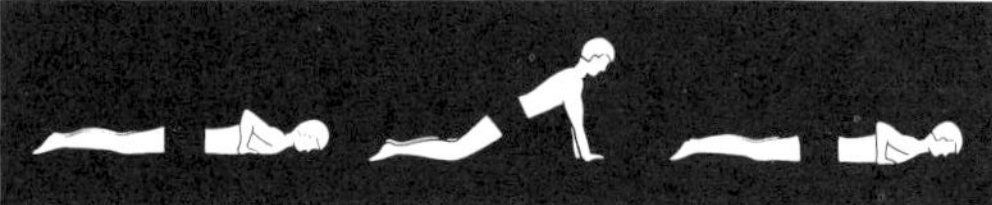

4 MODIFIED PUSH·UP

Figure 12.8. Calisthenic exercises to improve muscle strength.

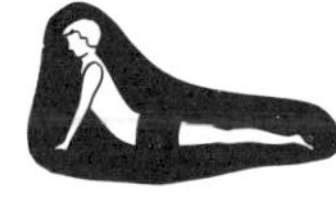

1 UPPER TRUNK STRETCHER

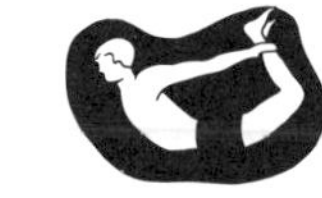

2 LOWER TRUNK STRETCHER

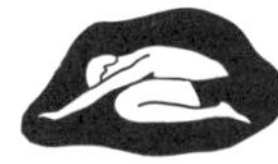
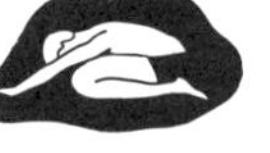

3 KNEELING LOW BACK STRETCHER

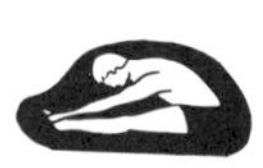
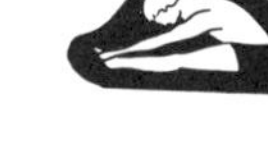

4 LOWER BACK STRETCHER

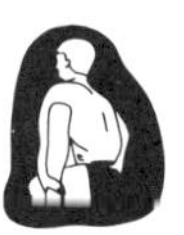
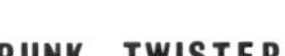

5 TRUNK TWISTER

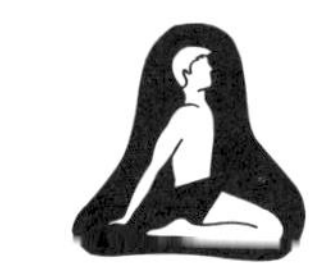

6 TOE POINTER

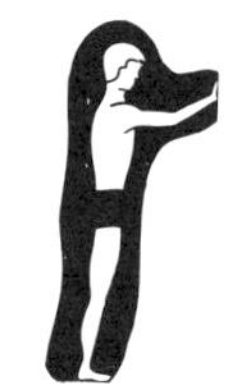

7 GASTROCNEMIUS STRETCHER

Figure 12.9. Static stretching exercises to improve flexibility.

minute, (c) alternate leg raisers, eight per minute, and (d) modified push-ups, four per minute (33). Figure 12.9 illustrates the static stretching exercises recommended for completing the cool-down phase of the workout. Each position should be held for 30-60 seconds to provide the safest possible means for improving flexibility in the elderly. The author has also provided laboratory evidence that suggests relief (36) and prevention (37) of muscle soreness, which often follows unaccustomed exercise, by use of these procedures.

CHRONIC ADAPTATIONS TO TRAINING

There seems little doubt that the PWC of the older individual can be significantly improved. While increased PWC may not add years to life, it most certainly adds "life to years." The improvement of PWC is tantamount to increasing the vigor of the older individual, and this can make an important contribution to the later years of life, certainly in terms of life-style and possibly even general health.

The physiological basis for the improvement in PWC is still very much in question. The literature indicates that the older organism is trainable and that relative improvement in cardiorespiratory function is probably comparable with that of the young. As to the mechanisms by which improved PWC is brought about, results reported by Saltin and colleagues (38) and Hartley and coworkers (39) suggest differences in the physiologic adaptations to endurance exercise training between young and middle-aged adults (34 to 55 years) in that the former respond with increases of (a) cardiovascular dimensions (heart size), (b) better redistribution of blood flow to the active tissues, perhaps augmenting the arterial-venous oxygen difference, and (c) increased stroke volume and cardiac output. In middle-aged men, increases in maximal stroke volume and cardiac output seem to account primarily for the improvement of aerobic capacity. Whether this is also true for the older population (60 and over) remains unanswered at this time. Available data suggest that improvement of respiratory function may also contribute to the postconditioning increase in PWC observed in older men.

For the healthy elderly the best documented data with respect to chronic adaptations to endurance exercise conditioning are: (a) decreased HR at any submaximal workload, (b) improvement in submaximal and maximal O_2 pulse, and (c) increased $\dot{V}O_2$max. There is also suggestive evidence that blood pressure and serum cholesterol may be reduced, but further investigation is needed to confirm this notion.

Improvement in respiratory function has been reported with respect to vital capacity (2) and maximal minute ventilation during exercise (2, 6, 40, 41), whereas the ventilatory equivalent for O_2 ($\dot{V}E/\dot{V}O_2$) has been found to decrease, suggesting a more efficient lung ventilation (6).

Muscular strength increases in the older individual as it does in the young with heavy resistance exercise, but the improvement is not accompanied by hypertrophy in the elderly (42).

Important effects of physical conditioning on bony tissues have also been reported. Two different groups of investigators have reported increases in bone mineral composition as a result of a walk training program (43, 44). Further work is needed to confirm these findings.

One of the more interesting findings in the author's laboratory has been the reduction in resting neuromuscular tension by exercise in elderly subjects with anxiety tension complaints (45). Recent investigations using changes in the Hoffman Reflex (46, 47) have corroborated our early work, which used electromyography to measure resting muscle action potentials. Whether these short-term changes observed over hours become chronic is not yet known.

SPECIAL EXERCISE PRECAUTIONS, LIMITATIONS, AND PROBLEMS

Rate of Progress

It is important for both physician and patient to recognize that although the ultimate percentage improvement in such fitness parameters as $\dot{V}O_2$max and muscular strength is not greatly different in the elderly, the rate at which improvement occurs is markedly attenuated. For example, Figure 12.10 shows the training curve for five older men who were monitored over 42 weeks in the author's laboratory. The training curve is exponential with the rate of improvement expressed as the half-time ($t_{1/2}$), or time to achieve one-half the potential improvement as expressed by oxygen pulse. The half-time for the elderly shown in Figure 12.10 is approximately 12 weeks compared with a half-time of 1.3 weeks for a healthy deconditioned young male (48). Thus, the elderly must be cautioned not to expect the rate of improvement they may remember from their youth. The data in Figure 12.10 also suggest the need for initial laboratory retesting at about 6 weeks and at 6-month intervals thereafter for healthy normals.

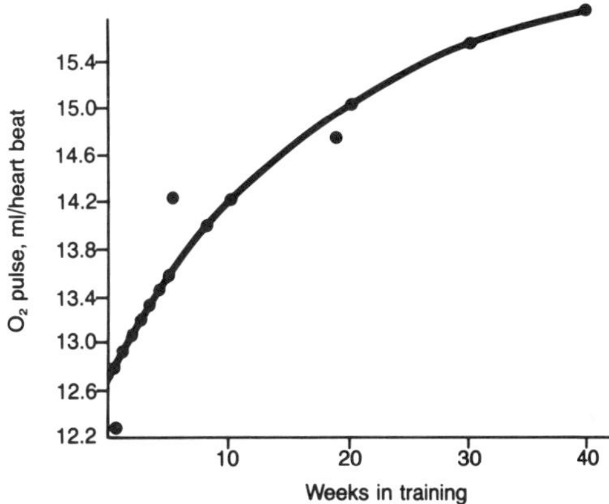

Figure 12.10. Training curve for older men (N = 5) who achieved a 29% improvement in O_2 transport ($P<.05$) (From deVries, HA: Physiological effects of an exercise training regimen upon men aged 52–88. J *Geron* 25:325–336, 1970).

Soft-Tissue Problems

Objective laboratory analyses of stiffness (examination of hysteresis loops of the plots of displacement versus force required) have shown a three- to fourfold greater elastic stiffness in joint movement of the elderly compared with that of the young (49). This is probably attributable to the reported changes in collagen-elastin ratios (50).

These changes highlight the need for warm-up in the elderly to prevent muscular tears and ruptures. Moreover, they suggest the need to caution the elderly against a too rapid acceleration-deceleration of movement since jerky movements can exceed the force required to rupture fascial investments of muscle in the elderly.

Medical Consultation and Examination

Elderly individuals should check with their physician before initiating significant increases in physical activity, particularly if such practices may result in excessive or sudden demands on the circulatory system.

Progress Gradually

Elderly persons should always start with a low level of exercise and progress slowly, using heart rate response and perceived exertion as intensity guidelines. Rest periods should be included when comfortable fatigue occurs.

Recognize Signs of Overtraining

Generally, signs of overtraining may include any one of the following: exercise heart rate is above limit values as defined earlier; sleep is not as sound as usual; or excessive fatigue occurs on the day following the workout.

Warm-up

It is essential to the welfare of older persons' muscles, bones, joints, and ligaments that any workout begin with exercise designed to bring about gradual increases in blood flow with concomitant increases in local tissue and general body temperature. This is necessary for prevention of muscular aches, pains, and injuries. Generally, no very vigorous movements should be made until sweating has begun. Muscles and connective tissues are most easily injured when they are cold. The older the individual, the more important the warm-up procedure becomes.

Cool-down

The need to make a gradual transition from vigorous exercise back to the resting state is as important as warm-up because of the adjustments that the circulatory system must make. The reflexes that promote vasodilatation during vigorous exercise are not reversed quickly upon cessation of exercise. Further, when a person abruptly stops strenuous exercise and remains motionless, he loses the activity of the "skeletal muscle pump," a natural means of making the circulatory adjustment. As a result there is a transient decrease in venous return and cardiac output falls, causing a rapid drop in blood pressure. In many persons, this is enough to compromise blood flow to the brain—causing them to become dizzy or lightheaded. To avoid this, we recommend a slow and gradual transition from vigorous exercise to the resting state. After jogging, for example, the elderly exerciser should walk for a period of time—at least 2 to 3 minutes.

Postworkout Shower

Since a hot shower also promotes peripheral vasodilatation, it is important that the postworkout shower be delayed until the circulatory system has returned to the normal, resting state. Depending on the weather, it is recommended waiting a minimum of 5 to 10 minutes. Even then, the shower should be only comfortably warm, not hot.

Breath-holding

Avoid any activity that requires breath-holding. Exercises that involve "straining" may evoke an excessive blood pressure response.

Competition

Elderly individuals should avoid competition during conditioning workouts. The excitement of competition may increase sympathetic activity and catecholamine levels, lowering the threshold to ventricular arrhythmias (51).

Illness

Certain illnesses cause dehydration and reduction of blood volume, whereas others may predispose to arrhythmias. Elderly individuals should be cautioned against exercise during illness or when unduly fatigued. Moreover, the exercise dosage should be decreased following a period of inactivity due to illness or injury.

SUMMARY AND CONCLUSION

Increasing experimental evidence indicates that healthy older individuals can improve their functional capacity through physical conditioning programs. In relative terms, their improvement is comparable with that in the young, although they start at and progress to lower achievement levels and probably require a lower training stimulus to bring about the desired response. In general, the effects of physical conditioning upon middle-aged and older individuals are opposite to those commonly associated with the aging process.

REFERENCES

1. Cunningham DA, Rechnitzer PA, Howard JH, et al.: Exercise training and the cardiovascular fitness of man at retirement. *Med Sci Sports Exerc* 17:270, 1985 (Abst).
2. deVries HA: Physiological effects of an exercise training regimen upon men aged 52–88. *J Geront* 25:325–336, 1970.
3. Seals DR, Hagberg JM, Hurley BF, et al.: Endurance training in older men and women. I. Cardiovascular responses to exercise. *J Appl Physiol* 57:1024–1029, 1984.
4. Seals DR, Hurley BF, Schultz J, et al.: Endurance training in older men and women. II. Blood lactate response to submaximal exercise. *J Appl Physiol* 57:1030–1033, 1984.
5. Sidney KH, Shephard RJ: Frequency and intensity of exercise for elderly subjects. *Med Sci Sports* 10:125–131, 1978.
6. Yerg JE, Seals DR, Hagberg JM, et al.: Effect of endurance exercise training on ventilatory function in older individuals. *J Appl Physiol* 58:791–794, 1985.
7. American College of Sports Medicine: *Guidelines for Exercise Testing and Prescription*, ed 3. Philadelphia, Lea & Febiger, 1986.
8. Ambe KS, Adams GM, deVries HA: Exercising the aged. *Med Sci Sports* 5:63, 1973 (abst).
9. Wright GR, Sidney K, Shephard RJ: Variance of direct and indirect measurements of aerobic power. *J Sports Med Phys Fitness* 18:33–42, 1978.
10. deVries HA, Tichy MW, Housh TJ, et al.: A method for estimating physical working capacity at the fatigue threshold (PWC_{FT}) *Ergonomics* 30:1195–1204, 1987.
11. Wasserman K, Van Kessel AL, Burton GG: Interaction of physiological mechanisms during exercise. *J Appl Physiol* 22:71–85, 1967.
12. Wiswell RA, deVries HA: Time course of O_2 pulse during the various tests of aerobic power. *Eur J Appl Physiol* 41:221–232, 1979.
13. Åstrand PO, Ryhming I: Prediction of max O_2: A nomogram for calculation of aerobic capacity (physical fitness) from pulse rate during submaximal work. *J Appl Physiol* 7:218–221, 1954.
14. Von Dobeln W, Åstrand I, Bergstrom A: An analysis of age and other factors related to maximal oxygen uptake. *J Appl Physiol* 22:934–938, 1967.
15. Friedman DB, Ramo BW, Gray GJ: Tennis and cardiovascular fitness in middle-aged man. *Phys Sportsmed* 12:87–92, 1984.
16. Bassett DR, Smith PA, Getchell LH: Energy cost of simulated rowing using a wind-resistance device. *Phys Sportsmed* 12:113–118, 1984.
17. Foster C: Physiological requirements of aerobic dancing. *Res Q* 46:120–122, 1975.
18. Pollock ML, Miller HS, Janeway R, et al.: Effects of walking on body composition and cardiovascular function of middle-aged men. *J Appl Physiol* 30:126–130, 1971.
19. Roberts JA, Morgan WP: Effects of type and frequency of participation in physical activity upon physical working capacity. *Am Correct Ther J* 25:99–104, 1971.
20. Pollock ML, Miller HS: Frequency of training as a determinant for improvement in cardiovascular function and body composition of middle aged man. *Arch Phys Med Rehabil* 56:141–145, 1975.
21. deVries HA, Adams GM: Effect of the type of exercise upon the work of the heart in older men. *J Sports Med Phys Fitness* 17:41–48, 1977.
22. deVries HA, Adams GM: Total muscle mass ac-

tivation vs relative loading of individual muscle as determinants of exercise response in older men. *Med Sci Sports* 4:146–154, 1972.
23. Adams GE, Bonner EA, Ribisl PM, et al.: Blood pressure during heavy work on the treadmill and bicycle ergometer. *Med Sci Sports* 10:50, 1978 (Abst).
24. Hartung GH, Smolensky MH, Harrist RB, et al.: Effects of varied durations of training on improvement in cardiorespiratory endurance. *J Hum Ergol* 6:61–68, 1977.
25. Pollock ML: How much exercise is enough? *Phys Sportsmed* 6:50–64, 1978.
26. Pollock ML, Gettman LR, Milesis CA, et al.: Effects of frequency and duration of training on attrition and incidence of injury. *Med Sci Sports* 9:31–36, 1977.
27. Pollock ML, Cureton TK, Greninger L: Effects of frequency of training on working capacity, cardiovascular function and body composition of adult men. *Med Sci Sports* 1:70–74, 1969.
28. Gettman LR, Pollock ML, Durstine JL, et al.: Physiological responses of men to 1, 3, and 5 day per week training programs. *Res Q* 47:638–646, 1976.
29. Atomi Y, Ito K, Iwasaki H, et al.: Effects of intensity and frequency of training on aerobic work capacity of young females. *J Sports Med Phys Fitness* 18:3–9, 1978.
30. Hickson RC, Rosenkoetter MA: Reduced training frequencies and maintenance of increased aerobic power. *Med Sci Sports* 13:13–16, 1981.
31. Karvonen MJ, Kentala E, Mustala O: Effects of training on heart rate: A longitudinal study. *Ann Med Exp Biol Fenn* 35:307–315, 1957.
32. deVries HA: Exercise intensity threshold for improvement of cardiovascular-respiratory function in older men. *Geriatrics* 26:94–101, 1971.
33. deVries HA: Prescription of exercise for older men from telemetered exercise heart rate data. *Geriatrics* 26:102–111, 1971.
34. Porcari J, McCarron R, Kline G, et al.: Is fast walking an adequate aerobic stimulus for 30-to-69-year-old men and women? *Phys Sportsmed* 15:119–129, 1987.
35. Adams GM, deVries HA: Physiological effects of an exercise training regimen upon women aged 52–79. *J Geront* 28:50–55, 1973.
36. deVries, HA: Quantitative electromyographic investigation of the spasm theory of muscle pain. *Am J Phys Med* 45:119–134, 1966.
37. deVries HA: Prevention of muscular distress after exercise. *Res Q* 32:177–185, 1961.
38. Saltin B, Hartley H, Kilbom A, et al.: Physical training in sedentary middle aged and old men. II. Oxygen uptake, heart rate, and blood lactate concentration at submaximal and maximal exercise. *Scand J Clin Invest* 24:323–334, 1969.
39. Hartley LH, Grimby G, Kilbom A, et al.: Physical training in sedentary middle aged and older men. III. Cardiac output and gas exchange at submaximal and maximal exercise. *Scand J Clin Invest* 24:335–349, 1969.
40. Barry AJ, Daly JW, Pruett EDR, et al.: The effects of physical conditioning on older individuals. I. Work capacity, circulatory-respiratory function, and work electrocardiogram. *J Geront* 21: 182–191, 1966.
41. Badenhop DT, Clearly PA, Schaal SF, et al.: Physiological adjustments to higher- or lower-intensity exercise in elders. *Med Sci Sports* 15: 496–502, 1983.
42. Moritani T, deVries HA: Potential for gross muscle hypertrophy in older men. *J Geront* 35:672–682, 1980.
43. Smith EL, Reddan W: Physical activity—a modality for bone accretion in the aged. Ann J Roentgenol 126:1297, 1976.
44. Brewer V, Meyer BM, Keele MS, et al.: Role of exercise in prevention of involutional bone loss. *Med Sci Sports* 15:445–449, 1983.
45. deVries HA, Adams GM: Electromyographic comparison of single doses of exercise and meprobamate as to effects on muscular relaxation. *Am J Phys Med* 51:130–141, 1972.
46. deVries HA, Wiswell RA, Bulbulian R, et al.: Tranquilizer effect of exercise: Acute effects of moderate aerobic exercise on spinal reflex activation level. *Am J Phys Med* 60:57–66, 1981.
47. Bulbulian R, Darabos BL: Motor neuron excitability: The Hoffman reflex following exercise of low and high intensity. *Med Sci Sports Exerc* 18:697–702, 1986.
48. deVries HA: *Physiology of Exercise*, ed 4. Dubuque, Wm C Brown, 1986, p 288.
49. Wright V, Johns RJ: Physical factors concerned with the stiffness of normal and diseased joints. *Johns Hopkins Hosp Bull* 106:215–231, 1960.
50. Kao KT, McGavack TH: Changes in connective tissue with aging. *W Va Med J* 59:123–125, 1963.
51. Lown B, Verrier RL, Rabinowitz SH: Neural and psychologic mechanisms and the problem of sudden cardiac death. *Am J Cardiol* 39:890–902, 1977.

CHAPTER 13

Wheelchair-Dependent Individuals

Roger M. Glaser, Ph.D.
Glen M. Davis, Ph.D.

INTRODUCTION

Recently, increased attention has been directed towards the role of exercise for improving the health, physical fitness, and rehabilitation potential of patients who are wheelchair-dependent because of neuromuscular dysfunction or lower-limb amputations. Common medical conditions such as stroke, multiple sclerosis, muscular dystrophy, and traumatic injury to the central nervous system can directly result in muscle paralysis, paresis, or spasticity. However, a sedentary life-style may cause wheelchair users to experience secondary complications such as reduced cardiorespiratory fitness, muscle atrophy, osteoporosis, and impaired circulation to the lower extremities leading to eventual thrombus formation or decubitus ulcers. In addition, a diminished self-concept, greater dependence upon others for daily living, and reduced ability for normal societal interactions can have drastic psychological impact.

To improve their general health and fitness, many tetra- and paraplegics regularly participate in arm exercise programs, and an increasing number are also active in wheelchair sporting events. Numerous beneficial physiologic and psychologic sequelae have been reported for wheelchair-dependent individuals who engage in habitual physical activity (1–8). Considering the success that many of these individuals have achieved with respect to their functional independence and life-styles, it appears that regular exercise can greatly contribute to the rehabilitation process.

Although leg exercise (e.g., walking, running, cycling) is the standard for stress testing and training of ambulatory patients, arm exercise is common for wheelchair-dependent patients. Many of the established principles for stress testing using leg exercise may also apply to arm tests, but the clinician should be aware of some crucial differences when lower-limb disabled individuals undertake arm exercise. These include differences in the (a) exercise intensity levels used, (b) physiologic (metabolic, cardiovascular, and pulmonary) response patterns elicited, and (c) nature and degree of possible risks encountered.

Exercise Capability of Neuromuscularly Impaired Patients

The central nervous system (CNS) and its outflow from its somatic and autonomic components are illustrated in Figure 13.1. Generally, the higher the level and extent of the CNS damage, the greater the concomitant somatic and autonomic dysfunction. In the case of spinal cord injury (SCI), lesions in the cervical region can cause tetraplegia, whereas lesions in the thoracic or lumbar regions can result in paraplegia. Skeletal muscle paralysis, of course, limits the muscle mass available for exercise and restricts the absolute fitness level that may be achieved through exercise training. In addition, most patients with neuromuscular impairments experience occasional spasms in the afflicted muscles ranging from mild to hazardous in severity. Pharmacotherapy is often employed to help control these unwanted contractions, but such agents may also cause consequent weakness of functional muscles and CNS side effects (9).

In addition to skeletal muscle paralysis, CNS lesions can disrupt the autonomic re-

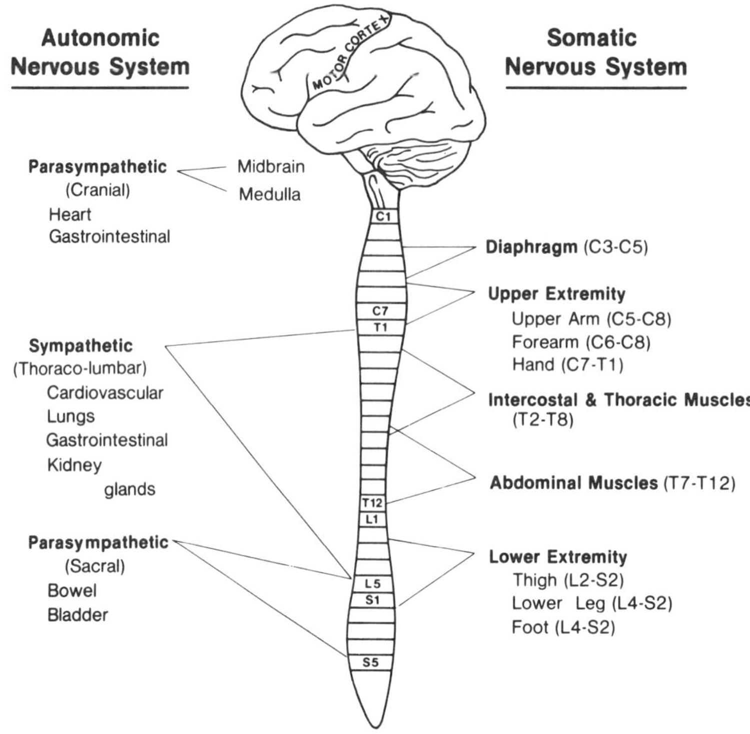

Figure 13.1. Diagram of the central nervous system, and the neuronal outflows for the somatic nervous system (skeletal muscle innervation) and autonomic nervous system (internal organ innervation). General innervations from each spinal cord level are indicated. (From Glaser RM: Exercise and locomotion for the spinal cord injured. In Terjung RL (ed): *Exercise and Sports Sciences Reviews*, Vol. 13. New York, MacMillan Publishers, 1985, p 269.)

flexes required for normal exercise responses. Diminished sympathetic outflow limits aerobic exercise capacity since adrenergic sympathetic stimulation is required for appropriate cardiovascular adjustments (e.g., to provide increased blood flow to active skeletal muscles for delivery of O_2 and fuel substrates, and for removal of metabolic by-products). In the intact person, vasoconstriction in inactive tissues and increased cardiac output both contribute to increased muscle blood flow. However, these cardiovascular reflexes may be reduced or nonexistent in CNS-damaged patients. Lesions above T1 interrupt the sympathetic outflow to the heart, which severely reduces maximal cardiac output by limiting normal exercise-induced cardioacceleration and myocardial contractility. Consequently, insufficient muscle blood flow often leads to early onset of peripheral fatigue resulting from limited aerobic energy supply, and a greater dependence upon anaerobiosis with a concomitant accumulation of lactic acid in the muscles. Additionally, thermoregulatory capacity during exercise may be impaired by an inappropriate blood flow distribution, and by an inability to activate a sufficient sweating response (via cholinergic sympathetic stimulation) for adequate cooling.

It is thus evident that many wheelchair-dependent patients manifest severely limited exercise performance resulting from the direct effects of skeletal muscle dysfunction, as well as the loss of autonomic sympathetic control of the cardiovascular and other organ systems during exercise. Pharmacotherapy often further reduces exercise capacity, as can the diminished physical fitness that results from insufficient or inappropriate exercise. These problems can discourage many wheelchair-dependent patients from leading active lives, which may lead to further loss of fitness. Objective fitness evaluation and regular exercise are essential for breaking the *sedentary lifestyle-loss of fitness* cycle, and enhancing rehabilitation outcome.

It is the purpose of this chapter to present some basic principles related to exercise testing and training of wheelchair users. Topics addressed include: exercise stress-testing for physical fitness assessment; exercise prescription for physical fitness improvement; physiologic adaptations to chronic exercise; and special exercise precautions, limitations, and problems. Additionally, a section is included that presents some recent techniques and data using functional electrical stimulation to exercise muscles weakened or paralyzed by neuromuscular impairments. Throughout, our fundamental approach will be to present an overview of basic principles, followed by a more in-depth analysis of pertinent research information.

EXERCISE TESTING

Classification of Disability

Medical practitioners and health-care professionals need to be aware that the nature and severity of SCI may play a role in the interpretation of cardiorespiratory and muscular strength data gained from fitness tests and used for the purposes of exercise prescription. We have previously advanced the view (10, 11) that neurologic disorders may be classified on either an anatomic (the site of causal lesion and degree of CNS dysfunction), a functional (quantity and quality of active musculature), or a dynamic (pattern of habitual physical activity or associated level of daily energy expenditure) basis. The common anatomic approach (12–17) has been to numerically define the vertebral segment receiving trauma (e.g., third thoracic segment or T3), and suffix that definition with an adjective describing the nature of neurologic disruption (e.g., complete, incomplete, poliomyelitic, etc.). A functional classification (such as the International Stoke Mandeville Games Federation grading scheme, Fig. 13.2) has the advantage of estimating both the quality and quantity of functioning musculature in individuals with tetraplegia, paraplegia, spina bifida, or poliomyelitis (18–21). However, a large body of evidence points to the interpretation of physiologic data in wheelchair users on the basis of dynamic activity patterns (22–29) as superior to the previous systems, since these patterns often reflect the total consequences of the disorder, including possible psychological sequelae (10, 11, 16, 18).

Cardiorespiratory Fitness

There are many well-established stress-testing protocols available to clinicians and exercise specialists for the assessment of cardiorespiratory fitness and physical performance in ambulatory individuals. These protocols typically utilize leg exercise because the large muscles of the lower limbs are usually stronger and less fatigable than the smaller muscle mass of the arms. By using a large muscle mass, it is more likely that the limiting factor during maximal exercise (especially maximal oxygen uptake, $\dot{V}O_2$ max) will be central circulatory in nature (insufficient delivery of blood and oxygen to the exercising muscles) rather than peripheral (local fatigue of the exercising muscles despite the availability of adequate blood and oxygen) (14, 30–36).

Unfortunately, relatively little research has been conducted into the development of arm exercise stress-testing protocols that can be used clinically for patients with lower-limb disabilities, and such tests are not currently in widespread use. These tests can potentially improve patient care since they usually provide objective information concerning: (a) physical fitness as indicated by maximal exercise performance and cardiorespiratory function; (b) the risks encountered during strenuous arm exercise due to cardiopulmonary impairments; (c) wheelchair locomotive capability; and (d) how these factors change over time (e.g., following exercise training or with altered medical status).

Since the highest oxygen uptake obtained during maximal effort arm exercise is lower than the true physiologic maximum (i.e., approximately two-thirds of maximal leg exercise data) (9, 10, 37), the term "$\dot{V}O_2$ peak" is usually employed instead of "$\dot{V}O_2$max" to describe aerobic met-

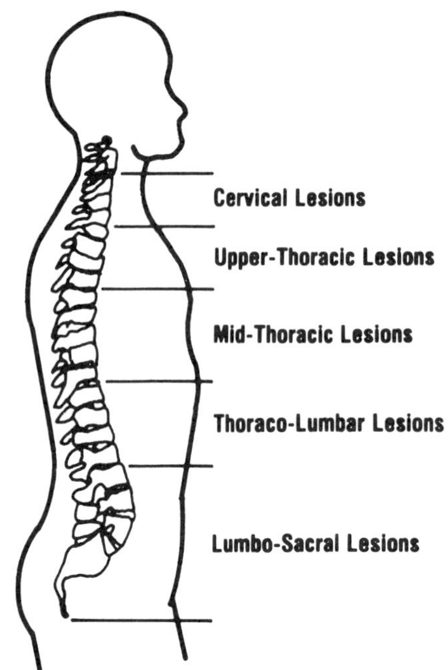

Figure 13.2. The International Stoke Mandeville Games Federation medical grading scheme. (From Davis GM, Jackson RW, Shephard RJ: Sports and recreation for the physically disabled. In Strauss RH (ed): *Sports Medicine.* Philadelphia, WB Saunders Co., 1984, p 290.)

abolic values achieved during upper-body exercise. Similar terminology has been applied to other cardiorespiratory variables (e.g., "peak heart rate," "peak pulmonary ventilation," etc.). Glaser and coworkers (38) demonstrated that during maximal effort arm-crank ergometry and concurrent knee-extension exercise induced by electrical stimulation, a 28% higher $\dot{V}O_2$ peak was elicited compared to arm exercise alone. Furthermore, it has been shown that paraplegic individuals highly acclimated to strenuous arm exertion are more capable of utilizing the capability of their oxygen delivery system to achieve a higher percentage of their physiologic $\dot{V}O_2$max during arm effort (15).

To objectively assess the stressfulness of specific exercise protocols in terms of metabolic and cardiopulmonary performance, physiologic monitoring has been employed at rest and during steady-rate exercise and recovery from exercise. Physiologic variables typically monitored include: $\dot{V}O_2$, respiratory exchange ratio (RER), pulmonary ventilation ($\dot{V}_E$), heart rate (HR, derived from the ECG), arterial blood pressure (BP), and blood lactate concentration (LA). In addition, some researchers have estimated cardiac output ($\dot{Q}$), ventricular stroke volume (SV), and arteriovenous O_2 difference ($a-\bar{v}O_2$) using noninvasive techniques such as CO_2-rebreathing or impedance cardiography to assess myocardial performance and peripheral oxygen extraction (14, 39–42). The interpretation of these physiologic variables will be discussed below.

Arm Exercise Modes

The two modes of arm exercise most frequently used to assess the cardiorespiratory fitness of lower-limb disabled individuals are arm-crank and wheelchair ergometry. Both exercise modalities elicit similar $\dot{V}O_2$peak values, but maximal power output (PO), $\dot{V}_E$, and HR for arm cranking are usually substantially higher (24, 25, 43). In contrast, at given PO levels, $\dot{V}O_2$, $\dot{V}_E$, and HR tend to be lower for arm cranking (41). For basic cardiorespiratory fitness assessment, arm-crank ergometry appears to be a satisfactory and practical exercise technique. However, if the purpose of the stress-test is to evaluate not only aerobic fitness but also wheelchair locomotive capability, then the wheelchair-type activity is superior. This is because the concept of exercise specificity (44–48) suggests that the same muscles and joint movements used for daily ambulation should also be used during stress-testing.

Actual Wheelchair Locomotion

A direct mechanism to evaluate the fitness of lower-limb disabled patients is to assess their abilities for propulsion of their own wheelchairs over a predetermined test course (49–52). Patients are paced at standard wheelchair velocities (e.g., 1.0, 2.0, and 3.0 km·h^{-1}) during which steady-rate physiologic responses are monitored using portable data collection equipment (Fig. 13.3). Glaser and associates (51, 52) developed one such technique whereby the subject (Fig. 13.3a) attempts to maintain a preset wheelchair velocity by following a technician pushing a speedometer-equipped (53) pace cart (Fig. 13.3b). A second technician (Fig. 13.3c) supports a Plexiglass board on which metabolic data collection instrumentation is mounted. Subjects breathe through a two-way respiratory valve and, at specified times, expired gases are collected for later calculation of $\dot{V}_E$, $\dot{V}O_2$, RER, and the energy cost of locomotion (kJ). If desired, the net locomotive energy cost (NLEC; kJ·kg^{-1}·km^{-1}) may also be estimated, providing a relative index that is inversely related to the efficiency of locomotion (51, 52). Examples of NLEC data, which have been reported for actual wheelchair propulsion over tile and carpet at 3.0 km·h^{-1}, are 1.9 and 3.3 kJ·kg^{-1}·km^{-1} (approximately 0.46 and 0.80 kcal·kg^{-1}·km^{-1}), respectively (51). Higher NLEC values might be expected for propelling wheelchairs up inclines or over uneven surfaces. Major fac-

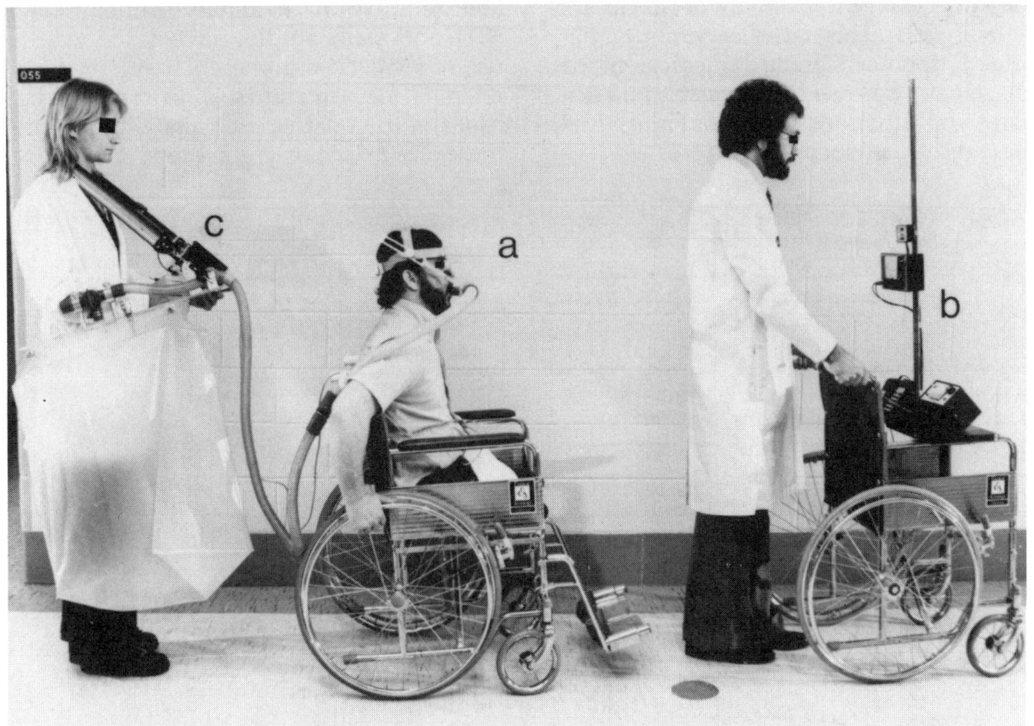

Figure 13.3. Technique used to monitor physiologic responses during wheelchair locomotion: (*a*) subject in wheelchair, (*b*) pace cart, (*c*) data collection instrumentation. (From Glaser RM, Sawka MN, Wilde SW, et al.: Energy cost and cardiopulmonary responses for wheelchair locomotion and walking on tile and carpet. *Paraplegia* 19:222, 1981.)

tors that influence the oxygen uptake (and efficiency) of locomotion are the physical characteristics of the wheelchair and the biomechanics of the patient's propulsion technique. This field-testing method can be used as an aid to wheelchair prescription, as well as a means to improve the instruction of operating techniques on the basis of reducing energy costs. The lowering of $\dot{V}O_2$ for a given locomotive task will also lower cardiopulmonary and muscular stresses.

To better understand the exercise intensity encountered, the PO requirements of actual wheelchair locomotion for given velocities, floor surfaces, and inclines have been estimated by (a) measuring the force necessary to keep a weight-loaded wheelchair in a stationary position on a motor-driven treadmill (54–56), (b) measuring the distance and elapsed time a weight-loaded wheelchair coasts after the cessation of pushing force (57), and (c) measuring the average force (with a strain-gauge transducer) necessary to push a wheelchair and its user (53). This latter technique, performed upon a standard medical model wheelchair, was used to calculate the linear regression equations shown in Figure 13.4. The product of locomotive force and velocity provides an estimate of the PO required (kpm·min^{-1} or watts) for wheelchair operation over tiled or low-pile carpeted surfaces (if the total mass of the patient plus wheelchair and the degree of incline are known). For example, if a 70-kg person operates a 20-kg wheelchair up a 2° tiled incline at 3.0 km·h^{-1}, the estimated PO would be 32 watts (197 kpm·min^{-1}). If the surface were carpeted, PO would be approximately 42 watts (260 kpm·min^{-1}).

Arm-Crank and Wheelchair Ergometry

Arm-crank and wheelchair ergometers have been used in laboratory and clinical settings to evaluate the physiologic responses of disabled individuals. These stationary devices can be calibrated to ensure an accurate and reproducible setting of the PO necessary for graded intensity exercise assessments, physical conditioning, or comparative stress studies. Ergometers for arm-crank exercise are commercially available (e.g., Monark Rehab Trainer model 881), and many studies have described the use of leg cycle ergometers that have been adapted for arm cranking. In contrast, because of the relative unavailability of commercial wheelchair ergometers, most have

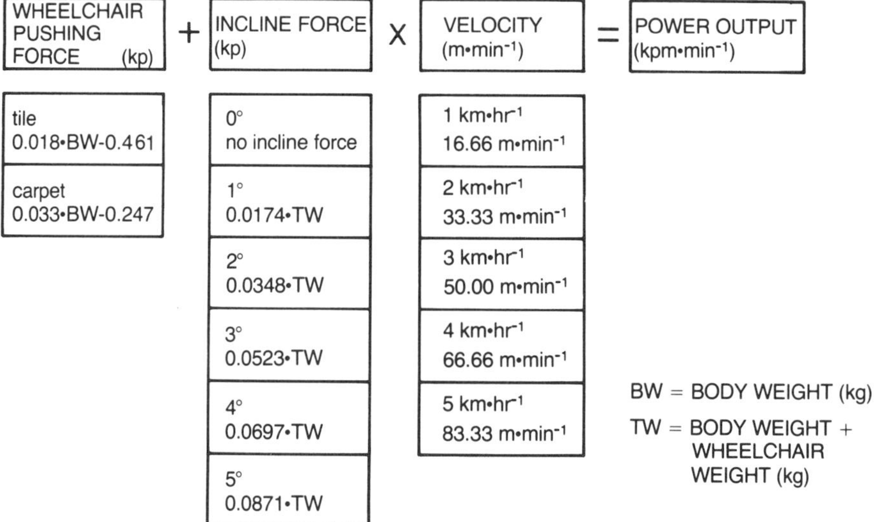

Figure 13.4. Composite summary of linear regression equations used to predict power output requirements (kpm·min^{-1}) for wheelchair locomotion over given terrains. (From Glaser RM, Collins SR, Wilde SW: Power output requirements for manual wheelchair locomotion. *Proc IEEE National Aerospace and Electronics Conference* 2:507, 1980.)

been specially designed and constructed (24, 43, 58–65).

The ergometer illustrated in Figure 13.5 enables both arm-crank and wheelchair-type exercise to be performed by disabled individuals (43). A standard mechanically-braked bicycle ergometer (e.g., Monark model 868) serves as the basis of this arm-crank/wheelchair exercise device. Conventional wheelchair wheels are mounted on a solid steel axle supported by low friction ball bearings. A chain and sprocket couple this axle to the bicycle flywheel, which has been fitted for an additional sprocket. A steel bar, welded to the arm-crank unit, is inserted into the seat support of the bicycle and secured by a bolt and clamp. A chain and sprocket couple the arm crank to the other sprocket of the flywheel. The height and forward and backward position of the seats are fully adjustable to enable proper positioning of the patient with respect to the wheelchair handrims and arm crank. Seat belts should be used to help support severely immobilized patients. The PO ($kpm \cdot min^{-1}$, watts) for wheelchair or arm-crank ergometry is determined by multiplying the flywheel braking force (kp, N) by its velocity ($km \cdot min^{-1}$). The wheelchair ergometer component has been shown to provide valid (ability to simulate actual wheelchair locomotion) and reliable (high test-retest repeatability) results (66).

Other methods of providing wheelchair-type exercise in a clinical setting include operating the patient's wheelchair over rollers (59) or on a motor-driven treadmill (12, 13, 54, 56, 67, 68). Although wheelchair rollers can provide an appropriate and relatively inexpensive solution for exercise assessments, it may be difficult to accurately quantify the PO level for duplicating the test at a future time or for comparing patients of disparate body mass. Operating a wheelchair on a motor-driven treadmill is probably the best method of simulating actual wheelchair locomotion in the laboratory, and augmented cardiorespiratory responses have been obtained in comparison to other arm ergometers (12, 13). But this exercise mode requires special equipment, skill by the wheelchair user, numerous safety precautions, and can be quite expensive.

Exercise Testing Protocols

The basic principles employed for upper body exercise stress-testing are quite similar to those described in previous chapters for lower body exercise assessments. These tests are typically progressive with respect to exercise intensity, and have well-defined criteria for termination. Protocols may be designed using either continuous or discontinuous (alternating exercise and recov-

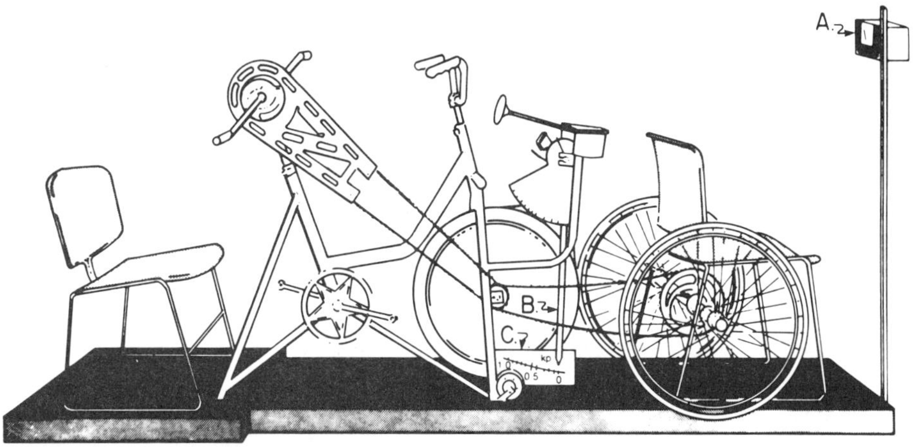

Figure 13.5. Diagram of the combination wheelchair-arm crank ergometer: (*A*) electronic speedometer, (*B*) lengthened pendular arm, (*C*) expanded braking force scale. (From Glaser RM, Sawka MN, Brune MF, et al.: Physiological responses to maximal effort wheelchair and arm crank ergometry. *J Appl Physiol* 48:1061, 1980.)

ery periods) exercise, as PO is incrementally increased to a point of submaximal or maximal stress at the termination of the test. For neuromuscularly impaired patients, discontinuous exercise protocols of submaximal intensities may be preferable (46, 50). Such tests are relatively safe and are task-specific since the range of exercise intensity is usually similar to that encountered during daily wheelchair activity.

Fitness evaluation for exercise testing is usually based upon: (a) the magnitude of physiologic responses at each power output, and (b) the maximal power output achieved. Generally, the oxygen consumption at a given submaximal PO indicates the level of aerobic energy expenditure, and thus the efficiency for performing that task. In contrast, $\dot{V}E$ and HR are more related to the relative stress encountered by the patient during exercise (unless the degree of neurological impairment affects these variables). So individuals who exhibit lower metabolic and cardiorespiratory responses during steady-rate exertion are usually considered to be more fit and possessing a greater cardiorespiratory reserve (i.e., a given task is accomplished at lower percentages of peak $\dot{V}O_2$, $\dot{V}E$ and HR). These physiologic data can be compared to previous results for the same individual to determine changes in aerobic fitness over a period of time, or to norms that have been established (by testing many individuals) for the appropriate patient population (46). End-points for terminating an exercise test include: a) voluntary cessation, b) symptoms of cardiovascular or pulmonary abnormalities (e.g., chest discomfort, ECG changes, marked hypertension, dyspnea), c) completion of the maximal PO level required for the test, and d) attainment of a predetermined heart rate (e.g., 75% of age-adjusted HR reserve) (30, 46).

As indicated previously, basic exercise testing can be accomplished by having the patient operate his or her own wheelchair over an established test course at self-selected or paced velocities. A discontinuous, submaximal exercise protocol is often desirable, each locomotive task being performed at a constant velocity and lasting approximately 4–6 minutes in duration. Steady-rate physiologic responses are normally monitored during the last minute of wheelchair propulsion, and 5–10-minute recovery periods are typically permitted between locomotive bouts. For subsequent exercise levels, wheelchair velocity is increased by 0.5–1.0 $km \cdot h^{-1}$.

During wheelchair ergometry, an initial power output of 5 watts provides a good starting point for exercise stress tests, as this intensity is frequently encountered during daily wheelchair operation (53). Incremental PO progressions of 5–10 watts are usual for wheelchair-dependent patients, while maximal PO is normally limited to 25–35 watts (41, 46, 50, 69). The PO increment and maximal PO achieved can be substantially greater when testing highly fit, disabled individuals. Most wheelchair ergometer protocols hold velocity constant while the braking force of the instrument is increased. A few researchers have experimented with protocols that maintain a constant braking force while the propulsion velocity is increased (24, 25), but these are perceived to be more stressful by the wheelchair user. Glaser and coworkers (46) have developed a graded wheelchair ergometer test employing up to five submaximal 4-minute exercise bouts (with 5-minute recovery periods). The steady-rate relationships they obtained between power output and $\dot{V}O_2$, $\dot{V}E$, or HR (over a range of 5–25 W) are illustrated in Figure 13.6. Peak oxygen uptake and maximal PO could later be predicted by extrapolating the submaximal HR data (usually linear with respect to $\dot{V}O_2$ and PO) to estimated maxima (with the additional caveat cited below) (70).

Submaximal, discontinuous arm-crank ergometry to predict aerobic fitness can also be based upon the steady-rate HR responses achieved at fixed PO levels. For clinicians or rehabilitation specialists with access to arm-crank devices, a "cookbook" approach has been developed by Kofsky and colleagues (29, 71), which utilizes submaximal exercise to accurately predict $\dot{V}O_2$ peak values. In brief, three submaximal power outputs are attempted (each lasting 4–6 minutes), and the HR responses are entered into gender- and age-specific regression equations for the prediction of $\dot{V}O_2$peak (Fig. 13.7). Due to the greater mechanical efficiency of arm cranking, a lower

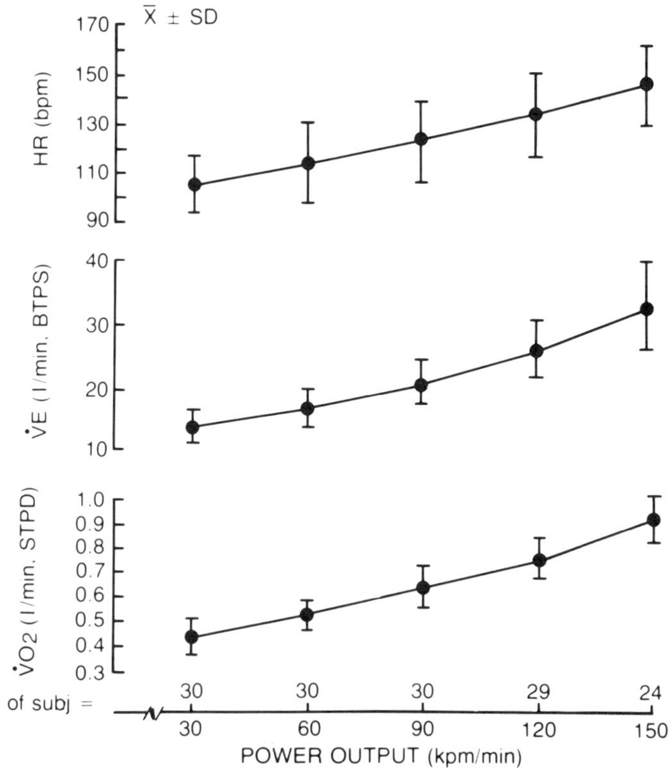

Figure 13.6. Steady-rate relationships between wheelchair ergometer power output and oxygen uptake ($\dot{V}O_2$), pulmonary ventilation ($\dot{V}_E$), and heart rate (HR) for 30 able-bodied female subjects. (Modified from Glaser RM, Foley DM, Laubach LL, et al.: An exercise test to evaluate fitness for wheelchair activity. *Paraplegia* 16:344–345, 1978–79.)

physiologic stress is elicited than for wheelchair testing at comparable power outputs, and higher PO levels (approximately 2X) must normally be employed while performing arm-crank ergometry (41, 43). In addition, the maximal HR for arm exercise (using either wheelchair or arm-crank modalities) has been reported to be 10-20 beats·min^{-1} lower than for strenuous leg effort (70, 72, 73). This should be taken into account when predicting maximal HR by the usual formula: HRmax = 220 beats·min^{-1} minus age in years. Of course, the use of exercise HR as an index of fitness cannot be effectively employed in those with damaged autonomic control of the heart, or with patients who are taking medications that inhibit cardioacceleration.

Maximal exercise testing permits direct determination of $\dot{V}O_2$peak and physical performance during wheelchair or arm-crank ergometry. For either technique, the discontinuous submaximal exercise protocol (described above) can be modified by increasing the number of exercise bouts until a point of volitional fatigue (or limiting symptoms) is reached. A disadvantage of such an exercise design is the extensive time that may be required to complete the test. In addition, numerous exercise bouts may contribute to peripheral fatigue, possibly causing $\dot{V}O_2$peak and maximal PO to be lower than for the shorter duration exercise of continuous protocols. Therefore, if actual peak data are desired and the patient is at low risk, continuous exercise protocols are advantageous. An example of such a wheelchair protocol is one whereby the patient begins to exercise at a relatively low PO (e.g., 50% predicted $\dot{V}O_2$peak), and exercise intensity is subsequently increased (by raising braking force, velocity, or both) by predetermined increments every 1–2 minutes until maximal effort is achieved (5,

STEP 1: DISCONTINUOUS FOREARM ERGOMETER TEST

THREE 5-MINUTE SUBMAXIMAL POWER OUTPUTS AT 40 %, 60 % AND 80 % OF PREDICTED AGE-ADJUSTED MAXIMAL HEART RATE.

STEP 2: POWER OUTPUT - $\dot{V}O_2$ EQUIVALENCY CALCULATION

$\dot{V}O_2$ (ML) = POWER OUTPUT (WATTS) x 18.2 - 395.2

$\dot{V}O_2$ (ML) = POWER OUTPUT (WATTS) x 17.6 + 352.8

STEP 3: ÅSTRAND-RYHMING NOMOGRAM

$$\dot{V}O_2\text{MAX (ML)} = \dot{V}O_2\text{(ML)} \times \frac{(195 - 61)}{(\text{HR} - 61)} \times \text{AGE CORRECTION}$$

$$\dot{V}O_2\text{MAX (ML)} = \dot{V}O_2\text{(ML)} \times \frac{(198 - 72)}{(\text{HR} - 72)} \times \text{AGE CORRECTION}$$

WHERE HR IS THE SUBMAXIMAL STEADY-STATE HEART RATE,
$\dot{V}O_2$(ML) IS THE CALCULATED SUBMAXIMAL STEADY-STATE VO_2 (FROM STEP 2), AND,
AGE CORRECTION IS THE ASTRAND-RYHMING AGE CORRECTION FACTOR.

Figure 13.7. The University of Toronto protocol for estimating $\dot{V}O_2$peak in wheelchair users. (From Davis GM, Jackson RW, Shephard RJ: Sports and recreation for the physically disabled. In Strauss RH (ed): *Sports Medicine*. Philadelphia, WB Saunders Co., 1984 p 294).

6, 24, 29, 32, 74–78). Power output increments of 4–8 $W \cdot min^{-1}$ have been used for wheelchair ergometry, whereas increments of 8–12 $W \cdot min^{-1}$ have been used for arm-crank testing. A short submaximal pretest may be useful to adjust the initial PO level and magnitude of the resistance increment so that the maximal test can be completed in 8–12 minutes.

Fitness Status of the Disabled

Individuals who use wheelchairs often vary widely in their levels of cardiorespiratory fitness and muscular strength; some are seriously incapacitated, while others achieve fitness levels that compare favorably with moderately trained able-bodied adults. In a classic study, Zwiren and Bar-Or (15) compared the maximal exercise responses of wheelchair athletes (WA) and wheelchair sedentary (WS) individuals with able-bodied (AB) athletic subjects. They noted that although there were no intergroup differences of heart rate during maximal arm-crank ergometry, the $\dot{V}O_2$peak of WA subjects was only 8% below that of the AB individuals, and fully 44% greater than that of the WS group. In addition, WA subjects exhibited higher peak $\dot{V}$E and peak oxygen pulse ($\dot{V}O_2 \cdot HR^{-1}$), and lower submaximal HR at fixed PO intensities. Kofsky and coworkers (29) observed that paralytic subjects of "athletic" or "active" (regular exercise at least once per week) backgrounds were similar in terms of maximal aerobic power (2.52 and 2.42 $l \cdot min^{-1}$, respectively), but that both were significantly more fit than inactive subjects (1.63 $l \cdot min^{-1}$).

The finding of such high aerobic fitness levels in elite wheelchair athletes, nearly comparable to those of sedentary, able-bodied individuals of similar age, has been confirmed by other researchers (12, 64, 79–81). Cameron and colleagues (23) noted that $\dot{V}O_2$peaks observed during wheelchair ergometry were highest in track (37.4 $ml \cdot kg^{-1} \cdot min^{-1}$) and swimming (34.6 $ml \cdot kg^{-1} \cdot min^{-1}$) athletes competing in international sports competitions. Gandee et al. (81) observed a forearm crank $\dot{V}O_2$peak of 64 $ml \cdot kg^{-1} \cdot min^{-1}$ in a bilateral above-knee amputee who was a "world class" wheelchair marathon racer. The highest reported values for traumatic tetraplegia have been 17–20 $ml \cdot kg^{-1} \cdot min^{-1}$ (82), although tetraplegics of a traumatic etiology may develop cardiorespiratory fitness levels analogous to their paraplegic counterparts (24, 25).

In contrast, the $\dot{V}O_2$peak of sedentary or deconditioned disabled adults is usually quite low. Middle-aged (50–60 yr) and elderly (80–90 yr) wheelchair users in one study displayed peak cardiorespiratory fitness levels in the range of 5–12 $ml \cdot kg^{-1} \cdot min^{-1}$ (83). Even lower values have been reported for spinal injured adults confined to bed during the postacute phase of rehabilitation (84, 85). As commented upon by several clinicians (8, 86–88), such low levels of cardiorespiratory fitness make difficult the prescription of fitness training, as these individuals often display orthostatic or exercise intolerance.

The results of submaximal fitness tests are sometimes difficult to interpret in subjects with lower-limb disabilities. Both the arm-crank and wheelchair ergometers require the use of relatively small muscle groups (10, 89, 90), resulting in low mechanical efficiencies of work (50, 63, 68, 69, 90). In consequence, the heart rate may be high for a given power output at a submaximal intensity of effort (9, 50, 63, 91). One further difficulty encountered when assessing cardiorespiratory fitness at submaximal levels is the tendency of tetraplegic and paraplegic subjects to display a marked circulatory "hypokinesis" compared to their able-bodied counterparts (14, 85, 92–95). This may reflect venous pooling in the lower extremities, secondary to a disruption of the central sympathetic vasomotor and cardioacceleratory outflow below the level of spinal cord trauma (14, 96). In contrast, tetraplegics sustaining complete cord damage above the second thoracic vertebra in addition to vasomotor dysfunction are dependent upon the withdrawal of vagal activity for increases of exercise heart rate (97, 98).

Central hemodynamic data generally confirm the preceding theoretical limitations to exercise in wheelchair users (Fig. 13.8). Davis and coworkers (99, 100) observed that during exercise intensities ranging from light to severe exertion, stroke volumes were 76–80 ml in sports participants, but only 55–56 ml in sedentary men. The authors suggested that venous pooling was likely responsible for circulatory "hypokinesis" in both groups, but might be lessened by regular participation in exercise or sports training regimens. VanLoan and associates (101) estimated maximal cardiac outputs during arm cranking of 17.2 $l \cdot min^{-1}$, 10.5 $l \cdot min^{-1}$ and 5.7 $l \cdot min^{-1}$ in able-bodied, paraplegic, and tetraplegic subjects, respectively. Stroke volumes for the disabled subjects (52–58 ml) were only one-half that of their able-bodied counterparts. Figoni (93, 94, 102, 103) also found significantly reduced exercise stroke volumes in tetraplegics (36–54 ml) compared to able-bodied men (68–78 ml), matching dramatically diminished cardiac outputs. Other researchers (84, 85, 92, 96) have provided suggestive evidence supporting the view that restrictions of exercise capacity in wheelchair users are secondary to reduced stroke volume and cardiac output arising from moderate to severe venous pooling in paralyzed muscles.

Upper-Body Strength Assessment

Early work on the muscular strength and daily energy requirements of those acquiring neuromuscular impairments was accomplished at the Danish Infantile Paralysis Association (104–107). Its research sought to define the minimal levels of muscular strength required by poliomyelitis victims to perform daily tasks, assessed by handgrip force and cable tensiometry. Since that time, many popular techniques have been used to assess the muscular performance of disabled adults, including handgrip dynamometry (15, 25, 108), the repetitive lifting of free weights (5, 109, 110), static cable tensiometry upon upper-limb musculature (11, 111, 112), and, more recently, measurements of isokinetic moment and power at the shoulder, elbow, and wrist joints (25, 79, 80).

In healthy, able-bodied subjects, static handgrip force has been reported to be a good predictor ($r = 0.80$) of overall muscle strength (10). A single measure of dominant handgrip force was similarly well correlated ($r = 0.79$) with total upper-body isokinetic strength in 49 wheelchair-dependent adults (100). Japanese researchers (113) reported that among 280 disabled factory workers, the grasping force of traumatic paraplegics (382 N) was slightly greater than that of able-bodied (363 N) or poliomyelitic (313 N) subjects. The average grip forces of cerebral palsied, muscular dystrophic, or tetraplegic individuals were considerably lower. In contrast, highly fit wheelchair marathon racers may record values in excess of 700 N (12, 114, 115)! Although few differences in handgrip strength have been observed among paraplegics classified on the basis of anatomic or functional disability gradings (25), several authors have noted that marked dif-

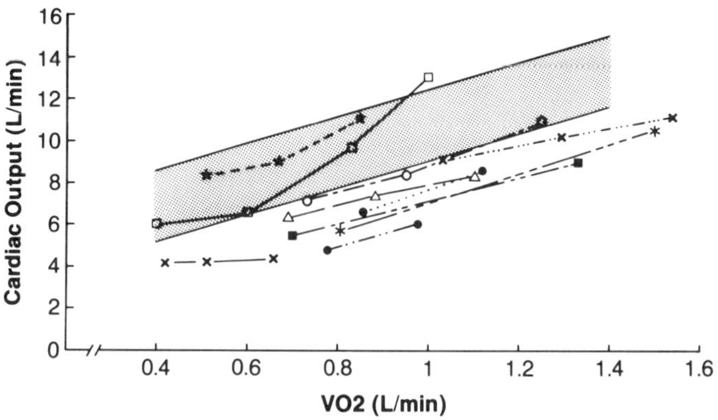

Figure 13.8. Cardiac output versus oxygen consumption during steady-state arm crank exercise for disabled subjects from several studies. Shaded area represents normal range for able-bodied adults performing arm ergometry (consisting of 181 observations cited in Davis GM: *Cardiovascular Fitness and Muscular Fitness in Lower-Limb Disabled Males*. Toronto, University of Toronto Press, 1985). Symbols represent data from studies cited in text: (■) reference 14; (□) reference 41; (★) reference 42; (●) reference 84; (✖) references 93, 94, 102, 103; (○, △) references 99, 100; (∗) reference 101.

ferences of grip force exist among wheelchair users classified according to their gender and level of habitual physical activity (26, 27, 29). Thus, for the clinician or health professional lacking more sophisticated strength testing equipment, handgrip dynamometry provides a fair basis for assessment of upper-limb strength in the wheelchair-dependent population (for normative standards see reference 71).

Strength measurements based upon cable tensiometry have many advantages in a nonlaboratory setting, including ease of use, portability, and low cost. When precautions are taken to minimize possible sources of intra- and interobserver measurement error (usually 9–13%) (112), isometric dynamometry offers a reliable and acceptable strategy for assessing the upper-body strength of paralyzed individuals. Kofsky and associates (29, 116, 117) demonstrated that the sum of isometric elbow flexion, elbow extension, and shoulder extension was most effective in predicting isokinetic total upper-body strength ($r = 0.82$) or $\dot{V}O_2$peak ($r = 0.65$) in wheelchair users. Furthermore (as illustrated in Fig. 13.9), the total static strength of inactive subjects was significantly lower than that of recreational sports participants or elite disabled athletes (23, 80, 111, 114, 118). In contrast, there are few differences among individuals classified according to ana-

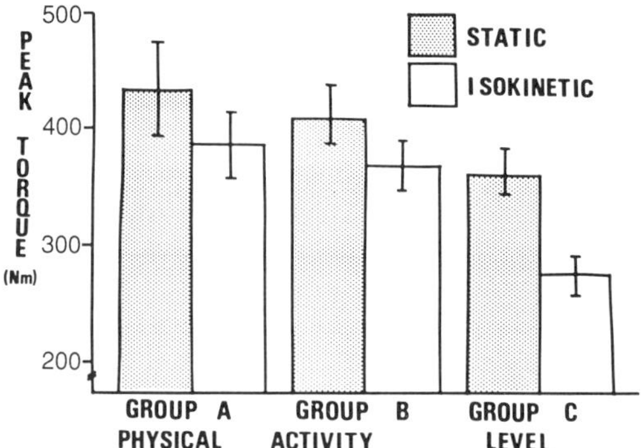

Figure 13.9. Static and isokinetic strength in wheelchair users with varying activity levels. Static measurements were evaluated as the sum of four forces (N) using cable tensiometry. Isokinetic measurements were evaluated as the sum of six peak torques (Nm) during CYBEX dynamometry at 1.05 rad·sec^{-1}. Group A = national caliber athletes; Group B = recreational sportsmen, and Group C = sedentary. (From Davis GM, Jackson RW, Shephard RJ: Sports and recreation for the physically disabled. In Strauss RH (ed): *Sports Medicine*. Philadelphia, WB Saunders Co., 1984, p 296).

tomic or functional disability criteria, supporting the view that in paraplegics there seems to be a poor correlation between the site of spinal cord lesion and isometric strength (26, 117).

Although not without its critics, isokinetic testing is probably the most advanced laboratory technique for the assessment of muscle function. However, only recently has this procedure been applied to upper-extremity testing in a wheelchair-dependent population (27, 29, 89). The basic methodology comprises the calculation of peak torque (a.k.a. moment), peak power, average power, and total work of shoulder and elbow flexion/extension over joint-specific velocities ranging from 1.05–5.24 rad·sec^{-1} (114). Davis and others (10, 26) observed a positive relationship between the level of habitual physical activity and upper-body isokinetic strength in 42 paraplegic males (Figure 13.9). Tupling and coworkers (119, 120) further noted that wheelchair impulse generation (assessed using a force platform) was strongly related to the isokinetic strength of upper-body musculature. For the medical practitioner, therapist, or exercise scientist with access to such equipment, isokinetic strength and endurance testing is the optimal choice for the assessment of muscle function in the wheelchair-dependent population (see references 10 and 26 for testing methodology).

EXERCISE PRESCRIPTION

General Principles

Need for Exercise Training

The elevated physiologic stresses and rapid fatigue encountered during wheelchair locomotion may be due in part to the patient's poor fitness for arm exercise (15, 46, 50, 54, 121). Such stresses can discourage wheelchair use of sufficient intensity and duration to maintain muscular or cardiorespiratory fitness, eventually leading to a sedentary life-style. Inactivity subsequently results in further loss of fitness, compounding rehabilitation problems (121). Engel and Hildebrandt (54) have stated that typical daily wheelchair activity was an insufficient stimulus to tax the cardiorespiratory system, and supplementary arm exercise training is required for fitness gains. Higher physical fitness normally lowers the relative stresses for wheelchair locomotion and permits greater societal participation by wheelchair users.

Basic Principles of Arm Exercise Training

The development of upper-body strength and cardiorespiratory fitness is a desirable goal for all wheelchair users. Generally, the principle of training "overload" should be followed (33, 44, 45, 47, 122), whereby exercise is performed at an intensity beyond that normally encountered during daily activities. With improved physical fitness and performance, exercise intensity or duration may be further increased until desired fitness goals are attained. To maintain optimal fitness levels, exercise training must be continued, but further "overload" is unnecessary. If exercise is discontinued, detraining will occur and fitness gains will be lost in several weeks (45, 47, 123, 124).

Strength conditioning of the upper-body musculature can be accomplished using high-resistance, low-repetition dynamic exercises. Isotonic weight training has been used extensively for this purpose, and much equipment is readily available. Recently, specialized devices have become available to permit isokinetic training, and this may improve muscle function to a greater degree throughout a larger range of motion than traditional strength training modalities (47, 99). Isometric exercise for wheelchair users is not recommended because such training is not effective throughout the full range of movement, blood flow through the muscles is occluded during the contractions, and blood pressure responses may become excessive (122, 125).

The "specificity of exercise" concept suggests that activities that employ the same muscles and joint movements as those used during wheelchair propulsion may be the most effective for improving daily wheelchair performance (91, 121). However, vigorous, prolonged wheelchair-type exercises may also lead to "over-use syndrome" (a general feeling of malaise and/or orthopaedic problems), especially in disabled athletes. To deter this, arm cranking and alternative exercises (e.g., rowing, swimming) have been widely practiced as a supplement to physical fitness conditioning (118, 126). Although arm exercise has been reported to increase cardiorespiratory fitness in wheelchair users (indicated by significant increases of maximal PO and $\dot{V}O_2$peak), arm training cannot promote the high aerobic fitness levels that are accomplished by leg exercise in able-bodied individuals. Additionally, the small muscle mass employed rarely elevates oxygen consumption to sufficiently high levels for long enough durations for marked central circulatory training effects to take place (15, 32, 54, 68, 127, 128). Instead, major improvements in exercise performance are primarily due to peripheral adaptations within the active musculature such as hypertrophy, increased vascularity, higher mitochondrial density, and enhanced concentrations of oxidative enzymes.

Exercise Training Protocols

Endurance (aerobic) training protocols can be either discontinuous or continuous in nature. Initially, exercise intensity is set at a certain percentage of the HR range (e.g., 60–90% of maximal HR reserve corresponding to 50–85% of $\dot{V}O_2$peak), determined from cardiorespiratory stress tests (6, 33, 39, 45, 47, 122, 123). However, with improved fitness, target HR is normally achieved at higher PO levels, permitting a greater training stimulus. As previously noted, HR is a poor criterion to indicate relative exercise stress in patients with diminished autonomic function (e.g., tetraplegics). The exercise duration for continuous training protocols is optimally 15–60 minutes per session (6, 61, 129, 130). In contrast, exercise bouts for discontinuous (a.k.a. "interval") training programs are shorter (approximately 3–5 minutes), and are typically separated by recovery periods of equal duration. Guidelines for construction of interval training programs have previously been described by Fox and Mathews (45). Briefly, the intensity, duration, and number of exercise bouts, as well as the duration of recovery periods and the number of exercise sets, can all be selectively manipulated to train the desired energy system (aerobic and/or anaerobic). The following sections present an overview of recent research assessing the fitness levels and effects of chronic arm exercise in wheelchair users.

The "Fitness Factors"

Although comprehensive reviews describing the interrelationship of frequency, intensity, duration, and exercise modality (the so-called "Fitness Factors") have been undertaken with reference to the able-bodied (131–135), few researchers have yet to address similar questions in the wheelchair-dependent population. In wheelchair users possessing only a marginal aerobic reserve, subtle differences in the intensity and duration of an exercise task may result in quite dissimilar training effects. Huang and coworkers (76) noted that in a single training session, a fixed amount of work (5 W·hr) could be completed by unfit wheelchair users with lower physiologic stress using continuous (30 W for 10 min) or interval (60 W for 0.5 min followed by 0.5 min recovery, repeated 10 times) exercise patterns than for incremental, graded effort (10, 20, 30, 40, 50 W for 2 min each). Graded exercise resulted in severe physiologic disturbance; heart rates were 11–16 beats·min^{-1} greater than for interval or continuous exercise, with oxygen consumptions and serum lactates averaging 24% higher. Thus, interval training would seem to be more tolerable for the majority of nonathletic wheelchair users.

The majority of able-bodied training studies have pointed to exercise duration (or daily training volume) as the preeminent factor for cardiorespiratory fitness improvements when effort exceeds a minimum threshold intensity (31). However, an important exception to this rule must be noted in cases in which subjects have very low initial fitness levels or restricted daily energy expenditures. Shephard (135) found that the intensity of exercise may assume a larger role when the initial fitness level or training status of the participants is very low. In support of this view, Davis and associates (99, 118) observed that among sedentary paraplegics undertaking fitness conditioning, subjects employing higher intensity programs realized the largest gains of $\dot{V}O_2$peak, muscular strength, and physical performance. Wheelchair users who trained at 70% of their $\dot{V}O_2$peak for 40 minutes achieved nearly 19% increases of maximal aerobic power, primarily due to marked augmentation of cardiac output and stroke volume (Fig. 13.10). Subjects following fitness programs of shorter duration or lower intensity generally realized smaller improvements. The authors suggested that in wheelchair users of very low fitness level (especially immediate posttraumatic paraplegics), training intensity is initially a more important determinant of improved cardiovascular performance than exercise duration.

Training in a wheelchair or with a wheelchair ergometer has proven useful when the task specificity is important to everyday ambulation or sports performance (136, 137). Several authors have quantified the advantages of wheelchair training in reducing submaximal energy expenditure and physiologic stress (50, 54, 121). However, in tetraplegics and high-lesion paraplegics, some researchers (56, 68) have taken a less optimistic view of the benefits of wheelchair exercise by suggesting that the limited effective muscle mass becomes fatigued too quickly to permit the circulatory system to be taxed adequately for a conditioning response. The clinician or exercise specialist recommending this modality of physical activity must also stress the importance of maintaining proper exercise intensity (greater than 60% $\dot{V}O_2$peak monitored via externally palpated heart rate) and duration (exceeding 30 minutes) (30, 31).

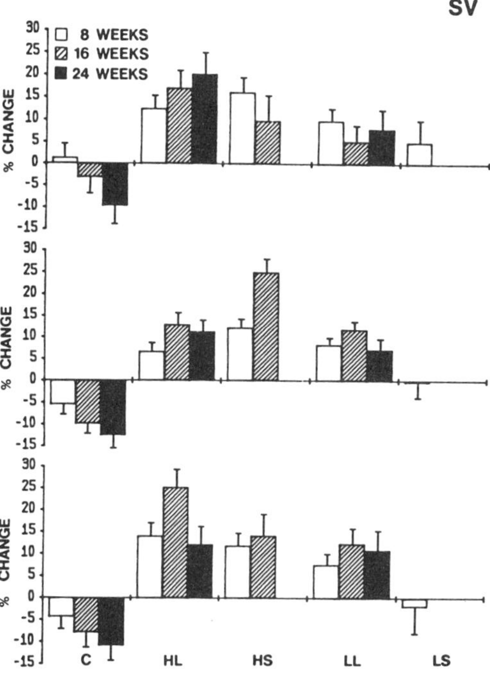

Figure 13.10. Per cent change of stroke volume (*SV*) in control (C), *HL* (High Intensity, Long Duration), *HS* (High Intensity, Short Duration), *LL* (Low Intensity, Long Duration), and *LS* (Low Intensity, Short Duration) groups after 8, 16, and 24 weeks of arm-crank training (See text for explanation of training programs). *Top, middle,* and *bottom* panels are low submaximal (115–126 beats·min^{-1}), moderate submaximal (130–140 beats·min^{-1}), and heavy submaximal (145–155 beats·min^{-1}) arm-crank ergometry. Values are mean per cent change ± SE. (From Davis GM: *Cardiovascular Fitness and Muscular Fitness in Lower-Limb Disabled Males.* Toronto, University of Toronto Press, 1985, p 181.)

The arm-crank ergometer has also traditionally been a popular rehabilitation and training apparatus, since its power output can be precisely monitored and the device makes efficient use of available space (77, 138, 139). A secondary advantage for the clinician or therapist is the ability to carefully monitor a patient's physiologic responses and daily progress to the training regimen. Early researchers (5, 6) demonstrated that experienced wheelchair users were able to increase their $\dot{V}O_2$peak by 12–19% after 7–20 weeks of training. In tetraplegics of very low initial fitness level, DiCarlo (140) quantified even larger gains of cardiorespiratory fitness (67%) and maximal power output (55%) following only 5 weeks of arm cranking. However, clinicians and physical therapists critical of arm-crank training have focused on its lack of specificity to everyday locomotion (48, 121, 141), inconsistent gains of fitness (142), or minimal increments of physical performance in patients with severely restricted usable muscle mass (76, 143).

Upper-body calisthenics, weight training, swimming, and sports participation constitute a third modality for fitness conditioning with particular merits and drawbacks. Like wheelchair training, these "mixed modes" usually have direct specificity to the daily activities and interests of wheelchair users (137). Calisthenics and weight training can augment upper-body strength as well as maximal aerobic capacity (8, 144). Swimming may enhance cardiorespiratory fitness (145, 146). Sports participation (e.g., tennis, basketball, downhill amputee skiing) can be a positive force to improve overall body kinesthesis and wheelchair mobility (8, 87). On the other hand, the intermittent nature of these activities may make them less desirable than arm-crank ergometry as a means of eliciting gains of cardiovascular fitness.

Strength Training

Despite the obvious practical importance of upper-extremity strength and endurance for wheelchair users, there have been few studies of strength training in these individuals. Both Gairdner (109) and Walsh and Steadward (147) have recommended specific strength training exercises for disabled persons based on common principles of muscle physiology in the able-bodied (148) or specific biomechanical studies of wheelchair users (119, 120, 141). However, lacking specific research into strength training determinants as applied to the disabled population, we are constrained to propose only modifications of conventional wisdom (149).

As a general rule, a muscle group worked near its maximal force-generating capacity will increase in strength (150, 151). This "overload" can be applied using free weights, pulleys and springs, immovable bars and cables, or by manipulating a variety of isokinetic devices. The important point is that unlike cardiorespiratory fitness gains, improvements of muscle function are generally governed by the relative *intensity* of the "overload" and not by the specific strength training modality (149, 151). Certain methods make more efficient use of time, lend themselves to precise "overload" application, or stress the muscle over a wider range of joint motions. In the wheelchair-dependent population, three strength and endurance conditioning techniques have been used most frequently: a) progressive resistance strength training; b) isometric training; and c) isokinetic training. While we will deal with the scientific evidence surrounding the efficacy of each modality in a later section, the medical practitioner and physical therapist may prescribe any or all of these techniques with reasonable safety.

Prior research has essentially focused upon *progressive resistance isotonic training* in terms of establishing the optimal number of sets and repetitions of a strength task, and the weekly frequency and intensity of exercise necessary to elicit gains of muscular performance (151). McArdle and associates (152) summarized the basic principles of strength conditioning prescription: a) In the first 6 weeks of a conditioning program, as little as one repetition of a maximal effort each week will increase a muscle's force-generating capacity. b) Performing between three and nine repetitions of a maximal effort is optimal for each set. c) There seems to be no difference in the sequence of weight training with different percentages of a maximal effort as long as at least one set includes 10 repetitions of a maximal effort. d) More than one set of multiple repetitions is necessary for strength increases especially after the first 6 weeks. e) When strength conditioning involves several different muscle groups, training four to five times per week is less effective than training two to three times per week. f) For a given weight load, there is some evidence that "fast lifting" is superior to "slow lifting" for strength improvements. g) One specific exercise modality is not inherently superior to another in terms of eliciting performance gains.

Both *isometric* and *isokinetic exercise* have been less well studied as far as the determinants of a training effect are concerned (149). However, isokinetic strength conditioning bears many similarities to progressive resistance isotonic exercise, and the guidelines listed above are likely analogous. Conversely, isometric training is highly task-specific; that is, a muscle group trained statically presents largest strength gains when tested statically, especially at the specific joint angle and body position at which training occurred (152). This characteristic of high task-specificity and, occasionally, excessive blood pressure responses makes isometric strength training less desirable from a rehabilitation point of view than dynamic exercise modes.

CHRONIC ADAPTATIONS TO TRAINING

Cardiorespiratory Alterations to Upper-Body Training

The concept that regular physical activity enhances cardiorespiratory fitness and provides some defense against coronary artery atherosclerosis has become generally accepted by the public. This viewpoint, which has been actively promoted by physical educators, clinicians, and researchers, has received major funding from healthcare organizations, governments, and the private sector (37, 153). That endurance training significantly enhances the cardiorespiratory function of healthy, able-bodied adults is beyond dispute. Scientific evidence for the "exercise hypothesis" has been competently reviewed by Haskell (154). Less well defined are the possible immediate and long-term sequelae of an active life-style for wheelchair-dependent individuals (10, 87, 155–158).

Some investigators have suggested that spinal cord-injured persons who follow adequate training regimens make very good physiologic and psychologic adjustment to their disability (159–161). However, such evidence is based largely upon cross-sectional or anecdotal comparisons between untrained and highly trained wheelchair users. A study of college-aged wheelchair basketball players and their able-bodied cohorts revealed no differences in their ability to work with the upper trunk and arm muscles, suggesting that the disabled athletes had adjusted quite well to their disability (75). Competitors in wheelchair marathon events routinely expend 33–54 $kJ \cdot min^{-1}$ (depending on the participant's skill and fitness level), comparable to a 6–8 $km \cdot hr^{-1}$ walk/run pace or a 16 $km \cdot hr^{-1}$ cycling pace for able-bodied subjects (115, 162). Yet, while it is interesting to compare disabled athletes to their able-bodied counterparts, the cross-sectional approach is plainly limited by possible genetic predisposition for superior performance among athletes, lack of quantification of their training programs, and the cumulative effects of long periods of physical conditioning begun at an early age when dimensional and morphological changes are more apt to occur.

The arm-crank ergometer (ACE, Fig. 13.5) has been a popular choice for those laboratories undertaking clinical exercise testing and rehabilitation programs for persons with spinal cord trauma (24, 77, 88, 138). Nilsson and colleagues (5) found that after only 7 weeks of training, disabled men were able to perform maximal ACE at a 12% higher $\dot{V}O_2$peak and a 31% greater physical working capacity. Comparable studies (6, 84–86, 138, 140, 163) have demonstrated similar increments of peak aerobic power ranging from 19–61%. Davis and coworkers (99, 100) compared four ACE training programs differing in the daily intensity (50% or 70% $\dot{V}O_2$peak) or duration (20 or 40 minutes) of exercise stress. The authors noted that wheelchair users following the high-intensity, long-duration (70% $\dot{V}O_2$peak for 40 minutes) training regimen developed the greatest gains of cardiorespiratory fitness as assessed by cardiac output, stroke volume (Fig. 13.10) and $\dot{V}O_2$peak. Other training groups developed smaller increments of fitness. Training-induced alterations of central hemodynamics were perceived to be due to increased venous return (decreased lower-limb blood pooling) or enhanced muscle utilization of oxygen following training, as no changes of myocardial dimensions or performance were observed (126).

The temporal changes of maximal aerobic power and physical work capacity with wheelchair or wheelchair ergometer (WERG; Fig. 13.5) training are quite similar to ACE fitness programs. After training regimens of 4–20 weeks' duration, $\dot{V}O_2$peak was improved from 9–35%, and performance ability augmented by 31–44% (39, 54, 74, 121). Glaser and associates (50, 121) have found WERG interval training to be particularly well suited to wheelchair users since it mimics the periodicity of normal, daily wheelchair propulsion and may produce nearly 30% increments of submaximal PO for given levels of physiologic stress. As yet, we are unaware of any studies that have investigated the hemodynamic alterations consequent upon WERG training, so augmented $\dot{V}O_2$peak may be due to either "central" and/or "peripheral"adaptations.

Swimming has also been a popular exercise regimen for the disabled since it requires little lower-limb involvement for satisfactory force generation in the water (146, 164, 165). In a 3-year clinical rehabilitation program (145), a 300% increase in fitness score was observed in 60 paraplegics following therapeutic swimming programs. In contrast, Ornstein et al. (166) noted $\dot{V}O_2$peak was unchanged after 8 weeks of aerobic swimming in previously sedentary disabled males. Their lack of improvement may have been the result of testing cardiorespiratory fitness via ACE, as there is evidence that swim training is task-specific, and possible fitness gains may not be detected using arm ergometry (167).

Muscle Strength Training

An important consideration in the daily life-style of wheelchair users is their proficiency in overcoming the many physical limitations of the external environment such as street curbs, ramps, and uneven terrain. Yet, despite the obvious practical importance of strength and endurance to the everyday life of paraplegics, there have been few studies of strength conditioning in such individuals (144, 147). Nilsson and colleagues (5) observed that whereas limb girth was unchanged after training, dynamic strength and muscular endurance (repetitive lifting of free weights) were augmented by 19% and 80%, respectively. Other researchers (23, 79, 114, 168) have determined that elbow flexion and extension peak forces are strongly associated with the type of physical training performed by disabled athletes. Participants in sports activities requiring upper-body strength display isokinetic muscle forces 50% higher than other athletes. As we have previously noted (114, 118), sedentary wheelchair users following conditioning programs of high intensity (arm-crank ergometry at greater than 70% $\dot{V}O_2$peak) improved isokinetic strength of shoulder flexors and elbow extensors more than those training at lower exercise intensities (Fig. 13.11).

Muscle biopsy studies (80, 169) have also demonstrated that disabled athletes have skeletal muscle fiber diameters two to three times anticipated normal values with an overwhelming predominance of fast-twitch types (170). Some elite wheelchair athletes have morphological characteristics and muscle enzyme activities equal to those of their able-bodied counterparts (169).

The Psychosocial Benefits of Exercise

The psychic reaction of the individual to spinal cord injury, deformity, and eventual lower-limb impairment results from a complex interaction of many contingent factors. These naturally include the postmorbid body image, feelings of self-esteem, and awareness of physical disability as it affects current life-style. However, the attitudes and beliefs held prior to injury are also important (171), as is the extent of their modification by trauma. Ultimately, societal stereotypes and the degree of acceptance of the disabled as fully functional members of society probably most affect the disabled individual's psychosocial outcome.

Previous authors have commented upon the effect of a neuromuscular disorder upon the individual's psychological adjustment (172–175), although this may be as dependent upon age, gender, locus and etiology (175, 176) of the lesion as upon perception of the handicap (177). Harper (173) observed no differences in personality traits between adolescents with traumatic versus congenital etiology of disability, although both groups were prone to emotional problems of poor self-perception and negative body-image during physical rehabilitation. In contrast, Shephard and associates (175, 178) found that more than 86% of wheelchair-dependent men and women could be correctly classified as to severity of injury (having cervical, thoracic, or low-level spinal cord lesions) using a variety of psychosocial attributes and attitudes towards physical activity (Fig.13.12).

Current societal stereotypes of "accept-

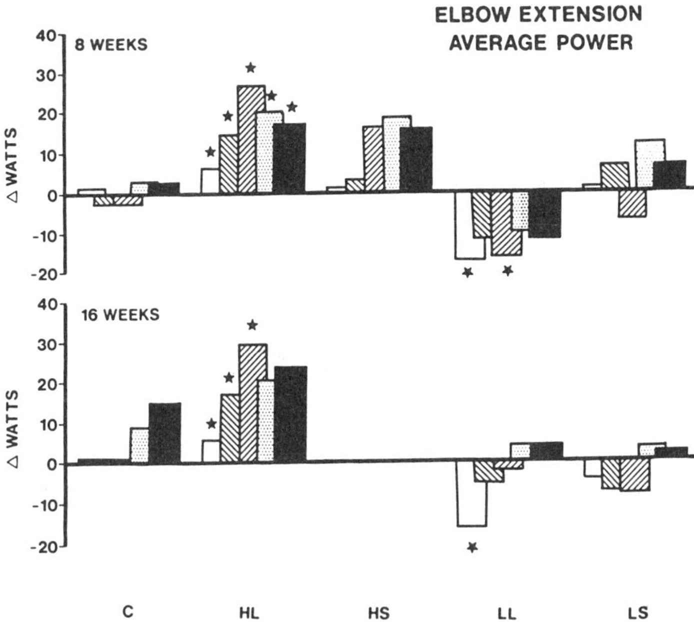

Figure 13.11. Change of elbow extension average power in control (C), *HL* (High Intensity, Long Duration), *HS* (High Intensity, Short Duration), *LL* (Low Intensity, Long Duration), and *LS* (Low Intensity, Short Duration) groups after 8 and 16 weeks of arm-crank training. (See text for explanation of training programs.) Values are mean change from initial scores ± SE. Bar clusters denote isokinetic velocities of 1.05 (open), 2.09 (right diagonal), 3.14 (left diagonal), 4.19 (screen) and 5.24 (solid) rad·sec^{-1}. * indicate significant differences from pretraining scores ($p \leq .02$). (Cited in Davis GM, Shephard RJ, Ward GR: Alteration of dynamic strength following forearm crank training of disabled subjects. *Med Sci Sports Exerc* 16:147, 1984.)

able" disability sometimes place an additional burden upon the physically handicapped. Able-bodied individuals seem to react more favorably to wheelchair-dependent military veterans than to those who have acquired their disabilities in work or sporting accidents (176). Furthermore, this positive perception appears to improve the veterans' self-esteem relative to disabled individuals of nonmilitary background. Lazar and associates (179) found no appreciable differences of social adjustment or attitudes towards physical disability between paraplegic and able-bodied college students, but the former generally were more ambitious toward achieving cognitive goals. In a thorough review of current psychosocial theory as applied to wheelchair users, Sherrill (180) discussed the implications of stigmatization, stereotyping, and discrimination upon the individual's feelings of self-concept.

If sports participation or fitness training has any basis in improving the physical fitness of disabled individuals, it seems reasonable to anticipate some positive psychological benefits in terms of perceptions of self-worth and body image. Several authors (159, 160, 175, 178) have documented significant increases of skill, self-concept, and self-acceptance among wheelchair users who participate in recreational exercise or endurance training programs. Interestingly, Godin and coworkers (171) observed that the intention to future exercise was governed more by premorbid exercise pattern and nature of physical disability (traumatic versus congenital) than present exercise habit, gender, or subjective norms.

Despite suggestive evidence that fitness conditioning and sports participation can alter posttraumatic psychosocial adjustment, categorical proof of the "exercise hypothesis" does not yet exist. Further careful research is necessary to document the interactions between current exercise behav-

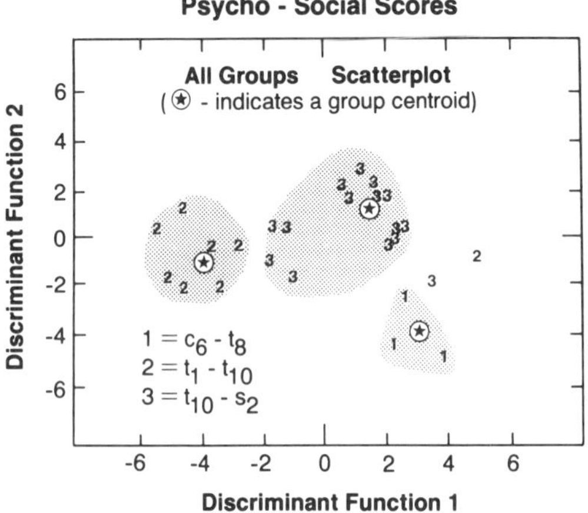

Figure 13.12. Discrimination of site of spinal cord injury based on self-reported psychosocial scores. Subjects were 49 male and female wheelchair users aged 19 to 59 years with cervical, thoracic, or low-level lesions. (Modified from Shephard RJ, Davis GM, Kofsky PR, et al.: Interactions between attitudes, personality and physical activity in the lower-limb disabled. *Can J Appl Sport Sci* 8:173, 1983.)

iors and the underlying personality traits, attitudes, and beliefs of the disabled individual.

SPECIAL EXERCISE PRECAUTIONS, LIMITATIONS, AND PROBLEMS

Besides the usual risks encountered by able-bodied individuals performing strenuous exercise, paralyzed patients may be exposed to additional peril depending upon the level and completeness of their CNS damage, and the resulting motor, sensory, and autonomic dysfunction. Common risks that may be encountered by paraplegics and tetraplegics undertaking exercise programs include autonomic dysreflexia (i.e., inappropriate or unexpected blood pressure responses), orthostatic hypotension, trunk instability, and pressure sores (77, 181–183). Thermoregulation can also be a problem for some disabled patients. However, taking adequate precautions can minimize the risks of exercise for these individuals and many positive benefits can be derived.

Autonomic dysreflexia during arm exercise can be quite hazardous since it can result in extreme hypertension. The condition can be alleviated by appropriate health habits and medical treatment aimed at eliminating noxious stimuli associated with bowel impaction, bladder overdistension, and skin tissue trauma. It is advisable for wheelchair users to empty their bladder prior to exercise, and for a technician to monitor blood pressure and heart rate at regular intervals (77). The occurrence of orthostatic hypotension in an upright posture or during exercise can be reduced by regular orthostatic training (e.g., tilting, standing, ambulation), proper hydration, compression stockings, and physical conditioning. Of course, exercise should be terminated immediately if irregular responses are observed.

To prevent falls due to trunk instability and poor sitting balance, a security belt around the patient's trunk during arm exercise is recommended. It is also essential to incorporate conscientious techniques for pressure relief to prevent decubitus ulcers. These include the use of effective cushions under ischial tuberosities and other weight-bearing areas, and periodically (i.e., every 20–30 minutes) raising the body off the cushion(s) for a short period of time (e.g., 30–60 seconds). Finally, ambient temperature, relative humidity, and patient attire should be carefully considered before permitting strenuous exercise of prolonged duration. The possibility exists that some patients may possess impaired thermoregulatory capacity due to inadequate secretion by sweat glands or impaired cardiovascular system control. Exercise should be terminated if there are signs of overheating.

EXERCISE OF PARALYZED MUSCLES VIA FUNCTIONAL ELECTRICAL STIMULATION

For over 25 years, research aimed at restoring purposeful movements to muscles paralyzed by upper motor neuron impairments (e.g., spinal cord injury, head trauma, stroke) has been conducted using functional electrical stimulation (FES) (184–

186). With the application of recent technologies to this research, more advanced FES systems are emerging with the potential for improving the rehabilitation process. Although single-channel, hand-held stimulators have been used with paralyzed patients for some time, more complex instrumentation has recently become commercially available to permit FES-induced exercise of multiple lower-limb muscles. Still, much research is needed to better understand the role of FES in rehabilitation, and to solve numerous problems for the development of FES instrumentation and protocols that can be used safely.

Besides the enormous bioengineering problems of using FES for precise control of multiple muscles, there are also considerable physiologic problems that can markedly limit FES task performance capability. These are related to the deteriorated condition of the musculoskeletal and cardiorespiratory systems, the nonphysiologic activation pattern of the paralyzed muscles, and the probability that organ system adjustments that normally accompany voluntary exercise may not occur to the same extent with FES-induced exercise (187–189).

Candidates for FES use must have intact and functional motor units (lower motor neurons and the muscle fibers they innervate). This is usually indicated by the presence of the stretch reflex and occasional muscle spasms. FES will probably not be useful in cases of lower motor neuron damage. To be most effective, skin surface electrodes should be located directly over motor points (where motor nerves enter the muscle) of the muscles to be exercised. Motor points can be found by moving an exploratory electrode around the muscle while stimulating at a level that is just above the threshold level of the muscle. At motor points, greater contraction force can be obtained for a given stimulation level. Many of the same principles that have been well established for voluntary exercise can also be used for FES exercise.

Precautions

To prevent injury to the deteriorated muscles, bones, and joints, FES-induced contractions and limb movements should be as smooth as possible. In some patients, this may be difficult to achieve because severe spasms and reflex contractions of other muscles can be triggered by the stimulation. On the other hand, if these patients take pharmacologic agents to relax muscles, the effectiveness of FES may be reduced because of rapid muscle fatigue (187, 188). The maximal force of contraction should be limited to a safe level (e.g., 15 kg for knee extension exercise) because it appears possible to increase muscle strength beyond levels that the bones and joints can withstand. Ramped dynamic contractions of a few seconds' duration (with both concentric and eccentric components) may be safer and more effective than using abrupt forceful isometric contractions. Dynamic movements may result in performance gains throughout the range of motion, enhanced circulation in active muscles, and less severe arterial blood pressure responses (122, 125). With increases in strength and endurance, load resistance progressions should be gradual (187, 188). Since many patients have sensory loss in the paralyzed limbs and cannot experience pain, it is important to check for signs of damage on a regular basis.

It has been suggested that the organ system adjustments normally accompanying voluntary exercise may not occur to the same extent during FES-induced muscular contractions. This is because the FES is peripherally induced, and in effect bypasses the CNS. As a result, normal ANS sympathetic outflow may be deficient (because of inappropriate stimulation and/or CNS damage), leading to a lack of cardioacceleration during FES knee extension exercise in SCI patients (187–189). Thus, exercise performance may be limited by insufficient blood flow to the muscles. Additionally, the potential exists that the active muscles can be overheated because mechanisms that alter blood flow patterns and induce sweating for heat dissipation may not be operative (187, 188). In certain patients (e.g., high-level SCI), autonomic dysreflexia can result in high (>175 mm Hg) blood pressure during FES-induced contractions, indicating that the patient is at risk and the exercise should be discontinued (187, 188). Therefore, it is recommended that blood pressure be monitored during (at least) the initial FES exercise bouts.

Exercise Training with FES

Muscle paralysis typically results in subsequent muscle atrophy, bone demineralization, and diminished cardiorespiratory fitness. FES training of paralyzed muscles has been reported to markedly increase muscle strength and endurance for this form of exercise (188, 190–192). Physiologic mechanisms for improved muscle performance appear to be mostly peripheral in nature, and may include muscle hypertrophy, conversion of fast- to slow-twitch muscle fiber characteristics, increased levels of oxidative enzymes, and higher capillary density (193–202). There is currently no convincing evidence that FES exercise training by itself reverses osteoporosis or significantly improves cardiorespiratory fitness. However, there may be other health benefits, including improved circulation in the exercising limbs (192), temporary alleviation of muscle spasms (192, 203), and improvement of self-image (9, 188).

The scientific literature contains little information about specific protocols and procedures for safe and effective FES exercise training. Most previous FES exercise studies simply involved on-off patterns of stimulation for inducing rhythmic isometric contractions or dynamic contractions without external load resistance (190, 191, 204). Although these techniques have resulted in improved performance of hand and leg muscles, more dramatic results have recently been obtained by using well-established weight training principles in conjunction with FES (188, 192). This has been demonstrated with knee-extension exercise, which was induced by FES of the quadriceps muscles with specially constructed instrumentation. Figure 13.13 illustrates FES knee-extension exercise being conducted with a weight-lifting lever system and closed-loop (feedback) electrical stimulators constructed by Glaser and coworkers (205). By progressively increasing the load resistance imposed and the number of repetitions attempted over a several-

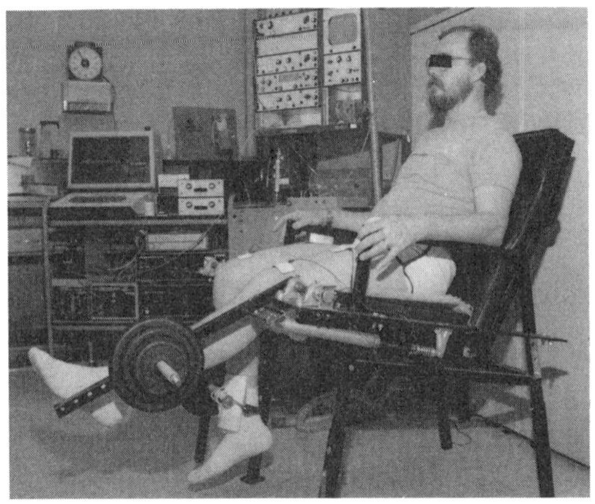

Figure 13.13. Closed-loop electrical stimulator systems used to provide knee-extension exercise. Limb position sensors are coupled to the shaft of the afterload weight levers. (Modified from Glaser RM, Collins SR, Strayer, JR, et al.: A closed-loop stimulator for exercising paralyzed muscles. *Proc Eighth Annual RESNA Conference on Rehabilitation Engineering*. 1985, p 390.)

week period, strength and endurance can gradually be increased toward the desired end-point goals. Figure 13.14 illustrates the load weight progression that was used for knee-extension training of six SCI subjects over a 12-week period (3X per week) by Gruner and colleagues (188). SCI patients who respond well to this FES exercise can commonly lift load weights in excess of 9 kg for two sets of 20 contractions each.

By using a computer to control FES of several lower-limb muscle groups (e.g., quadriceps, hamstrings, gluteus maximus), paraplegics and tetraplegics have been able to pedal bicycle ergometers (206). Figure 13.15 illustrates an SCI patient pedalling a commercial version of this FES exercise device. Such pedalling exercise brings in more muscles and stimulates them to contract at a considerably higher rate (up to 50X per minute) than does the previously described knee-extension exercise (6X per minute). However, less force is developed during the pulsed contractions, and the duty cycle is quite short. Thus, FES bicycle ergometer exercise seems better suited for improving muscular endurance than strength. Higher oxygen uptakes (approximately three to four times resting levels) have been reported for this exercise mode

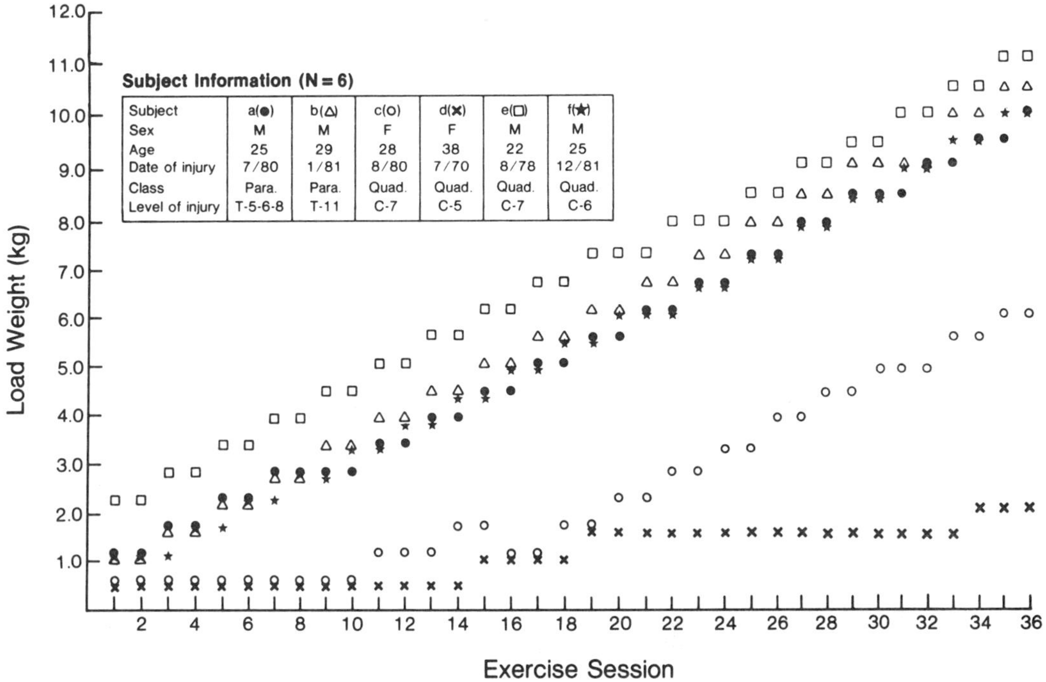

Figure 13.14. Individual subject load weight progression data (right leg) during 12 weeks (3X/wk) of functional electrical stimulation knee-extension exercise-conditioning. (Modified from Gruner JA, Glaser RM, Feinberg SD, et al.: A system for evaluation and exercise-conditioning of paralyzed leg muscles. *J Rehabil R D* 20:27, 1983.)

compared to knee-extension exercise (207). Several weeks of exercise training using this device (3X per week) resulted in substantial gains in endurance time, from an initial 1–2 minutes per session to over 30 minutes (206, 208). A protocol, which has been described, uses power output levels that result in fatigue after 15–30 minutes of pedalling. As resistance to fatigue improves, PO is increased slightly (by 20 kpm·min^{-1}) to maintain the desired exercise duration.

Hybrid Exercise

Improved training effects may be obtained by using hybrid exercise (combinations of FES and voluntary exercise performed simultaneously). One such technique has been described by Glaser and associates (38) whereby FES-induced contractions of paralyzed leg muscles (knee extension) accompany voluntary arm exercise (arm cranking). This exercise has several theoretical advantages over either training modality performed alone including: a) utilization of greater muscle mass, b) higher elicited aerobic metabolic rates, which can improve aerobic training capability, c) reduced pooling of blood in the lower extremities due to activation of the venous muscle pump, d) improved arm exercise performance because of greater availability of blood, and e) improved FES leg performance, possibly because the ANS sympathetic stimulation induced by the voluntary arm exercise increases blood flow to the active paralyzed muscles. Davis and coworkers (209) have provided strong evidence for reduced venous pooling coincident with augmented cardiac output and stroke volume during hybrid (arm-cranking and simultaneous FES-induced leg contractions) exercise in paraplegics.

FES exercise training is not believed to cause neural regeneration, thereby return-

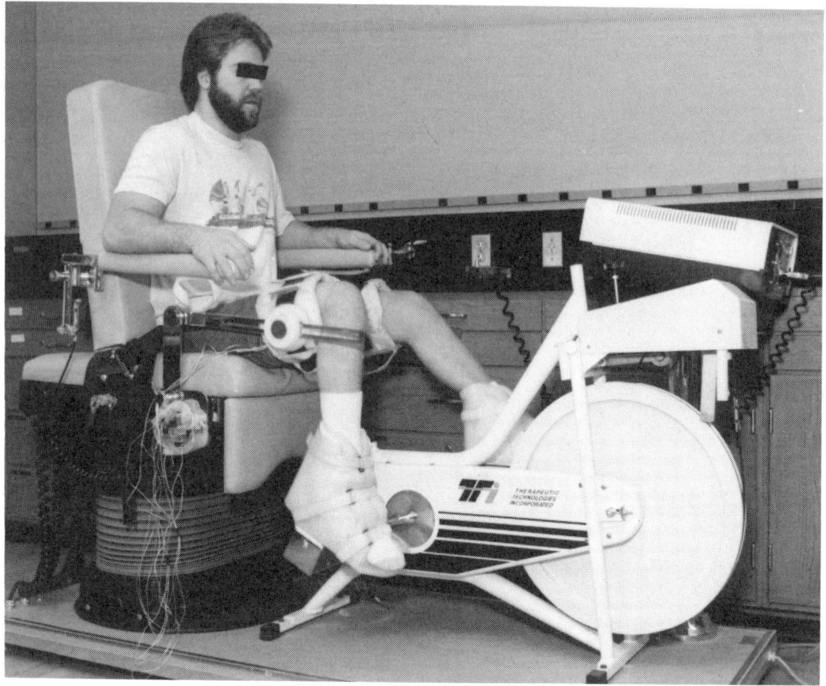

Figure 13.15. Functional electrical stimulation-induced bicycle ergometer exercise being performed on a commercially available instrument. The quadriceps, hamstrings, and gluteus maximus muscles are activated during appropriate angles of the crank cycle.

ing voluntary function to patients with complete motor loss. However, this exercise may contribute to improved voluntary function of paretic muscles in cases of incomplete paralysis. To enhance muscle force output, a form of hybrid exercise has been described by Servedio and colleagues (210) whereby FES-induced contractions were superimposed upon the voluntary contractions of weak muscles. The combined contractions were stronger than the voluntary efforts alone, suggesting that more effective strength and endurance training of muscles could be achieved in a hemiparetic population using hybrid exercise. By improving the performance of muscles with this training technique, stroke patients may be better able to take advantage of intact neural pathways and achieve greater voluntary function. Since those with incomplete motor dysfunction usually have some sensory capability, the maximal tolerable level of electrical stimulation should be determined before commencing hybrid exercise. Much more research is needed to develop FES exercise techniques that can provide optimal fitness and function for patients with neuromuscular impairments.

SUMMARY AND CONCLUSIONS

The goal of this chapter was to acquaint the health-care professional and exercise scientist with current information related to arm exercise stress testing and training of wheelchair-dependent patients. Neuromuscular impairments often lead to a highly sedentary life-style, resulting in diminished physical and psychological fitness. However, there is convincing evidence that disabled individuals who participate in regular physical activities possess higher exercise capacity, greater cardiorespiratory reserve, and improved psychological status. In these more fit individuals, activities of daily living can be achieved with lower stress and more vigor. We believe that regular physical activity or fitness training for wheelchair users should be encouraged to promote optimal rehabilitation outcome.

Ultimately, objective fitness evaluation and exercise training programs should be made available to all patients on a routine basis. Although there has been an increase in exercise-oriented research for disabled individuals during the last decade, more information is necessary to further develop safe and effective fitness equipment and protocols. This research must be both interdisciplinary in nature and involve interactions between exercise scientists, biomedical engineers, and health-care professionals. Innovative rehabilitative techniques to improve the independence and quality of life for disabled patients should be the norm—not the exception!

REFERENCES

1. Adams RC, Daniel AN, Rullman L: *Games, Sports and Exercises for the Physically Handicapped.* Philadelphia, Lea & Febiger, 1981, p 24.
2. Clark MW: Competitive sports for the disabled. *Am J Sports Med* 8:366–369, 1980.
3. Corcoran PJ, Goldman RF, Hoerner EF, et al.: Sports medicine and the physiology of wheelchair marathon racing. *Orthop Clin North Am* 11:697–716, 1980.
4. Guttmann L: *Textbook of Sport for the Disabled.* Aylesbury Bucks, England, H.M. & M. Publishers, 1976, p 1.
5. Nilsson S, Staff D, Pruett E: Physical work capacity and the effect of training on subjects with long standing paraplegia. *Scand J Rehabil Med* 7:51–56, 1975.
6. Pollock M, Miller H, Linnerud A, et al.: Arm pedalling as an endurance training regimen for the disabled. *Arch Phys Med Rehabil* 55:418–423, 1974.
7. Stauffer ES: Long-term management of traumatic quadriplegia. In DS Pierce, VH Nickel (eds): *The Total Care of Spinal Cord Injuries.* Boston, Little, Brown, 1978, p 81.
8. Weiss M, Beck J: Sport as a part of therapy and rehabilitation of paraplegics. *Paraplegia* 11:166–172, 1973.
9. Glaser RM: Exercise and locomotion for the spinal cord injured. In Terjung RL (ed): *Exercise and Sports Sciences Reviews,* Vol. 13. New York, MacMillian Publishers, 1985, p 263.
10. Davis GM, Jackson RW, Shephard RJ: Sports and recreation for the physically disabled. In Strauss RH (ed): *Sports Medicine.* Philadelphia, WB Saunders, 1984, p 286.
11. Davis GM, Kofsky PR, Kelsey JC, et al.: Cardiorespiratory fitness and muscular strength of wheelchair users. *Can Med Assoc J* 125:1313–1323, 1981.
12. Gass CG, Camp EM: Physiological characteristics of trained Australian paraplegic and tetraplegic subjects. *Med Sci Sports Exerc* 11:256–265, 1979.
13. Gass CG, Camp EM, Davis HA, et al.: The effects of prolonged exercise on spinally injured subjects. *Med Sci Sports Exerc* 13:277–283, 1981.
14. Hjeltnes N: Oxygen uptake and cardiac output in graded arm exercise in paraplegics with low level spinal lesions. *Scand J Rehabil Med* 9:107–113, 1977.
15. Zwiren L, Bar-Or O: Responses to exercise of paraplegics who differ in conditioning level. *Med Sci Sports Exerc* 7:94–98, 1975.
16. Long C, Lawton EB: Functional significance of spinal cord lesion level. *Arch Phys Med Rehabil* 36:249–255, 1955.
17. McDonald JJ, Chusid JG: *Correlative neuroanatomy and functional neurology.* California, Lange Medical, 1952, p 1.
18. Jackson RW, Fredrickson A: Sports for the physically disabled: The 1976 Olympiad (Toronto). *Am J Sports Med* 7:293–298, 1979.
19. Biering-Sorensen F: Classification of paralyzed and amputee sportsmen. In Natvig H. (ed): *The First International Medical Congress on Sports for the Disabled.* Oslo, Royal Ministry of Church and Education, 1980, p 44.
20. Grosfield IN: Classification of asymmetrical quads in swimming and track. In Natvig H (ed): *The First International Medical Congress on Sports for the Disabled.* Oslo, Royal Ministry of Church and Education, 1980, p 55.
21. McCann BC: Classification of the locomotor disabled for competitive sports: Theory and practice. *Int J Sports Med* 5:167–170, 1984.
22. Daniels L, Worthingham C: *Muscle Testing: Techniques of Manual Examination.* New York, WB Saunders, 1982, p 1.
23. Cameron BJ, Ward GR, Wicks JR: Relationship of type of training to maximum oxygen uptake and upper limb strength in male paraplegic athletes. *Med Sci Sports Exerc* 9:58, 1978.
24. Wicks J, Lymburner K, Dinsdale S, et al.: The use of multistage exercise testing with wheelchair ergometry and arm cranking in subjects with spinal cord lesions. *Paraplegia* 15:252–261, 1977.
25. Wicks JR, Oldridge NB, Cameron NB, et al.: Arm cranking and wheelchair ergometry in elite spinal cord injured athletes. *Med Sci Sports Exerc* 15:224–231, 1983.
26. Davis GM, Kofsky PR, Shephard RJ, et al.: Fit-

ness levels in the lower limb disabled. *Can J Appl Sport Sci* 5:21, 1980.
27. Jackson RW, Davis GM, Kofsky PR, et al.: Fitness levels in the lower limb disabled. *Transactions of the 27th Annual Meeting of the Orthopaedic Research Society* 6:12, 1981.
28. Kofsky PR, Davis GM, Shephard RJ, et al.: Cardio-respiratory fitness in the lower limb disabled. *Can J Appl Sport Sci* 5:65, 1980.
29. Kofsky PR, Davis GM, Jackson RW, et al.: Field testing—assessment of physical fitness of disabled adults. *Eur J Appl Physiol* 51:109–120, 1983.
30. American College of Sports Medicine: *Guidelines for Graded Exercise Testing and Exercise Prescription*. Philadelphia, Lea and Febiger, 1980, p 1.
31. American College of Sports Medicine: The recommended quantity and quality of exercise for developing and maintaining fitness in healthy adults. *Med Sci Sports Exerc* 10:VII–X, 1978.
32. Bar-Or O, Zwiren LD: Maximal oxygen consumption test during arm exercise—reliability and validity. *J Appl Physiol* 38:424–426. 1975.
33. Magel JR, McArdle WD, Toner M, et al.: Metabolic and cardiovascular adjustments to arm training. *J Appl Physiol* 45:75–79, 1978.
34. McArdle WD, Glaser RM, Magel JR: Metabolic and cardiorespiratory responses during free swimming and treadmill walking. *J Appl Physiol* 30:733–738, 1971.
35. Reybrouck T, Heigenhauser GF, Faulkner JA: Limitations to maximum oxygen uptake in arm, leg and combined arm-leg ergometry. *J Appl Physiol* 38:774–779, 1975.
36. Sawka MN, Foley ME, Pimental MM, et al.: Determination of maximal aerobic power during upper body exercise. *J Appl Physiol* 54:113–117, 1983.
37. Shephard RJ: *Physiology and Biochemistry of Exercise*. New York, Praeger Scientific, 1983, p 63.
38. Glaser RM, Strayer RS, May KP: Combined FES leg and voluntary arm exercise of SCI patients. *IEEE/Seventh Annual Conference of Eng in Med Biol Soc*. Chicago, 1985, p 308.
39. Miles DS, Sawka MN, Wilde SW, et al.: Pulmonary function changes in wheelchair athletes subsequent to exercise training. *Ergonomics* 25:239–246, 1982.
40. Miles DS, Sawka MN, Glaser RM, et al.: Assessment of central hemodynamics during arm-crank exercise. *Proc IEEE National Electronics and Aerospace Conference* 3:442–448, 1982.
41. Sawka MN, Glaser RM, Wilde SW, et al.: Metabolic and circulatory responses to wheelchair and arm crank exercise. *J Appl Physiol* 49:784–788, 1980.
42. Wilde SW, Miles DS, Durbin RJ, et al.: Evaluation of myocardial performance during wheelchair ergometer exercise. *Am J Phys Med* 60:277–291, 1981.
43. Glaser RM, Sawka MN, Brune MF, et al.: Physiological responses to maximal effort wheelchair and arm crank ergometry. *J Appl Physiol* 48:1060–1064, 1980.
44. Brooks GA, Fahey TD: *Exercise Physiology: Human Bioenergetics and Its Applications*. New York, John Wiley and Sons, 1984, p 405.
45. Fox EL, Mathews DK: *Interval Training: Conditioning for Sports and General Fitness*. Philadelphia, WB Saunders, 1974, p 35.
46. Glaser RM, Foley DM, Laubach LL, et al.: An exercise test to evaluate fitness for wheelchair activity. *Paraplegia* 16:341–349, 1978–79.
47. McArdle W, Katch F, Katch V: *Exercise Physiology: Energy, Nutrition, and Human Performance*. Philadelphia, Lea and Febiger, 1986, p 349.
48. McCafferty WR, Horvath SM: Specificity of exercise and specificity of training: A subcellular response. *Res Q* 48:358–371, 1977.
49. Clarke KS: Caloric costs of activity in paraplegic persons. *Arch Phys Med Rehabil* 47:427–435, 1966.
50. Glaser RM, Laubach LL, Sawka MN, et al.: Exercise stress fitness evaluation and training of wheelchair users. In Leon AS, Amundson GJ (eds): *Proceedings of the First International Conference on Lifestyle and Health*. Minneapolis: University of Minnesota, 1978, p 167.
51. Glaser RM, Sawka MN, Wilde SW, et al.: Energy cost and cardiopulmonary responses for wheelchair locomotion and walking on tile and on carpet. *Paraplegia* 19:220–226, 1981.
52. Glaser RM, Simsen-Harold CA, Petrofsky JS, et al.: Metabolic and cardiopulmonary responses of older wheelchair-dependent and ambulatory patients during locomotion. *Ergonomics* 26:687–697, 1983.
53. Glaser RM, Collins SR, Wilde SW: Power output requirements for manual wheelchair locomotion. *Proc IEEE National Aerospace and Electronics Conference* 2:502–509, 1980.
54. Engel P, Hildebrandt G: Long term spiro-ergonometric studies of paraplegics during the clinical period of rehabilitation. *Paraplegia* 11:105–110, 1973.
55. Gass GC, Watson J, Camp EM, et al.: The effects of physical training on high level spinal lesion patients. *Scand J Rehabil Med* 12:61–65, 1980.
56. Voight ED, Bahn D: Metabolism and pulse rate in physically handicapped when propelling a wheelchair up an incline. *Scand J Rehabil Med* 1:101–106, 1969.
57. Brauer RL: *An Ergonomic Analysis of Wheelchair Wheeling*. Ph.D. Dissertation, University of Illinois, 1972.
58. Brattgard SO, Grimby G, Höök O: Energy expenditure and heart rate in driving a wheel-chair ergometer. *Scand J Rehabil Med* 2:143–148, 1970.
59. Brouha L, Krobath HD: Continuous recording of

cardiac and respiratory functions in normal and handicapped people. *Hum Factors* 9:567–572, 1976.
60. Brubaker C, Wood J, Gibson J, et al.: Wheelchair propulsion studies. In Stamp WG (ed): *Rehabilitation Engineering*. Charlottesville, University of Virginia, 1979, p 1.
61. Dreisinger TE, Londeree BR: Wheelchair exercise: A Review. *Paraplegia* 20:20–34, 1982.
62. Glaser RM, Barr SA, Laubach LL, et al.: Relative stresses of wheelchair activity. *Hum Factors* 22:177–181, 1980.
63. Glaser RM, Sawka MN, Laubach LL, et al.: Metabolic and cardiopulmonary responses to wheelchair and bicycle ergometry. *J Appl Physiol* 46:1066–1070, 1979.
64. Lundberg A: Wheelchair driving: Evaluation of a new training outfit. *Scand J Rehabil Med* 12:67–72, 1980.
65. Skrinar GS, Evans WJ, Ornstein LJ, et al.: Glycogen utilization in wheelchair-dependent athletes. *Int J Sports Med* 3:215–219, 1982.
66. Glaser RM, Collins SR: Validity of power output estimation for wheelchair locomotion. *Am J Phys Med* 60:180–189, 1981.
67. Bennedik K, Engel P, Hildebrandt G: *Der Rollstuhl: experimentelle Grundlagen zsu technischen and ergometrischsen Beuteilung handbetriebener Krankenfahrzeuge*. Rheinstetten, Schindele-Verlag, 1978, p 91.
68. Hildebrandt G, Voigt ED, Bahn D, et al.: Energy costs of propelling a wheelchair at various speeds: Cardiac responses and effect on steering accuracy. *Arch Phys Med Rehabil* 51:131–136, 1970.
69. Glaser RM, Sawka MN, Miles DS: Efficiency of wheelchair and low power bicycle power ergometry. *Proc IEEE National Aerospace and Electronics Conference* 2:946–953, 1984.
70. Sawka MN, Glaser RM, Wilde SW, et al.: Submaximal test to predict peak oxygen uptake for wheelchair exercise. *Fed Proc* 39:287, 1980.
71. Kofsky PR, Shephard RJ, Davis GM, et al.: Classification of aerobic power and muscular strength for disabled individuals with differing patterns of habitual physical activity. In Sherrill C (ed): *1984 Olympic Scientific Congress—Sport and Disabled Athletes*. Champaign, Illinois, Human Kinetics, 1986, p 147.
72. Stenberg J, Åstrand PO, Ekblom B, et al.: Hemodynamic response to work with different muscle groups, sitting and supine. *J Appl Physiol* 22:61–70, 1967.
73. Bevegard S, Freyschüss U, Strandell T: Circulatory adaptation to arm and leg exercise in supine and sitting positions. *J Appl Physiol* 21:37–46, 1966.
74. Ekblom B, Lundberg A: Effect of physical training on adolescents with severe motor handicaps. *Acta Paediatr Scand* 57:17–23, 1968.
75. Emes C: Physical work capacity of wheelchair athletes. *Res Q* 48:209–212, 1978.
76. Huang CT, McEachran AB, Kuhlemeier KV, et al.: Prescriptive arm ergometry to optimize muscular endurance in acutely injured paraplegic patients. *Arch Phys Med Rehabil* 64:578–582, 1983.
77. Knutsson E, Lewenhaupt-Olsson E, Thorsen M: Physical work capacity and physical conditioning in paraplegic patients. *Paraplegia* 11:205–216, 1973.
78. Whiting RB, Dreisinger TE, Abbott C: Clinical value of exercise testing in handicapped subjects. *South Med J* 76:1225–1227, 1983.
79. Gandee R, Porterfield J, Narraway A, et al.: Somatotype and isokinetic strength profile of an elite wheelchair marathon racer. *Med Sci Sports Exerc* 13:132, 1981.
80. Grimby G: Aerobic capacity, muscle strength and fiber composition in young paraplegics. In Natvig H (ed): *1st International Medical Congress on Sports for the Disabled*. Oslo, Royal Ministry for Church and Education, 1980, p 13.
81. Gandee R, Winningham M, Deitchman R, et al.: The aerobic capacity of an elite wheelchair marathon racer. *Med Sci Sports Exerc* 12:142, 1980.
82. Ward GR, Fraser LN: Fitness characteristics of Canadian national wheelchair athletes. *Med Sci Sports Exerc* 16:142, 1984.
83. Sawka MN, Glaser RM, Laubach LL, et al.: Wheelchair exercise performance in the young, middle aged, and elderly. *J Appl Physiol* 50:824–828, 1981.
84. Hjeltnes N: Control of medical rehabilitation of para- and tetraplegics. In Natvig H (ed): *1st International Medical Congress on Sports for the Disabled*. Oslo, Royal Ministry for Church and Education, 1980, p 162.
85. Hjeltnes N: Control of medical rehabilitation of para- and tetraplegics by repeated evaluation of endurance capacity. *Int J Sports Med* 5:171–174, 1984.
86. Hjeltnes N, Vokac Z: Circulatory strain in everyday life of paraplegics. *Scand J Rehabil Med* 11:67–73, 1979.
87. Joacheim KA, Strohkendl H: The value of particular sports of the wheelchair disabled in maintaining health of the paraplegic. *Paraplegia* 11:173–178, 1973.
88. Marion C, Berg K, Meyer K, et al.: Effects of arm ergometry training in an adolescent with myelodysplasia. *Phys Ther* 66:59–63, 1986.
89. Davis GM, Shephard RJ, Jackson RW: Cardiorespiratory fitness and muscular strength in the lower-limb disabled. *Can J Appl Sport Sci* 6:159–165, 1981.
90. Clinkingbeard JR, Gersten JW, Hoehn D: Energy cost of ambulation in the traumatic paraplegic. *Am J Phys Med* 43:157–164, 1964.

91. Golding LA, Horvat MA, Beutel-Horvat T, et al.: A graded exercise test protocol for spinal cord individuals. *J Cardiopul Rehabil* 6:362–367, 1986.
92. Heigenhauser GF, Ruff CL, Miller B, et al.: Cardiovascular responses of paraplegics during graded arm ergometry. *Med Sci Sports Exerc* 8:68, 1976.
93. Figoni SF: Comparison of cardiovascular responses of quadriplegic and able-bodied men during dynamic arm exercise at an equivalent rate of oxygen uptake. *Am Correct Ther J* 40:118, 1986.
94. Figoni SF: Cardiac function curves for quadriplegic men during dynamic arm exercise. *Med Sci Sports Exerc* 18 (Suppl):S8, 1986.
95. Haller RG, Lewis SF, Cook JD, et al.: Hypokinetic circulation during exercise in neuromuscular disease. *Neurology* 33:1283–1287, 1983.
96. DiRocco P, Hashimoto A, Daskalovic I, et al.: Cardiopulmonary responses during arm work on land and in a water environment of nonambulatory, spinal cord impaired individuals. *Paraplegia* 23:90–99, 1985.
97. Freyschuss U, Knutsson E: Cardiovascular control in man with transverse cervical cord lesions. *Life Sci* 8:421–424, 1969.
98. Freyschuss U: Cardiovascular adjustments to somatomotor activation. *Acta Physiol Scand* 342 (Suppl):28–33, 1970.
99. Davis GM: *Cardiovascular Fitness and Muscular Fitness in Lower-Limb Disabled Males.* Toronto, University of Toronto Press, 1985, p 88.
100. Davis GM, Ward GR, Jackson RW, et al.: Cardiorespiratory fitness in the lower limb disabled. In Sherrill C (ed): *Proceedings of 1984 Olympic Scientific Congress-Sport and Disabled Athletes.* Champaign, Illinois, Human Kinetics, 1986.
101. VanLoan M, McCluer S, Loftin JM, et al.: Comparison of physiological responses to maximal arm exercise among able-bodied, paraplegics and quadriplegics. *Paraplegia* 25:397–405, 1987.
102. Figoni SF: Circulorespiratory responses of spinal cord injured, quadriplegic men to dynamic physical exercise. Ph.D. Dissertation, Champaign, Illinois, Dissertation Abstracts International 48:2015–A, 1988.
103. Figoni SF: Circulorespiratory effects of arm training and detraining in one C5-6 quadriplegic man. *Phys Ther* 66:779, 1986.
104. Asmussen E: *Correlation Between Various Physiological Test Results in Handicapped Persons.* Vol 4. Hellerup, Denmark, Communication of Testing and Observation Institute, 1968.
105. Asmussen E, Molbech SV: *Methods and Standards for Evaluation of the Physical Working Capacity of Patients.* Vol 4. Hellerup, Denmark, Communication of Testing and Observation Institute, 1954, p 9.
106. Asmussen E, Poulsen E: *A Battery of Physiological Tests Applied to Two Different Groups of Handicapped Persons.* Vol 13. Hellerup, Denmark, Communication of Testing and Observation Institute, 1966, p 11.
107. Asmussen E, Poulsen E, Bogh HE: *Measurements of Muscle Strength Necessary for Driving a Motor Car* Vol 19. Hellerup, Denmark, Communication of Testing and Observation Institute, 1964, p 1.
108. Beal DP, Glaser RM, Petrofsky JS, et al.: Static component of handgrip muscles for various wheelchair propulsion methods. *Fed Proc* 40:497, 1981.
109. Gairdner J: *Fitness for the Disabled: Wheelchair Users.* Toronto, Fitzhenry & Whiteside, 1983, p 31.
110. Wakim KG, Elkins EC, Worden RE, et al.: The effect of therapeutic exercise on the peripheral circulation of normal and paraplegic individuals. *Arch Phys Med Rehabil* 30:86–94, 1949.
111. Gersten J, Brown I, Speck L, et al.: Comparison of tension development and circulation in bicep and tricep in man. *Am J Phys Med* 42:156–165, 1963.
112. Wiles CM, Karni Y: The measurement of muscle strength in patients with peripheral neuromuscular disorders. *J Neurol Neurosurg Psychiatry* 46:1006–1013, 1983.
113. Nakamura Y: Working ability of the paraplegics. *Paraplegia* 11:182–193, 1973.
114. Davis GM, Tupling SJ, Shephard RJ: Dynamic strength and physical activity in wheelchair users. In Sherrill C (ed): *1984 Olympic Scientific Congress—Sport and Disabled Athletes.* Champaign, Illinois, Human Kinetics, 1986, p 139.
115. Asayama K, Nakamura Y, Ogata H, et al.: Physical fitness of paraplegics in full wheelchair marathon racing. *Paraplegia* 23:277–287, 1985.
116. Kofsky P, Davis G, Shephard RJ: Muscle strength and aerobic power of the lower-limb disabled. Ann ISEF-L'Aquila 2:201–208, 1983.
117. Kofsky PR, David GM, Shephard RJ, et al.: Strength and aerobic power in the wheelchair-bound. *Can J Appl Sport Sci* 7:5, 1982.
118. Davis GM, Shephard RJ, Ward GR: Alteration of dynamic strength following forearm crank training of disabled subjects. *Med Sci Sports Exerc* 16:147, 1984.
119. Tupling SJ, Davis GM, Pierrynowski MR, et al.: Arm strength and impulse generation: Initiation of wheelchair movement by the physically disabled. *Ergonomics* 29:303–311, 1986.
120. Tupling SJ, Davis GM, Shephard RJ: Arm strength and impulse generation in the physically disabled. *Can J Appl Sport Sci* 9:148, 1983.
121. Glaser RM, Sawka MN, Durbin RJ, et al.: Exercise program for wheelchair activity. *Am J Phys Med* 60:67–75, 1981.
122. Åstrand PO, Rodahl K: *Textbook of Work Physiology.* New York, McGraw Hill, 1986, p 420.

123. Pollock ML, Wilmore JH, Fox SM: *Exercise in Health and Disease: Evaluation and Prescription for Prevention and Rehabilitation*. Philadelphia, WB Saunders, 1984, p 23.
124. Thorstensson A: Observations on strength training and detraining. *Acta Physiol Scand* 100:491–493, 1977.
125. Tuttle W, Horvath SM: Comparison of effects of static and dynamic work on blood pressure and heart rate. *J Appl Physiol* 10:294–296, 1957.
126. Davis GM, Shephard RJ, Leenen FHH: Cardiac effects of short term arm crank training in paraplegics: Echocardiographic evidence. *Eur J Applied Physiol* 56:90–96, 1987.
127. Bergh U, Kanstrup IL, Ekblom B: Maximal oxygen uptake during exercise with various combinations of arm and leg work. *J Appl Physiol* 41:191–196, 1976.
128. Clausen JP, Klausen K, Rasmussen B, et al.: Central and peripheral circulatory changes after training of the arms or legs. *Am J Physiol* 225:675–682, 1973.
129. Cross DL: The influence of physical fitness as a rehabilitation tool. *Int J Rehabil Res* 3:163–175, 1980.
130. Simmons R, Shephard RJ: Effects of physical conditioning upon the central and peripheral circulatory responses to arm work. *Int Z Angew Physiol* 30:73–84, 1971.
131. Crews TR, Roberts JA: Effects of interaction of frequency and intensity of training. *Res Q* 47:48–55, 1976.
132. Davies CTM, Knibbs AV: The training stimulus: The effect of intensity, duration and frequency of effort on maximum aerobic power output. *Inter Z Angew Arbeitsphysiol* 29:299–305, 1971.
133. Fox EL, Bartels RL, Billings CE, et al.: Frequency and duration of interval training programs and changes in aerobic power. *J Appl Physiol* 38:481–484, 1975.
134. Pollock M, Ayres J, Ward A: Cardiorespiratory fitness: Response to differing intensities and durations of training. *Arch Phys Med Rehabil* 58:467–473, 1977.
135. Shephard RJ: Intensity, duration and frequency of exercise as determinants of the response to a training regime. *Inter Z Angew Arbeitsphysiol* 26:272–278, 1969.
136. Gettman L, Greninger L, Molnar S: Efficiency of wheeling after training. *Proc Ann Conv South Dist Amer Alliance Health, Phys Educ Rec* 7:83, 1968.
137. Marwick C: Wheelchair calisthenics keep patients fit. [Letter to the editor]. *JAMA* 251:303, 1984.
138. Franklin BA: Exercise testing, training and arm ergometry. *Sports Med* 2:100–119, 1985.
139. Marincék CRT, Valéncic V: Arm cyclo-ergometry and kinetics of oxygen consumption in paraplegics. *Paraplegia* 15:178–185, 1978.
140. DiCarlo SE, Supp MD, Taylor HC: Effect of arm ergometry training on physical work capacity of individuals with spinal cord injuries. *Phys Ther* 63:1104–1107, 1983.
141. Steadward RD: Analysis of wheelchair sports events. In Natvig H (ed): *The First International Medical Congress on Sports for the Disabled*. Oslo, Royal Ministry of Church and Education, 1980, p 184.
142. McDonell E, Brassard L, Taylor AW: Effects of an arm ergometer training program on wheelchair subjects. *Can J Appl Sport Sci* 5:71, 1980.
143. Stoboy H, Wilson-Rich B: Muscle strength and electrical activity, heart rate, and energy cost during isometric contractions in disabled and non-disabled. *Paraplegia* 8:217–222, 1971.
144. Cooney MM, Walker JB: Hydraulic resistance exercise benefits cardiovascular fitness of spinal cord injured. *Med Sci Sports Exerc* 18:522–525, 1986.
145. Pachalski A, Mekarski T: Effect of swimming on increasing of cardio-respiratory capacity of paraplegics. *Paraplegia* 18:190–196, 1980.
146. DiRocco P: Tethered swimming and the development of cardiopulmonary fitness for nonambulatory individuals. *Am Correct Ther J* 40:43–45, 1986.
147. Walsh CM, Steadward RD: *Get Fit: Muscular fitness exercises for the wheelchair user*. Edmonton, University of Alberta, 1984, p 20.
148. Chawla JC, Bar C, Creber I, et al.: Techniques for improving the strength and fitness of spinal injured patients. *Paralegia* 17:185–189, 1979.
149. Clarke DH: Adaptations in strength and muscular endurance resulting from exercise. In Wilmore, JH (ed): *Exercise and Sports Sciences Reviews* Vol 1, 1973, p 74.
150. DeLorme TL, Watkins AL: Techniques of progressive resistance exercise. *Arch Phys Med Rehabil* 29:263–267, 1948.
151. Clarke HH: Development of Muscular Strength and Endurance. *Phys Fitness Res Dig*. President's Council on Physical Fitness in Sports. Washington D.C., US Government Printing Office, 1974.
152. McArdle WD, Katch FI, Katch VL: *Exercise Physiology: Energy, Nutrition and Human Performance*. Philadelphia, Lea & Febiger, 1986, p 378.
153. Shephard RJ: *Endurance Fitness*. Toronto, University of Toronto Press, 1977, p 270.
154. Haskell WL: Cardiovascular benefits and risks of exercise: The scientific evidence. In Strauss R (ed): *Sports Medicine*. Toronto, WB Saunders, 1984, p 57.
155. Brenes G, Dearwater S, Shapera R, et al.: High density lipoprotein cholesterol concentrations in physically active and sedentary spinal cord injured patients. *Arch Phys Med Rehabil* 67:445–450, 1986.

156. Cowel LL, Squires WG, Raven PB: Benefits of aerobic exercise for the paraplegic: A brief review. *Med Sci Sports Exerc* 18:501–508, 1986.
157. Dearwater SR, Laporte RE, Robertson RJ, et al.: Activity in the spinal cord-injured patient: An epidemiologic analysis of metabolic parameters. *Med Sci Sports Exerc* 18:541–544, 1986.
158. Flandrois R, Grandmontagne M, Gerin H, et al.: Aerobic performance capacity in paraplegic subjects. *Eur J Applied Physiol* 55:604–609, 1986.
159. Ankenbrand LJ: *The Self Concept of Students Physically Handicapped and Non-handicapped Related to Participation in an Individual Sport.* Ph.D. Dissertation, University of Missouri, Columbia, Missouri, 1972.
160. Dalton RB: *Effects of Exercise and Vitamin B-12 Supplementation on the Depression Scores of a Wheelchair Confined Population.* Ph.D. Dissertation, University of Missouri, Columbia, Missouri, 1980.
161. Roberts K: Sports for the disabled. *Physiotherapy* 60:271–274, 1974.
162. Crews D, Purkett L, Wells CL, et al.: Cardiovascular characteristics of wheelchair marathon racers compared with marathon runners. *Int J Sports Med* 3:64, 1982.
163. DiCarlo SE: Improved cardiopulmonary status after a two-month program of graded arm exercise in a patient with C6 quadriplegia. *Phys Ther* 62:456–459, 1982.
164. Croucher N: Sports and disability. In Williams JGP, Sperry PN (eds): *Sports and Medicine,* ed 2. London, Arnold, 1976, p 1.
165. Rathbone JL, Lucas C: *Recreation in Total Rehabilitation.* Springfield, Illinois, Charles C Thomas, 1980, p 1.
166. Ornstein LJ, Skrinar GS, Garrett GG: Physiological effects of swimming training in physically disabled individuals. *Med Sci Sports Exerc* 15:110, 1983.
167. Andersen EC, Kasch FW: Maximum oxygen uptake of trained paraplegics during arm ergometry and tethered swimming. *Med Sci Sports Exerc* 16:148, 1984.
168. Francis RS, Nelson AG: Physiological and performance profiles of a world class wheelchair athlete. *Med Sci Sports Exerc* 13:132, 1981.
169. Taylor AW, McDonnell E, Royer D, et al.: Skeletal muscle analysis of wheelchair athletes. *Paraplegia* 17:456–460, 1979.
170. Tesch PA, Karlsson J: Muscle fiber type characteristics of M. Deltoideus in wheelchair athletes: Comparison with other trained athletes. *Am J Phys Med* 62:239–243, 1983.
171. Godin G, Davis GM, Shepard RJ, et al.: Prediction of leisure time exercise behavior among a group of lower-limb disabled adults. *J Clin Psychol* 42:271–279, 1986.
172. Flynn RJ, Salomon PR: Performance of the MMPI in predicting rehabilitation outcome: A discriminant analysis, double cross-validation assessment. *Rehabil Lit* 38:12–15, 1977.
173. Harper DC: Personality characteristics of physically impaired adolescents. *J Clin Psychol* 34:97–104, 1978.
174. Harper DC, Richman LC: Personality profiles of physically impaired adolescents. *J Clin Psychol* 34:636–642, 1978.
175. Davis GM, Kofsky PR, Shephard RJ, et al.: Classification of psycho-physiological variables in the lower limb disabled. *Can J Appl Sport Sci* 6:14, 1981.
176. Katz S, Shurks E, Florian V: The relationship between physical disability, social perception and psychological stress. *Scand J Rehabil Med* 10:109–113, 1978.
177. Simon JI: Emotional aspects of physical disability. *Am J Occup Ther* 25:408–410, 1971.
178. Shephard RJ, Davis GM, Kofsky PR, et al.: Interactions between attitudes, personality and physical activity in the lower-limb disabled. *Can J Appl Sport Sci* 8:173, 1983.
179. Lazar AL, Demos GD, Gaines L, et al.: Attitudes of handicapped and non-handicapped university students on three attitude scales. *Rehabil Lit* 38:49–52, 1978.
180. Sherrill C: Social and psychological dimensions of sport for disabled athletes. In Sherrill C (ed): *1984 Olympic Scientific Congress—Sport and Disabled Athletes.* Champaign IL, Human Kinetics, 1986, p 21.
181. Cole TM, Kottke FJ, Olson M, et al.: Alterations of cardiovascular control in high spinal myelomalacia. *Arch Phys Med Rehabil* 14:359–368, 1967.
182. Corbett JL, Frankel HL, Harris PJ: Cardiovascular reflexes in tetraplegia. *Paraplegia* 9:113–119, 1971.
183. Pierce DS, Nickel VH: *The Total Care of Spinal Cord Injuries.* Boston, Little, Brown, 1977.
184. Benton LA, Baker LL, Bowman BR, et al.: *Functional Electrical Stimulation—A Practical Guide.* The Professional Staff Association of the Rancho Los Amigos Hospital, Inc., Downey, CA, 1981.
185. Cybulski GR, Penn RD, Jaeger RJ: Lower extremity functional neuromuscular stimulation in case of spinal cord injury. *Neurosurgery* 15:132–146, 1984.
186. Mortimer JT: Motor Prostheses. In Brookhart JM, Mountcastle VB, Brooks VB, et al. (eds): *Handbook of Physiology. The Nervous System II.* Baltimore, American Physiological Society, 1981, p 155.
187. Glaser RM: Physiologic aspects of spinal cord injury and functional neuromuscular stimulation. *CNS Trauma* 3:49–62, 1986.
188. Gruner JA, Glaser RM, Feinberg SD, et al.: A system for evaluation and exercise-conditioning of paralyzed leg muscles. *J Rehabil R D* 20:21–30, 1983.
189. Collins SR, Glaser RM: Comparison of aerobic metabolism and cardiopulmonary responses for

electrically induced and voluntary exercise, *Proc Eighth Annual RESNA Conference on Rehabilitation Engineering.* 1985, p 391.

190. Kralj A, Bajd T, Turk R: Electrical stimulation providing functional use of paraplegic patient muscles. *Med Prog Technol* 7:3–9, 1980.
191. Peckham PH, Mortimer JT, Marsolais EB: Alteration in the force and fatigability of skeletal muscle in quadriplegic humans following exercise induced by chronic electrical stimulation. *Clin Orthop* 114:326–334, 1976.
192. Petrofsky JS, Phillips CA: Active physical therapy: A modern approach to rehabilitation therapy. *J Neurol Orthop Surg* 4:165–173, 1983.
193. Munsat TL, McNeal D, Waters R: Effects of nerve stimulation on human muscle. *Arch Neurol* 33:608–617, 1976.
194. Peckham PH, Mortimer JT, Van Der Meulen JP: Physiologic and metabolic changes in white muscle of cat following induced exercise. *Brain Res* 50:424–429, 1973.
195. Reddanna P, Moorthy CVN, Govindappa S: Pattern of skeletal muscle chemical composition during in vivo electrical stimulation. *Indian J Physiol Pharmacol* 25:33–39, 1981.
196. Riley DA, Allin EF: The effects of inactivity, programmed stimulation and denervation on the histochemistry of skeletal muscle fiber types. *Exp Neurol* 40:391–413, 1973.
197. Salmons A, Vrbova G: The influence of activity on some contractile characteristics of mammalian fast and slow muscles. *J Physiol* 201:535–549, 1969.
198. Buchegger A, Nemeth PM, Pette D, et al.: Effects of chronic stimulation on the metabolic heterogeneity of the fibre population in rabbit tibialis anterior muscle. *J Physiol* (London) 350:109–119, 1984.
199. Green HJ, Reichmann H, Pette D: Fibre type specific transformations in the enzyme activity pattern of rat vastus lateralis muscle by prolonged endurance training. *Pflugers Arch* 399:216–222, 1983.
200. Rhagnar M, Hudlicka O: Capillary growth in chronically stimulated adult skeletal muscle as studied by intravital microscopy and histological methods in rabbits and rats. *Microvasc Res* 16:730–790, 1978.
201. Salmons S, Gale DR, Steter FA: Ultrastructural aspects of the transformation of muscle fibre type by long term stimulation: Changes in Z discs and mitochondria. *J Anat* 127:17–21, 1978.
202. Vrbova G: Factors determining the speed of contraction of striated muscle. *J Physiol* (London) 185:17–18, 1966.
203. Kralj A, Bajd T, Turk R, et al.: Gait restoration in paraplegic patients: A feasibility study using multi-channel surface electrode FES. *J Rehabil R D* 20:3–20, 1983.
204. Crago PE, Peckham PH, Mortimer JT, et al.: The choice of pulse duration for chronic electrical stimulation via surface, nerve, and intramuscular electrodes. *Ann Biomed Eng* 2:252–264, 1974.
205. Glaser RM, Collins SR, Strayer JR, et al.: A closed-loop stimulator for exercising paralyzed muscles. *Proc Eighth Annual RESNA Conference on Rehabilitation Engineering.* 1985, p 388.
206. Petrofsky JS, Phillips CA, Heaton HH III, et al.: Bicycle ergometer for paralyzed muscle. *J Clin Eng* 9:13–19, 1984.
207. Phillips CA, Petrofsky JS, Hendershot DM et al.: Functional electrical exercise: A comprehensive approach for physical conditioning of the spinal cord injured patient. *Orthopedics* 7:1112–1123, 1984.
208. Petrofsky JS, Phillips CA: The use of functional electrical stimulation for rehabilitation of spinal cord injured patients. *CNS Trauma* 1:29–45, 1984.
209. Davis GM, Servedio FJ, Glaser RM, et al.: Hemodynamic responses during electrically-induced leg and voluntary arm crank exercise in lower-limb disabled males. *Proc Tenth Annual RESNA Conference on Rehabilitation Engineering.* 1987, p 591.
210. Servedio FJ, Servedio A, Davis GM, et al.: Voluntary strength gains in paretic muscle after hybrid (FNS-VOLUNTARY) exercise training. *Proc Tenth Annual RESNA Conference on Rehabilitation Engineering.* 1987, p 594.

CHAPTER 14

Pregnancy

James F. Clapp III, M.D.

This chapter has five educational goals. First, to introduce the subject of exercise testing and prescription during pregnancy by pointing out the reasons why the topic of exercise during pregnancy is one that currently presents a dilemma at a societal, medical, and personal level. Second, to acquaint the reader with some of the potentially important interactions between the physiology of exercise and the physiology of pregnancy. Third, to clearly identify the limitations of our knowledge concerning potential risks and benefits of exercise during pregnancy. Next, to familiarize the reader with both the available clinical information and the status of current guidelines and practices. Finally, to identify specific points that, in the author's opinion, should be frankly discussed with all physically active women prior to or during pregnancy. The latter should be of value in the formulation of testing procedures and individualized exercise prescription during pregnancy.

INTRODUCTION

Physical fitness and/or recreational athletic endeavor has become an integral part of leisure-time activity for a large number of women in our society. Most plan to continue their chosen activity without interruption throughout pregnancy. The societal magnitude of this practice and attitude is illustrated by survey data from Vermont where 50% of women in the reproductive age group exercise regularly and over 90% plan to continue their chosen fitness regimen or sport throughout pregnancy (1). This prevalence clearly makes exercise in pregnancy a societal reproductive issue of equal importance to those of nutrition, work, and environmental exposure.

While the health benefits of a regular fitness program are well recognized by the medical community, it is also clear that many types of physical activity carry some defined risk of temporary or permanent disability. This is the basic rationale for appropriate exercise testing and prescription. In this regard, pregnancy presents several unique problems, not the least of which is that the influence of maternal physical activity on the well-being and growth of the separate, yet dependent, developing organism within is ill-defined at present. It is further complicated by the multiple, well-recognized, ongoing maternal physiological changes of pregnancy (2–4) and by the paucity of objective information dealing with the interaction between physical activity and pregnancy (5). Thus, there is little but uncertainty and personal opinion to help the physician or athletic trainer design an appropriate exercise prescription for the physically active pregnant woman.

In today's society, with all its concerns about quality reproduction, this creates a real dilemma for the physically active woman contemplating pregnancy. On the one hand she feels a defined need to continue her exercise regimen, yet, on the other, she is concerned that it may have an adverse impact on the course and outcome of pregnancy. In the author's opinion, current information is insufficient to either allay or confirm this concern. Accordingly, it is strongly recommended that women who seek advice in this area be objectively counselled regarding the theoretical risks and benefits of exercise during pregnancy and that personal perspectives be clearly identified as such.

EXERCISE TESTING DURING PREGNANCY

The primary goals of exercise testing (assessment of fitness, physiological response, and function) are unchanged during pregnancy. However, its conduct, risk, and interpretation are complicated by several of the factors noted below.

Specific Problems Encountered During Pregnancy

First, the maternal physiological changes associated with pregnancy alter most baseline cardiorespiratory and metabolic parameters (2–4). Blood volume, pulse rate, cardiac output, minute ventilation, and metabolic rate all increase in a variable yet time-specific fashion, while hemoglobin, blood levels of multiple substrates, venous tone, and work efficiency decrease. Second, changes in autonomic tone, vascular reactivity, receptor levels, and vascular structure further complicate data collection and interpretation (2, 3). Third, several aspects of the physiological response to exercise appear to change in a time-specific fashion during pregnancy (5–8). For example, during pregnancy many women demonstrate a very variable and exercise-specific change in the relationship between pulse rate and exercise intensity so that, in most instances, pulse rate is no longer a valid measure of exercise intensity. This is most apparent in early and midpregnancy. Fourth, weight, its maternal and fetal components, and its gravitational effects are constantly changing, making morphometric and postural data normalization difficult, especially during antigravitational types of exercise. Fifth, the ligamentous laxity, lordosis, and change in the center of gravity characteristic of late pregnancy impact on the efficiency of specific muscular activity and may increase the risk of maternal injury during testing. Finally, the exercise-induced redistribution of cardiac output, rise in core temperature, and change in substrate levels place the fetus at theoretical risk, especially during high-intensity and/or prolonged episodes of endurance exercise (1, 4–6). Nonetheless, high-intensity exercise evaluation and $\dot{V}O_2$max testing have been carried out during pregnancy in both sedentary and physically active women without apparent ill effects (3, 6, 8–11).

General Indications for Exercise Testing During Pregnancy

For the reasons noted above, exercise testing during pregnancy is of limited clinical value unless it has a very specific medical indication. For example, the use of an exercise test to identify the source of atypical chest pain would clearly be of value and indicated in pregnancy. Likewise, its use during pregnancy to assess exercise tolerance, pulmonary function, or drug effectiveness could be of value in a variety of chronic disease states. In addition, it would be both helpful and indicated as a monitoring aid in rehabilitation following traumatic injury. However, at this point in time, routine fitness evaluation and $\dot{V}O_2$max testing are more rationally done either before or after pregnancy.

Although the clinical indications are limited, research exercise testing during pregnancy is essential if we are to clearly identify the risks and benefits of a variety of exercise regimens during pregnancy. As discussed in the following sections, this step is a prerequisite for developing definitive methods of exercise evaluation and prescription, which will allow the physician to accurately advise active women who wish to maintain an exercise program that is both safe and beneficial during pregnancy.

Exercise Testing for the Pregnant Athlete

Until the above is accomplished there is a specific group of women who should benefit from exercise testing during pregnancy. In the author's opinion, detailed and comprehensive, serial exercise testing should be an integral part of prenatal care for all female athletes who feel they must maintain an extensive training program during pregnancy. Ideally, the initial evaluation should occur prior to conception in order to have a valid reference for pregnancy-associated changes in the magnitude of the physiological responses to a specific exercise regimen. At a minimum, the testing should be repeated early in each trimester. Its format should be designed to mimic the individual athlete's field exercise regimen. It should include direct measurement of exercise intensity (oxygen consumption), several measures of cardiovascular, metabolic and thermal stress (arterial pressure, lactate, catecholamine and glucose levels, rectal temperature and recovery interval), a measure of fat deposition (skinfolds), and some assessment of the fetal response (heart rate pattern, activity, etc.) as well as general obstetrical evidence of normal fetal growth and development (including periodic ultrasound examination). In the author's opinion, this amount of information is essential to plan and maintain a regimen that will maximize maternal physiological benefit while avoiding physiological changes that indicate potential fetal compromise.

Helpful Hints for Exercise Testing During Pregnancy

There are several specific aspects of exercise testing during pregnancy that deserve special comment. First, due to the pregnancy-associated decrease in venous tone, dependent venous pooling with a decrease in venous return leading sequentially to a fall in cardiac output, postural hypotension, and syncope may occur during recovery unless a low level of muscular activity is maintained in the legs. This is particularly a problem late in pregnancy when a cycle ergometer is used for testing and pedalling is stopped abruptly and completely (3, 8). Thus, continued pedalling at a low rev·min^{-1} and zero load is recommended during recovery. Interestingly, the muscle tone present in the standing position is enough to maintain venous return at a level that avoids this complication in most runners and aerobic dancers during standing recovery (Clapp, JF, Unpublished data). However, evaluating their recovery in the sitting position creates a similar problem and should be avoided.

Second, unless the athlete trains under unusual field conditions, the testing environment should be maintained at an appropriate temperature (19–22°C) and humidity (less than 50%) in order to avoid a factitious hyperthermic response (12). For runners the use of a multispeed fan to mimic a headwind is often helpful in this regard. Conversely, the thermal impact of aerobic dancing may well be underestimated if the individual does not wear her usual costume for that activity (often synthetic fabric body tights are worn).

Third, make sure the subject is wearing appropriate footwear, that she is comfortable with the exercise surface, and that her bladder is empty at the start of the testing session. The former two are very important in terms of avoiding footstrike injuries on the treadmill or dancing area. The latter avoids two things. The risk of inadvertent urinary leakage and subsequently slipping on a wet surface, or the need to interrupt the testing session because of subject discomfort. This is especially important with antigravitational types of exercise such as aerobic dance and treadmill running.

Finally, the best measure of the time course of recovery is oxygen consumption. This is unfortunate in a practical sense but, for a variety of thermal and gravitational reasons, the usual cardiopulmonary measures of recovery are poor indicators during pregnancy (7, 8, 11).

There are several technical details that make monitoring easier during exercise testing. For example, a swivel device attached to the ceiling is often helpful in keeping a variety of leads and respiratory tubing out of the way. A 6-inch ace bandage, used as an abdominal binder, is very helpful in maintaining transducer contact when monitoring the fetal heart rate. Likewise, fixing a rectal thermocouple to a sanitary napkin worn by the subject during testing prevents shifting its position. Several of the commercially available heart-rate monitors are extremely helpful in defining the athlete's actual level of performance in the field. Obtaining these data makes it much easier to recreate field performance in the testing situation. Finally, with the variety of training aids available today, consultation with the subject or her trainer is often helpful in designing the actual testing protocol for a specific activity.

CHRONIC ADAPTATIONS TO PHYSICAL ACTIVITY DURING PREGNANCY

From a physiological point of view pregnancy is an ever-changing process. Therefore, one might anticipate that the body's physiological responses to physical activity would also change in an ongoing fashion during pregnancy. In addition, it is likely that the changes in response are exercise-specific due to the explicit morphometric and cardiopulmonary changes that occur during pregnancy. The remainder of this section will explore these issues in some detail by focusing on several of the important interactions between the physiology of pregnancy and that of exercise. In addition, how the interaction is and/or should be influenced by specific types of exercise will be discussed.

Physiological Interactions Between Pregnancy and Exercise

There are at least four major areas in which the physiological adaptations to exercise and pregnancy interact. In each instance, the physiological adaptations are additive. Thus, the combination of exercise and pregnancy should theoretically impact on both the pregnancy and the quality of the exercise performance. Clearly, the summation of these adaptations influences the testing data obtained and should be taken into account in exercise testing and prescription.

Cardiopulmonary

Physical exercise not only evokes an increase in cardiac output and heart rate but, at intensities greater than 25% of $\dot{V}O_2max$, it evokes a redistribution of absolute blood flow away from the splanchnic viscera to the exercising muscle and skin. Pregnancy also increases cardiac output by at least 40%, resting heart rate by 16 beats·min^{-1}, and evokes a redistribution of cardiac output in favor of the uterus, kidneys, breasts, and skin (2, 3, 13, 14). It also produces an increase in plasma volume that far exceeds that associated with either heat acclimation or training, increases peripheral venous compliance and capacitance (2, 15), and is associated with a variable change in body mass. As a result, the pregnancy-associated increase in basal function concomitantly decreases the cardiovascular reserve available for exercise.

The actual cardiac output and heart rate response are highly dependent on factors that influence venous return, such as the degree of antigravitational stress, the amount of muscle mass utilized, caval compression, and the thermal stress imposed both by the environment and the exercise. Therefore, with most exercise regimens, the relationship between heart rate and oxygen consumption needs to be periodically redefined under the actual exercise conditions if one wishes to use pulse rate as an index of exercise intensity.

Finally, the regional distribution of cardiac output associated with exercise is directly opposite to that associated with pregnancy in terms of the visceral circulation, but similar in terms of the cutaneous circulation. Thus, exercise during pregnancy may limit substrate delivery to the uterus and fetus because of its effects on uterine blood flow, while the pregnant woman's ability to dissipate heat may actually be improved (5, 6, 14). Theoretically, the magnitude of any reduction in uterine flow during exercise should be linearly related to exercise intensity. At usual training intensities it should approximate 50% (4). However, any potential impact that this flow reduction might have on the actual rate of oxygen and substrate uptake could easily be entirely compensated for by an increase in tissue extraction as the amount extracted at normal flow rates rarely exceeds 30%.

Both exercise and pregnancy increase oxygen consumption and minute ventilation (2, 7, 11, 16). During exercise ventilatory equivalents decrease, indicating an increased efficiency of pulmonary gas transfer. In contrast, during pregnancy, both at rest and with exercise, the ventilatory equivalents are increased by about 25%, denoting a significant decrease in the efficiency of pulmonary gas exchange. This is due to an increase in the sensitivity of the respiratory center to CO_2, which increases respiratory work and clearly limits the ventilatory reserve available for the demands of exercise. In one group of subjects (11), this restriction appeared to reduce symptom-limited maximum exercise performance in the third trimester of pregnancy.

Thermoregulation

Both physical activity and pregnancy increase metabolic rate and heat production (17). To dissipate the increased heat, cutaneous vasodilation with an increase in skin blood flow occurs and, if this is insufficient, core temperature rises and sweating begins (18).

During sustained physical activity the rise in core temperature begins at an intensity of 20% of $\dot{V}O_2$max and is linearly related to exercise intensity above that level. The slope of this relationship is increased quite dramatically by environmental factors, such as high temperature and humidity, that are known to decrease the efficiency of heat dissipation (18). Under normal environmental circumstances a training intensity of 60–70% of $\dot{V}O_2$max is associated with an increase of between 1.0 and 1.5°C in core temperature. However, under adverse environmental conditions, the rise in core temperature may exceed 2.5°C.

During pregnancy the growing, metabolically active fetus maintains a core temperature 0.5–1.0°C above that of the mother and dissipates its 15 watts of heat primarily through the umbilical and uterine circulations to the mother and then to the environment (17). At rest this increased thermal load is compensated for adequately by the pregnancy-associated increases in blood volume and skin blood flow, which are greater in magnitude than those associated with either training or heat acclimation (19).

When sustained physical activity and pregnancy are combined, the exercise-induced rise in maternal core temperature initiates heat storage in the fetus until the fetomaternal thermal gradient is reestablished. Thus, the rise in maternal core temperature produces a similar rise in fetal core temperature to a level 0.5–1.0°C higher than that of the mother. Accordingly, if thermoregulatory efficiency is not improved by pregnancy, then sustained exercise at usual training intensities could easily raise fetal or embryonic core temperature above the commonly accepted teratogenic threshold of 39.2°C, especially under adverse environmental conditions. In addition, the rise in temperature should increase fetal basal energy expenditure by 10% or more which, in turn, should decrease the energy available for growth. Clearly, these thermoregulatory factors have a distinct impact on pregnancy in a variety of animal models (20). However, in animals, both the mechanisms and efficiency of heat dissipation are quite different from those in the human (5, 18). Whether the same is true in human pregnancy is presently unknown. One study (21) found no difference in the thermal response to aerobic exercise during pregnancy which, although worrisome, suggests that the thermal effects of exercise and pregnancy are not additive. However, the findings from a separate investigation of runners (6) suggest that the thermal stress associated with that type of exercise may be significantly reduced by at least three factors that alter thermoregulation in pregnancy. Finally, the author is unaware of any epidemiological correlation suggesting that sustained exercise has any abortifacient or teratogenic effect.

Metabolic

Both exercise and pregnancy alter regional metabolism and circulating substrate levels and increase demands for energy substrate (2, 5–7). During exercise, substrate is diverted to the exercising muscle, and circulating levels of glucose and free fatty acids rise due to glycogenolysis, gluconeogenesis, and lipolysis. During pregnancy, substrate is diverted to the uterus and the growing fetoplacental mass within. The circulating levels of substrate fluctuate with the time in gestation but, in general, are lower than in the nonpregnant state (2, 6).

When exercise and pregnancy are combined, they create at least two theoretical problems. First is the specific issue of their combined effect on maternal blood glucose levels, which is a major factor governing fetal glucose availability. During pregnancy, the combined requirements for glucose of the maternal brain and exercising muscle along with those of the fetoplacental unit could result in a fall in maternal blood glucose similar to that seen with a simple overnight fast in the third trimester (22). As glucose is a major energy substrate whose availability for the fetus is dependent on the transplacental gradient, a fall in maternal levels should reduce its fetal availability. This should slow the rate of growth if its occurrence is either frequent or prolonged.

The second is the broader issue of the partitioning of energy expenditure between maintenance and productive processes, in this case fetoplacental growth. While the evidence from experimental animals is quite clear on this point, the slow velocity of growth in human pregnancy should modify its impact considerably (1, 2, 4, 20). In any case, the end points of concern are an exercise-induced decrease in maternal blood glucose and/or a diminution in the rate of fetoplacental growth.

Currently, the data are reassuring in that most of the reports have not noted a defined impact of a variety of exercises on birthweight (3, 4, 7–10, 20, 21). However, three reports note a hypoglycemic response to short episodes of jogging in late pregnancy (6, 23, 24) and one of the few prospective studies found a 500-gm reduction in the birthweight of offspring of women who continued antigravitational endurance exercise at or above a minimal conditioning level throughout pregnancy (1). Clearly more research is needed to definitively address these issues.

Endocrine

The endocrine response to physical exercise is complex and will not be dealt with in detail here. Briefly, the onset of exercise is accompanied by an acute stress response in which catecholamines, prolactin, glucagon, cortisol, and endorphins increase, while insulin and gonadotropins decrease. These responses are modified by the type, intensity, and duration of the exercise as well as the type and extent of training and other life-style stress factors. The hormonal adaptations to pregnancy are equally diverse and complex (2).

When exercise and pregnancy are combined, the main concern is that exercise will disrupt the endocrine milieu of pregnancy in a way that not only will alter the cardiovascular and metabolic parameters discussed above, but will activate the quiescent uterus by altering catecholamines, cortisol, prostaglandins, estradiol, or progesterone. Clearly, the combination of a reduction in oxygen availability and high levels of norepinephrine and cortisol, combined with surges in estradiol and low progesterone levels, would give cause for concern, especially if they were associated with objective evidence of an increase in myometrial activity or epidemiological evidence of preterm labor in women who exercise. Unfortunately, this is a poorly studied area in which only acute responses to very short-term exercise have been studied (24, 25). These studies both report an abrupt rise in catecholamines, and the latter notes an increase in estradiol with no change in either cortisol or progesterone during exercise. However, both hormonal levels fell significantly postexercise when irregular uterine activity was noted. A recent study that examined the effects of walking and cycle ergometer exercise on uterine activity in the latter portion of pregnancy is reassuring in that it found no evidence of increased myometrial activity postexercise (26). Likewise, the absence of an epidemiological association between preterm birth and exercise is reassuring. However, one study has noted a decreased incidence of postdatism in women who continued to perform antigravitational endurance exercise throughout pregnancy (1). This suggests that, under specific circumstances, exercise may shorten the overall duration of pregnancy by assuring the initiation of coordinate myometrial activity at or near term.

Specific Exercise Regimens and the Physiological Interaction

The physiological adaptations that occur during exercise are modified in both importance and magnitude by five exercise

effective. Simply put, the woman should listen carefully to the messages from her body and modify her behavior accordingly. If any question arises or if a competitive training program is planned, the laboratory evaluation discussed earlier should be utilized to avoid potential compromise. Second, the exercise prescription should include specific plans for rest periods and should explicitly address nutritional needs. Third, consideration should be given to maximizing hydration and utilizing postural, food intake, and environmental manipulation to minimize exercise-induced thermoregulatory, cardiopulmonary, and metabolic stress. In this regard, swimming in a cool environment with attention to fluid, electrolyte, and caloric intake may prove to be the ideal endurance training regimen for the pregnant athlete. Finally, attention should be given to preventing maternal injury by use of the best equipment; avoiding introducing new, coordinated, whole body tasks; and reducing activity that requires exceptional balance or range of motion in late pregnancy.

Specific Guidelines

Specific guidelines for monitoring the pregnant athlete who continues training during pregnancy are discussed in the first section of the chapter and will not be reiterated here. In other cases specific attention should be given to four parameters and they should be monitored periodically. The frequency should be individualized based on the perception of risk and the specific exercise regimen. The impact of the exercise regimen on maternal core temperature should be assessed objectively. This is easily accomplished by simply taking rectal temperature (oral is not accurate) immediately before and after exercise (6). Although there are little data on this point (6, 21), restricting the rise to less than 38.7°C seems reasonable.

Maternal weight gain and skinfolds should be monitored to assure adequate energy balance. Normally there should be evidence of significant fat deposition and at least a 2.5 kg weight gain in the first 16 weeks of pregnancy and continued weight gain with a minimal decrease in skinfolds in late pregnancy. The fetal response to the exercise regimen should also be periodically assessed. Fetal heart rate and activity should be relatively unaffected by the exercise regimen. Figure 14.1 illustrates the type of response that should generate concern until more is known. Note the brisk, postexercise elevation of heart rate and decrease in activity that persisted for over 20 minutes. Multiple reports suggest that the magnitude and duration of this response are unusual, suggest excessive fetal stress, and therefore should be handled with caution (10, 20, 23, 25, 26, 29, 31). However, postexercise changes in baseline heart rate of up to 20 beats·min^{-1} have been recorded and are of concern only if they persist beyond the 5th minute. The same is true for fetal activity.

Finally, the growth of the uterus and its tissue contents should be carefully monitored. This should include an initial baseline ultrasound to rule out multiple gestation and confirm normality, followed by usual clinical monitoring. If later deviation is noted, the ultrasound examination should be repeated. As long as these four parameters remain within the suggested range, the exercise prescription should be considered reasonable from a fetal point of view.

SPECIAL EXERCISE PRECAUTIONS, LIMITATIONS, AND PROBLEMS IN PREGNANCY

Many of the pregnancy-specific precautions, limitations, and problems associated with exercise testing and prescription have been appropriately dealt with in earlier sections and will not be restated here. The following will address only concerns that apply to specific types of athletic endeavor. First, in the author's opinion, despite the anecdotal reports of highly successful athletic competition in early pregnancy, our current level of knowledge dictates that serious competition should be discouraged and perhaps prohibited until we improve our understanding of its impact on embryonic development.

Second, the hyperbaric conditions as-

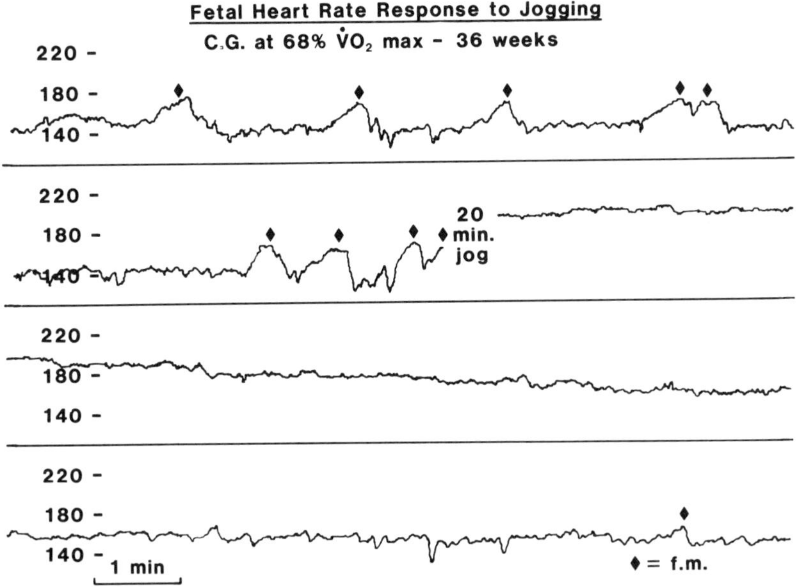

Figure 14.1. The fetal heart rate tracing obtained before and after a 20-minute jog in the 36th week of gestation at an intensity of 68% of $\dot{V}O_2$ max. Each of the four consecutive tracings represents 10 minutes. The superimposed diamonds indicate an epoch of perceived fetal motion. Note the immediate postexercise increase in baseline heart rate from 140 beats·min^{-1} to 200 beats·min^{-1} and the absence of perceived fetal activity until the heart rate had returned to near preexercise levels 20 minutes later.

sociated with scuba and deep-sea diving appear to place the embryo and fetus at defined risk of air embolus during decompression, and a teratogenic effect has been suggested in at least one retrospective study (32). Thus, diving to a depth and for a time that warrant decompression should be actively discouraged during pregnancy. Third, the hemodynamic effects of extreme and/or prolonged Valsalva maneuvers commonly associated with isometric exercise and weight lifting should be specifically avoided during pregnancy. The specific concerns are the profound reductions this should create in splanchnic blood flow as well as its extreme hypertensive effects. Given the morphometric vascular changes of pregnancy and the increased incidence of vascular rupture associated with pregnancy, the latter is best avoided. Currently this is a totally unstudied area.

Fourth, equally unconfirmed concern should at least be voiced about contact sports once the uterus becomes an abdominal organ as there are very real, documented fetal and maternal risks from both the blunt and/or penetrating abdominal trauma associated with automobile accidents in pregnancy. Similar risks should be present with sports such as hang gliding, horseback riding, and downhill skiing but, again, specific problems during pregnancy are yet to be reported.

SUMMARY AND CONCLUSIONS

In summary, the interaction between the physiology of exercise and that of pregnancy is poorly understood and is just beginning to be studied in a definitive fashion. Clearly, there are many exercise-specific and pregnancy-specific variables that must be considered in formulating and individualizing exercise prescriptions for pregnant women. Areas of concern are theoretical and include the potential risks associated with disturbances of the hormonal milieu, hyperthermia, hypoxia, hypoglycemia, reduced uterine blood flow, and the increased potential for maternal injury. Accordingly, routine detailed assessment of the physiological response to exercise is recommended for all athletes who wish to maintain a serious training program during pregnancy. Specific parameters should also be monitored less intensively in all women who wish to maintain an exercise regimen during pregnancy.

Other routine exercise testing for clinical purposes is not recommended, but testing for research purposes is badly needed. Likewise, well-controlled and exercise-specific data dealing with the impact of exercise on pregnancy outcome are badly needed. Although the currently available data do not support the theoretical concerns, they are sparse and by and large poorly controlled. Therefore, current guidelines emphasize the theoretical concerns and are probably overconservative.

It is anticipated that new information will lead to liberalization in the near future. Until that occurs the most important steps in exercise prescription are discussion, flexibility of thought, joint determination of goals and programs, and minimizing the impact of the exercise regimen on the physiological parameters of concern. There are specific contraindications to exercise during pregnancy. Likewise, there are obvious types of exercise that logically are best avoided during pregnancy.

REFERENCES

1. Clapp JF, Dickstein S: Endurance exercise and pregnancy outcome. *Med Sci Sports* 16:556–562, 1984.
2. Hytten F, Chamberlain G: *Clinical Physiology in Obstetrics*, ed 3. Oxford, UK, Blackwell Scientific, 1980, p 1.
3. Metcalfe J, McAnulty JH, Ueland K: *Heart Disease in Pregnancy*, ed 3. Boston, Little, Brown and Company, 1986, p 11.
4. Clapp JF: The effects of maternal exercise during pregnancy on uterine blood flow and pregnancy outcome. In Moawad AH, Lindheimer MD (eds): *Uterine and Placental Blood Flow*. New York, Masson Publishing, 1982, p 177.
5. Clapp JF: Physical exercise and sport during pregnancy. *Die Gynecol* 20:144–150, 1987.
6. Clapp JF, Wesley M, Sleamaker RH: Thermoregulatory and metabolic responses to jogging prior to and during pregnancy. *Med Sci Sports* 19:124–130, 1987.
7. Pernoll ML, Metcalfe J, Schlenker TL, et al.: Oxygen consumption at rest and during exercise in pregnancy. *Respir Physiol* 25:285–294, 1975.
8. Morton MJ, Paul MS, Campos GR, et al.: Exercise dynamics in late gestation: Effects of physical training. *Am J Obstet Gynecol* 152:91–97, 1985.
9. Dressendorfer RH: Physical training during pregnancy and lactation. *Phys Sportsmed* 6:74–80, 1979.
10. Collings CA, Curet LB, Mullin LB: Maternal and fetal responses to a maternal aerobic exercise program. *Am J Obstet Gynecol* 145:702–707, 1983.
11. Artal R, Wiswell RA, Greenspoon J, et al.: Pulmonary responses to exercise in pregnancy. In Artal R, Wiswell RA (eds): *Exercise in Pregnancy*. Baltimore, Williams & Wilkins, 1986, p 147.
12. Lind AR: A physiological criterion for setting thermal environmental limits for everyday work. *J Appl Physiol* 18:51–56, 1963.
13. Clapp JF: Maternal heart rate in pregnancy. *Am J Obstet Gynecol* 152:659–660, 1985.
14. Morton MJ, Metcalfe J: Changes in maternal hemodynamics during pregnancy. In Artal R, Wiswell RA (eds): *Exercise in Pregnancy*. Baltimore, Williams & Wilkins, 1986, p 113.
15. Fawer R, Dettling A, Weihs D, et al.: Effect of the menstrual cycle, oral contraception and pregnancy on forearm blood flow, venous distensibility and clotting factors. *Eur J Clin Pharmacol* 13:251–257, 1978.
16. Pernoll ML, Metcalfe J, Kovach PA, et al.: Ventilation during rest and exercise in pregnancy and postpartum. *Respir Physiol* 25:295–310, 1975.
17. Abrams RM, Caton D, Clapp JF, et al.: Thermal and metabolic features of life in utero. *Clin Obstet Gynecol* 13:549–564, 1970.
18. Rowell LB: Cardiovascular aspects of human thermoregulation. *Circ Res* 52:367–379, 1983.
19. Nadel ER, Pandolf KB, Roberts MF, et al.: Mechanisms of thermal acclimation to exercise and heat. *J Appl Physiol* 37: 515–520, 1974.
20. Lotgering FK, Gilbert RD, Longo LD: Maternal and fetal responses to exercise during pregnancy. *Physiol Rev* 65:1–36, 1985.
21. Jones RL, Botti JJ, Anderson WM, et al.: Thermoregulation during aerobic exercise in pregnancy. *Obstet Gynecol* 65:340–345, 1985.
22. Metzger BE, Ravnikar V, Vileisis RA, et al.: "Accelerated starvation" and the skipped breakfast in late normal pregnancy. *Lancet* 1:588–592, 1982.
23. Hauth JC, Gilstrap LC, Widmer K: Fetal heart rate reactivity before and after maternal jogging during the third trimester. *Am J Obstet Gynecol* 142:542–547, 1982.
24. Artal R: Hormonal responses to exercise in pregnancy. In Artal R, Wiswell RA (eds): *Exercise in Pregnancy*. Baltimore, Williams & Wilkins, 1986, p 139.
25. Rauramo I, Andersson B, Laatikainen T: Stress hormones and placental steroids in physical ex-

ercise during pregnancy. *Br J Obstet Gynecol* 89:921–925, 1982.

26. Vielle JC, Hohimer RA, Burry K, et al.: The effect of exercise on uterine activity in the last eight weeks of pregnancy. *Am J Obstet Gynecol* 151:727–730, 1985.
27. Åstrand PO, Rodahl K: *Textbook of Work Physiology: Physiological Basis of Exercise*, ed 3. New York, McGraw Hill, 1986, p 486.
28. Naeye RL, Peters ED: Working during pregnancy: Effects on the fetus. *Pediatrics* 69:724–727, 1982.
29. Sibley L, Ruhling RO, Cameron-Foster J, et al.: Swimming and physical fitness during pregnancy. *J Nurse Midwifery* 26:3–12, 1981.
30. Artal R, Wiswell RA: Exercise prescription in pregnancy. In Artal R, Wiswell RA (eds): *Exercise in Pregnancy*. Baltimore, Williams & Wilkins, 1986, p 225.
31. Clapp JF: Fetal heart rate response to running in midpregnancy and late pregnancy. *Am J Obstet Gynecol* 153:251–252, 1985.
32. Newhall JF: Scuba diving during pregnancy: a brief review. *Am J Obstet Gynecol* 140:893–894, 1981.

CHAPTER 15

Strategies to Enhance Patient Exercise Compliance

John E. Martin, Ph.D.

Regrettably, the demonstration of the efficacy of exercise in the prevention and rehabilitation of cardiovascular disease and other health problems, and subsequent prescription by a physician or other health-care professional, are not sufficient to ensure that the exercise will be effectively initiated and maintained. In fact, research suggests that the majority of people who eventually begin an exercise program will stop, generally within the first few months (1, 2). For example, approximately one-half of the participants in primary prevention studies will drop out within 3 to 6 months of program entry, while for secondary prevention programs, drop out approaches 50% by about 12 months (3, 4).

In particular, adherence is disappointingly low among those enrolled in structured exercise programs for rehabilitation following an acute coronary event. This is illustrated in a well-controlled study reported by Kentala (1) who found that only 77 of 298 postmyocardial infarction patients actually entered a prescribed exercise program. Moreover, 71% of these exercisers dropped out within 5 months, while only 13% continued to exercise through 1 year.

Clearly, poor adherence to prescribed exercise is a significant problem that necessitates specific interventional strategies rather than the too-often received "assumption neglect" (assuming compliance follows naturally from the prescription, especially when the benefits of exercise have been proven and explained to the patient). We know from ample clinical experience and countless studies in which exercise is employed as a treatment component that just because exercise may be highly efficacious (i.e., produces the desired treatment effect in those who actually take the treatment), it does not necessarily follow that it will be very effective (i.e., the efficacious treatment will be properly adhered to by those to whom it is offered). In light of the relatively disappointing data on the overall effectiveness (as opposed to efficacy) of exercise treatment, one must ask: Is it possible to get individuals to exercise over a long enough period to do any lasting good?

CAN NONEXERCISERS BE MADE INTO EXERCISERS?

We believe that the answer is "Yes," providing: (a) that the program is set up with adherence issues in mind; and (b) that individual programs are carried out in a fashion consonant with social learning principles and the techniques found effective in behavioral research on maximizing exercise adherence. In particular, the manner in which exercise programs are established is of paramount importance in determining patient adherence. The present chapter represents an effort to acquaint the reader with the findings from the research in this area, while suggesting strategies most likely to maximize adherence during the acquisition and maintenance phases of developing the lifetime habit of exercising.

Several bodies of research and clinical experience would seem to suggest that it is indeed possible to get physically underactive or inactive individuals to exercise on a consistent enough basis to produce (and maintain) desired health benefits (5). For example, coronary prevention and rehabilitation trials have accrued a large body of information on those individuals and exercise programs found successful in effectively establishing the exercise habit. In addition, a number of experimental studies have suggested techniques that are beneficial in enhancing exercise adoption and continuation (3, 5, 6). Finally, some approaches developed in our program have been found helpful in shaping and maintaining exercise behavior in sedentary hypertensives (7), as well as in dialysis and coronary patients, among others.

For example, in one clinical study, 77% of our hypertensive patients who were randomized completed the 10-week program, while 100% of those who crossed over to aerobic training following the ineffective control protocol completed the second 10-week program. To produce these high adherence rates in a group of very unfit hypertensives, we employed a variety of behavioral strategies that were developed from a series of studies we conducted on enhancing exercise adherence in community populations (7), and which will be described and interpreted later in the chapter.

In the following sections of this chapter, three bodies of evidence, including our study results, will be integrated to suggest strategies and pitfalls in implementing an exercise regimen in the sedentary patient—primary and secondary prevention trials, coronary rehabilitation studies, and exercise modification experiments. However, first it makes sense to summarize what we know about who is and is not likely to be a good candidate for exercise, and what that may suggest about the kind of physical conditioning program that will be necessary to promote and maintain adherence to the regimen. The conclusions are based on predominately male samples since we know much less about women in exercise programs because heart disease risk in females is only a relatively recent phenomenon.

MOST AND LEAST LIKELY TO EXERCISE: IMPLICATIONS FOR ADHERENCE

Exercise Adherence Predictors

Data from coronary prevention trials and cardiac rehabilitation programs have provided profiles of those more and less likely to begin and continue to engage in regular exercise (3–5, 8). Interestingly, the highest risk candidates for drop out are blue collar workers who smoke, are overweight, and unmotivated, and who have little or no support for their exercising from significant others in the home or work environments. On the other hand, those most likely to comply with an exercise prescription are nonobese, nonsmoking, white collar workers with active family support and encouragement for exercising, who have higher self-motivation to exercise (which may include having symptoms that might be alleviated or improved through regular exercise).

These are valuable findings, though they only just begin the process of suggesting the best approaches to ensuring compliance. Most importantly, they help identify to the clinician which individuals might need special programming or attention if the exercise treatment is to be effective over the long haul, and who might be put in more or less standard exercise programs (and perhaps what general form they should take) with good chances of success. For example, individuals who are poorer adherence risks for exercise might be targeted for closer supervision and more gradual increases in exercise intensity and complexity to prevent their greater likelihood of dropping out (approaches that will be detailed later).

Unfortunately, these high-risk dropouts have seldom been formally isolated (except retrospectively) for special treatment designed to retain them in exercise programs. Thus, we must fall back on our current knowledge about the most optimal conditions and techniques for shaping and maintaining the exercise habit in the general population. Whenever possible, it is recommended that programs tailor individualized treatment (as illustrated in this chapter) for these higher risk dropouts, rather than simply allowing them to eventually drop out. Indeed, it is good to develop individually tailored strategies to enhance the exercise adherence of all participants, and not just those identified as potential high-risk drop-out candidates.

Exercise Adherence Facilitators

A more in-depth look at the retrospective heart disease prevention and control trial data delineates selected program factors, some of which stem from the data on the dropout and adherer characteristics that seem to promote initial exercise participation as well as later program adherence. For example, the convenience, location, mode, and prescription of the exercise seem to significantly affect the probability that an individual will participate in exercise.

Most importantly, the exercise location must be convenient. That is, it should be either close to work, close to home, or conveniently in between. We actively discourage our clients from joining health spas or programs that require any significant amount of driving or other special preparation. A convenient location increases both the probability that an individual will make a commitment to participate and maintain the habit. Seemingly minor factors, such as difficulty finding parking spaces, can have a major negative impact on exercise program attendance and overall adherence.

In fact, the degree of available, active social support or reinforcement for exercise from the home environment has consistently been related to increased exercise adherence. For example, patients with spouses who support their exercise habit are two to three times more likely to have good adherence than those whose spouses are either neutral or negative toward exercising (9). Finally, the amount of social support during exercise is another critical factor in determining exercise adherence (2, 3, 5, 6). We tap into both these enhancers by encouraging family members to come to exercise sessions (and exercise) with their significant other, or at least provide praise and support during or after home exercise participation. For high-risk dropouts we specifically target the family for this type of coparticipation. Finally, long-term adherence can be enhanced for individuals participating in group exercise rather than exercising alone, and so we always encourage, if not organize, clinic and home exercise groups.

THE EXERCISE PRESCRIPTION AND ADHERENCE

Specification of the parameters of the exercise regimen should relate at least as much to the probability of future adherence as to the needed dose to produce the desired response. The mode or type of exercise, for example, should first and foremost be simple and convenient. It does little good to produce a rapid training effect if the individual eventually stops exercising because environmental restraints make long-term adherence too problematic. For example, most programs stress walking and jogging, as we do, because such activities can be performed with minimal preparation, cost, and equipment in almost any location and in all seasons (although some of our northern neighbors have turned by necessity to winter walking in the indoor shopping malls). Calisthenics are a poor choice, especially if performed alone and without other complementary aerobic exercises such as brisk walking. Most people prefer exercising in groups and will have up to twice the adherence rates than when they try to maintain an "individualized" exercise regimen.

The components of exercise prescription are also critical to adherence. The prescribed frequency, duration, and especially intensity will have a profound impact on the probability of exercise participation and longer-term adherence. If it even appears to people that they will be unable to perform the exercise regimen, they will be significantly less likely to fulfill the prescription. In one study performed at the Stanford Heart Disease Prevention Program, the very best predictor of 1-year adherence to a rigorous exercise program was the prospective participant's own confidence in being able to fullfill the requirements of the program. This points out the importance of setting easily attainable goals in at least the initial exercise prescription.

In addition to devising a simple, easily attainable prescription, the manner in which participants are encouraged and allowed to perform the exercise is of utmost importance to the probability of their developing and maintaining the exercise habit. Research has indicated that an exercise intensity greater than 85% of maximum heart rate (HR) or aerobic capacity, more than five sessions per week, and/or more than 45 minutes per session is associated with disproportionate drop-out and injury rates. In most cases, especially earlier in the regimen, less is better.

While enhancing adherence, a very modest exercise regimen may also be highly efficacious. For example, in studies of hypertensive individuals, only a minimal level of aerobic exercise was required to produce significant reductions in blood pressure (7). Generally, effective exercise regimens for blood pressure modulation consisted of 20 to 30 minutes, three sessions a week at approximately 70 to 75% of maximal HR, of an easy aerobic activity such as brisk walking—a minimal aerobic regimen that can have salutary effects for a number of people with chronic health problems.

At this point it will be instructive to discuss another important area closely tied to exercise prescription in its potential significant impact on later adherence—the exercise/fitness assessment.

ADHERENCE AND THE EXERCISE TEST

The type and especially the manner of exercise assessment can exert a significant influence on both immediate and eventual patient adherence/compliance to the exercise program. This is particularly true since the exercise/fitness testing is usually the first contact neophyte exercisers have with the exercise program, and it can set either a negative or positive tone for the upcoming experience in physical conditioning. The motivational aspects of the choice of certain graded exercise tests have been discussed elsewhere (10); however, it is important to note that pushing patients to exhaustion via maximal testing may bring the patient into contact with the most aversive aspects of exercise, and may model an approach to exercise ("no pain, no gain") that we initially take great pains to avoid. In fact, we switched our testing of asymptomatic individuals from a time-based test (in which many pushed to exhaustion despite our instructions to the contrary) to a response criterion (submaximal heart rate) that stopped them well short of strenuous levels of exercise. Whenever possible, we recommend avoiding maximal tests or time/distance tests before patients have sufficient capacity to sustain an intense effort without aversive (motivational) consequences. We do recognize the importance of maximal testing in certain populations, such as in myocardial infarction patients (we are also familiar with the use of maximal testing to demonstrate the safety of physical exertion to the patient and family).

In addition to basic testing, we strongly recommend that regular progress or maintenance checks be conducted to document fitness improvements and to serve as an adherence incentive. Whenever possible, these assessments should include other dependent variables targeted for change, such as weight/body fat/girth measures and mood or anxiety levels, as well as measures of baseline fitness level and activity.

This kind of thoroughness in the initial assessment, when followed by regular assessments during treatment, can be especially helpful in documenting improvements in health status for patients who do not experience changes in their primary goal (e.g., weight loss) as soon as they had hoped. This careful, multiple system tracking can then show at least some positive changes in other health indices, which may translate to reduced probabilities that slow responders will become discouraged drop-outs during those critical early weeks. Motivation can be maintained, for example, by being able to notify patients (graphs of these data are also excellent) that resting and exercise heart rates have significantly decreased, even though their weight or blood pressure has not yet changed during an initial phase of the program.

This comprehensive type of assessment and feedback appears to be extremely important to the majority of individuals undergoing exercise training. Moreover, a patient's failure to show any type of favorable change after a reasonable time can cue the program provider to several possibilities: a) the patient is not adhering well enough to the exercise prescription to produce the desired change, b) the exercise prescription itself is faulty or inadequate, or c) the measures are not sensitive enough to assess changes, and perhaps should be altered, supplemented, or replaced.

We try to employ submaximal exercise tests approximately every month to document (and reinforce) fitness changes and serve as an indirect check on home program adherence. On the latter point, while we recognized that this type of testing may not be a very accurate indicator of exercise adherence (one might be exercising but not improving in fitness), we used these tests as a "bogus pipeline," such that the patients were told that if they were not exercising as prescribed, the test would pick it up. At the very least, we felt the home self-monitoring data were more accurate because of our regular testing.

Our procedure was developed in collaboration with an exercise physiologist consultant (N. Oldridge) and included treadmill or cycle ergometer work for 5 minutes each at 1/3, 1/2, and 2/3 of their baseline maximum aerobic capacity. Heart rates were observed (and depicted graphically) from portable HR monitors during rest, at the conclusion of each 5-minute trial, and then again 5 minutes following cessation of the 15-minute exercise test. Evaluation might also be conducted using the step test (11, 12) or other submaximal exercise tests. Generally, the patients found this month-to-month feedback very motivational, and looked forward to each testing as an opportunity to demonstrate further fitness gains. Figure 15.1 illustrates a graph from this "adherence check" test.

MODIFYING EXERCISE BEHAVIOR

The final section of this chapter addresses the "meat" of adherence-enhancement strategies designed to directly modify exercise behavior. Before presenting and illustrating these specific techniques, a brief review of the literature on modification of exercise is appropriate.

Exercise Modification Studies

A number of studies have prospectively targeted the modification of exercise adherence in both clinical and, more typically, apparently healthy populations. These interventional studies have been presented and discussed elsewhere (3, 5, 8), and will not be repeated here, except to review their preliminary findings in more practical ways.

These studies are useful in that they suggest techniques that do not appear to be effective (e.g., health education alone), as well as those that seem to hold more promise (contracting, reinforcement, and stimulus control procedures). Generally, the studies indicate that exercise is a behavior that can be modified using consequent or reinforcement control, stimulus or antecedent control, and cognitive/self-control techniques. In particular, the use of reinforcement procedures, such as contracting and lotteries; praise and social support during exercise; cognitive self-control procedures, such as self-monitoring, self-contracting, and self-reinforcement; indi-

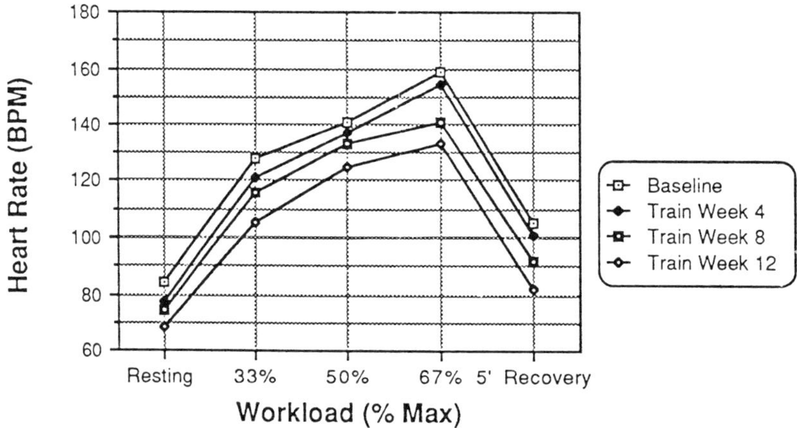

Figure 15.1. Submaximal graded exercise/adherence check.

vidualized and flexible goal-setting; and cognitive distraction have all been shown to be effective in increasing exercise adherence levels 25% to 100% above baseline or control group levels (2, 3, 5, 6).

The results of these investigations demonstrate at a minimum that exercise can be viewed as a behavior that is influenced by events that precede and follow it. The following listing and illustrations of the different behavioral and psychological strategies are designed to provide more detail with respect to implementing such a program, while emphasizing the behavioral habit aspects that are so important to laying an effective foundation for a lifetime of exercise.

Exercise Modification Techniques

In general, we employ and recommend a number of basic behavior modification and cognitive-behavioral techniques aimed at increasing adherence to an exercise program or prescription. These include shaping, positive reinforcement and feedback, contracting, cognitive/self-control training, relapse prevention/innoculation, fading, and generalization programming. These techniques will be described and illustrated.

Shaping the Exercise Habit

Shaping is perhaps the most vital procedure in establishing a long-term habit such as exercise. Shaping is the process by which behavior is directed into a series of successive goals that are very gradually and easily attained over time and repeated trials to achieve the desired end behavior. Probably the most common and destructive mistake made by exercise leaders or by exercisers themselves is in initiating the program at too high an intensity, frequency, or duration. For most individuals, it is far better to start at too low a level than a too challenging one. The program can always be accelerated as the habit is safely and comfortably established, but recovering the program after a major slip or relapse in adherence may be impossible.

We found shaping to be one of the essential elements in the success of our exercise programs for community sedentary adults (6) and hypertensives (7). Our primary emphasis in the first 3 to 4 weeks of exercise training, as well as throughout the treatment and maintenance period, is on effective shaping of the exercise *habit*. We stress three aspects of an effective exercise program: (a) comfort; (b) enjoyability; and (c) regularity. We tell patients that, unfortunately, the body "detrains," or loses fitness, even more quickly than it trains, and therefore it is vital to first establish a solid root system for the habit of exercising that can withstand transient minor injuries, loss of exercise partners, moving and travel, sickness, and seasonal/weather variations, which so frequently lead to exercise adherence slips, relapses, and program dropout.

Generally, in the laboratory sessions we gradually shape the exercise duration and intensity from 5 to 15 minutes at 60% maximal HR during the first 1 to 4 weeks, up to a maximum of 30 minutes at 75% to 80% maximal HR by the second or third month. Depending on their initial fitness level, enjoyment, perceived and actual exertion levels, as well as their stated goals, we can slow or speed up the progression in exercise duration and intensity. Importantly, to assist us in calibrating appropriately comfortable workloads, we carefully track exertional levels using the Borg Rating of Perceived Exertion (RPE) scale (13), and our own five-point exercise enjoyment scale shown in Table 15.1.

We find that an optimal exertional level from the standpoint of maximizing adherence to the exercise is between an RPE of 10 and 12 initially, and 11 to 13 eventually. Additionally, we use the breathing/talking rule that exercise is not to be done so intensely that one cannot exercise and talk comfortably at the same time. To enforce our rule of keeping beginning exercisers at an easy but effective level of exertion, we track (and eventually teach them to monitor) their breathing, enjoyment, and overall exercise intensity through RPE and HR monitoring on a special graph depicting what we term the "effective comfort zone (ECZ)." This scale represents an exercise level intense enough to be aerobic, but not so intense that it is aversive or even un-

Table 15.1
Exercise Enjoyment Scale

Very Unenjoyable	Somewhat Unenjoyable	Neutral	Somewhat Enjoyable	Very Enjoyable
1	2	3	4	5

comfortable. Regular feedback is ensured by plotting or (better) having exercisers plot their own exercise heart rates to assist them in maintaining between 60% and 75% of maximum HR, with corresponding RPEs between 10 and 13 and enjoyment levels between 3 and 5. Figure 15.2 illustrates one of these graphs.

For the most sedentary patients we recommend starting at an exercise intensity of 60% to 65% of aerobic capacity (or maximum heart rate) for at least the first several sessions, if not for the first 3 to 6 weeks. To assist in setting appropriate shaping goals, we regularly assess the individual's subjective reaction to the exercise. For example, we recommend monitoring the patients' rating of perceived exertion (13), and encourage patients to keep their exertion between 11 and 12, with a maximum of 13 for several weeks until the exercise is quite comfortable.

Along a similar vein, we recommend patients begin with two sessions of exercise per week (preferably in a laboratory or well-supervised program) of between 5 and 15 minutes (at 65% aerobic capacity and RPE of 11–12) for the first 2 weeks, while adding a third and fourth home exercise session at about weeks 2 and 4, respectively. This is intended to slowly shape the exercise habit while minimizing the potential for physical and psychological "burnout."

Instrumental to the success of the shaping program is the first session and week of exercise. These first sessions should be used to acquaint the individual with the program philosophy (exercise can and should be enjoyable and easy) as well as procedures to gradually and enjoyably shape the exercise habit. An important part of the shaping process in exercise acquisition is to do whatever is necessary to ensure that their first session is painless, easy, and fun (or, at worst, not unenjoyable).

Reinforcement Control

Any new behavior (and in the case of even a previously active person, the exer-

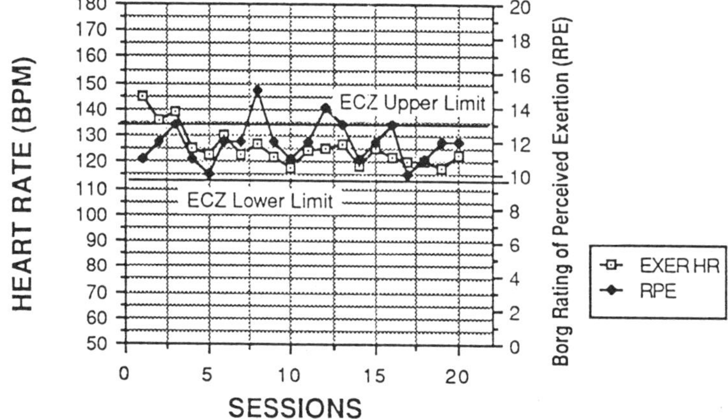

Figure 15.2. Effective comfort zone (ECZ) exercise graph.

cising must be considered a new behavior) requires a "fat" schedule of reinforcement to be effectively established in the person's behavioral repertoire. That is, it is essential that there be positive reinforcement both during and after the occurrence of the exercise behavior for it to be repeated and maintained. Studies have indicated that praise from the exercise leaders especially during the exercise, and social attention from fellow exercisers, can enhance levels of exercise adherence, presumably through increasing the enjoyability of the exercise bout. Other reinforcement procedures found effective in improving exercise adherence include lottery awards based on attendance at exercise class, and adherence-contingent return of deposited money or personal valuables.

Importantly, the rewards or reinforcement, to be effective, must be provided contingent on the exercise behavior. This reinforcement should also be gradually faded before the program is turned completely over to the individual so there is no abrupt cessation of rewards. Abrupt cessation of rewards may lead to exercise cessation if other more natural reinforcers, such as the good feeling and socializing with healthy people, do not first take over control of the behavior.

To ensure that the consequences of the exercise are positive, or at least not negative, we strongly advise keeping the exercise intensity below 75% of maximal heart rate for the first month or two to maximize enjoyment and minimize the potential for injury and "burnout." Gradual shaping of the exercise behavior, as noted previously, is a critical method of ensuring that the exercise will have more positive consequences for the individual. To enhance reinforcement during the potentially aversive exercise session, we provide music, group exercise, and a considerable amount of praise and positive encouragement from therapists and assistants during as well as after each session. Also, if either the subjective exertion or enjoyment scale deviates from the comfortable/enjoyable zone for more than two consecutive sessions, we discuss this with the patient and immediately reduce the intensity of exercise, and increase the laboratory and/or home exercise reinforcement.

Stimulus Control

Stimuli, events, cues, or prompts that reliably give rise to a subsequent behavior are said to exert stimulus control over that behavior. In the case of exercise, wearing exercise clothing, calling or being called by an exercise partner, driving to the exercise facility or location, and even viewing a graph of exercise performance can all serve as prompts to exercise and should be incorporated into exercise programs whenever possible. Exercisers should be trained to fill up their home and work environments with these exercise-cuing stimuli, while they should be made aware of and taught to avoid stimuli and events associated with nonexercise behavior (e.g., turning on TV just before exercise time, leaving exercise clothes at home rather than carrying them, etc.). One particularly effective stimulus control technique is to teach exercisers to encourage others to ask about how their exercise program is going, and to publicly post exercise-related data. Entering frequent fun runs and fitness events can also serve to cue appropriate exercise behavior.

Behavioral Contracting

People are most likely to respond positively to a behavior management program when they are made aware of the specific relationship between their behavior and positive and negative consequences (reinforcement and punishment). While these contingencies are usually verbally negotiated with the individual, an even more effective procedure is to put them down in writing. A written agreement specifies the behavior to be changed (exercise) and when and where and how often it will occur (the exercise mode and prescription), and the individual agrees, in writing, to abide by the specified behaviors. Written agreements have been shown to be effective in enhancing exercise adherence in cardiac rehabilitation populations. More effective is the behavioral contract, which adds to this written agreement positive and/or negative consequences. Thus, an individual may agree to exercise in a specified way in exchange for reinforcement (e.g., back rub or favorite meal). Figure 15.3 shows a sample behavioral contract.

Self-Monitoring

Self-monitoring has been shown to be one of the most effective ingredients of any self-managed health behavior change program, principally weight loss and smoking, and exercise appears to be no different in this respect. Our patients are required to monitor exercise in the clinic and at home. A home self-monitoring form is shown in Figure 15.4. We also require participants to self-monitor and graph their clinic and home levels of exercise and resting HR, enjoyment ratings, and RPEs, as shown in Figures 15.1 and 15.2.

While other health behavior change programs tend to drop the self-monitoring component during the home maintenance phase of training, except as a booster procedure for individuals in danger of, or who have experienced, a relapse, we recommend that exercise self-monitoring be a continuous part of both the acquisition and maintenance program.

Cognitive Strategies

An extensive body of research has indicated the importance of thoughts, beliefs, and imagery to behavior, and exercise is no exception. Studies on exercise performance and adherence suggest that a person's thoughts during exercise as well as their

1. Patient
I (patient name), ____________________ agree to perform the following:
(a) Health behavior change: ____________________ times per week. for __________ min, at a minimum intensity of __________ (HR/RPE/METS) and a maximum intensity of __________ (HR/RPE/METS).
(b) Record the behaviors on my weekly self-monitoring form.
(c) Keep my appointments or call in advance to reschedule:
(____________________ , X__________).
In return, ____________________ agrees to reinforce these changes in one of the following ways each week when I meet my goals.
(a) ____________________
(b) ____________________
(c) ____________________

2. Spouse or Helper
I, ____________________ agree to the following:
(a) Health behavior change: ____________________ times per week.
(b) ____________________
(c) ____________________
In return, I (patient) ____________________ agree to reinforce these changes in one of the following ways each week when I meet my goals.
(a) ____________________
(b) ____________________
(c) ____________________

3. Effective dates of the contract: ____________________

4. Signatures: PATIENT ____________________
SPOUSE or HELPER ____________________
CLINICAL PROFESSIONAL ____________________

Figure 15.3. Health improvement contract.

Name ______________________ **Exercise Goal** ______________________

date:	___ Sun	___ Mon	___ Tues	___ Wed	___ Thu	___ Fri	___ Sat	Avg/day
Activity Type								
Time								
Distance								
Heart Rate Before Exer.								
During Exer.								
After Exer.								
Enjoyment 1. Very Unenjoy.	1	1	1	1	1	1	1	
2. Unenjoyable	2	2	2	2	2	2	2	
3. Neutral	3	3	3	3	3	3	3	
4. Enjoyable	4	4	4	4	4	4	4	
5. Very Enjoy.	5	5	5	5	5	5	5	
RPE (6–20)								
Where Exercised								
With Whom Exer.								
Comments (number and list below)								
Comments (#):								

Figure 15.4. Home self-monitoring form.

exercise goal-setting behavior have an important influence on their maintenance of the exercise habit (5). For example, individuals who believed their own preferences were incorporated into their exercise prescription were more likely to have higher adherence levels; those who were encouraged to set flexible exercise goals daily and weekly (as opposed to having rigid goals set for them by trainers) also showed significantly higher exercise adherence levels. Further, a most interesting finding in one of our experiments (6) was that exercisers who set time-based goals (e.g., jog for 15 minutes) had superior adherence when compared to those who set distance-based goals (e.g., jog 1¼ miles).

In perhaps the most intriguing of our findings on cognitive control of exercise adherence, we discovered that exercisers who were taught to use distractional thoughts ("smell the roses"; think about anything but the exercise or how the body feels) showed significantly better exercise adherence through 6 months follow-up than did those who had thoughts associated with the exercise itself or the body's response.

The final two techniques that will be described relate more to the maintenance of the exercise habit rather than to the acquisition of the behavior that constitutes the primary focus of shaping, reinforcement and stimulus control, self-monitoring, behavioral contracting, and cognitive techniques.

Generalization Training

Generalization is the technical term for transferring a behavior from one setting to another (e.g., moving exercise from the clinic program to the home environment; stimulus generalization) or adding a new behavior in the same environment (cycle ergometry work to brisk walking around the program clinic; response generalization). Stimulus generalization of the exercise response is probably more critical and needs to be initiated early in the program for best results. We encourage home exercise sessions as early as possible (i.e., as soon as the second or third week of training) so as to ensure that the exercise program will be solidly established in (or generalized to) the environment in which it is to be maintained. One of the most common errors in exercise programs and in individual exercise programs that are based in a single facility (not the home or work environment) is that in the event the individual is "graduated" from the program or lets the health program membership lapse, he or she is then far more likely to encounter an exercise relapse.

The advantages of this early home intervention are basically threefold: First, even if exercisers miss one home session (which often occurs, especially early on), they have still met the aerobic criterion of three sessions per week; second, less program-personnel time is required; finally, and perhaps most critically, early home sessions help to more completely establish the exercise habit in the home environment, thereby maximizing stimulus (setting) generalization and increasing the probability of long-term maintenance of the exercise regimen once treatment has been completed.

Response generalization may also be important to establish if the exercise performed in the program or clinic is different (e.g., different equipment) from that in the home environment, where the exercise is to be maintained after program sessions are faded and then discontinued. Once the laboratory exercise is well-established (e.g., after 6 or 8 weeks), efforts should be directed to identifying the mode of exercise that will be used for home maintenance of the program. In our program, patients exercise from the start on both the treadmill and cycle ergometer for about equal time, and include brisk walking/jogging around the hospital grounds after about 6 weeks. This response generalization to the home exercise (patients did not have treadmills or ergometers at home, though they were very efficient for our early training purposes) was begun at least 4–6 weeks before graduating patients to the home maintenance phase of the program to ensure that there was sufficient time to "stamp in" the new exercise habit.

Relapse Prevention Inoculation

A last technique recommended for exercise programming that has some research support in the behavioral exercise literature targets the inevitable relapse situations which almost all exercisers will encounter sooner or later. We generally instruct participants that the question is not whether they will slip or relapse, since most will become sick or experience an injury or environmental change such as a move, trip, or loss of partner, but how they will cope with it when it happens.

After establishing the likelihood of at least a temporary slip or relapse, we teach our exercisers about what has been termed the "abstinence violation effect (AVE)." Generally referring to the tendency of those abstaining from a negative habit or addiction to return to former levels of the habit upon even the first minor slip, we explain that in the area of exercise, it would refer to stopping exercising altogether following the first temporary lapse. This AVE is usually accompanied by self-statements to the effect that "what's the use,. . . I blew it . . . might as well give up now . . ." After warning individuals that this may happen, and to protect themselves from these misleading and erroneous thoughts through counter, positive thoughts ("no problem . . . this was bound to happen . . . all I need to do is get back on my program . . . I've only gone from 100% adherence to 95% adherence with my 1-week absence rather than to 0% . . ."), we teach them how to gradually restart their program, calling an exercise friend and planning to exercise, and to use other stimulus and reinforcement-control procedures. In some cases we even put individuals through a planned relapse during treatment so that they can reinitiate their program on their own under more controlled circumstances, but we do not recommend this to any but the very ambitious (in some cases it backfired and some never came back; others refused to stop!).

SUMMARY AND CONCLUSIONS

The present chapter has reviewed the very common and difficult problem of noncompliance or nonadherence to prescribed exercise. Although the majority of those entered into an exercise program or for whom one is prescribed will drop out or adhere so poorly that the clinical benefit will be limited, research has indicated that their exercise patterns can be modified through specific programmatic and behavioral interventions. Strategies found to be effective include behavior shaping, reinforcement and stimulus control, behavioral contracting, self-monitoring, cognitive strategies, generalization training, and relapse inoculation. Suggestions were also provided with respect to the overall adherence-promoting program structure and prescription as well as testing recommendations and cautions.

The predominant finding, chief focus, and primary recommendation of the chapter is that exercise is a behavior, first and foremost, subject to the laws of learning, and that careful attention to the science of behavioral shaping and maintenance has the potential to minimize exercise drop out while ultimately maximizing the therapeutic effects of exercise. The primary goal of all exercise programs should be to establish the *habit* of exercise, even before efforts are directed toward producing the desired training effect. To reverse these priorities, as the data so overwhelmingly indicate, may result in a more immediate training effect but in a much greater probability that it will be in vain since the individual may be far more likely to stop exercising over the long run. Because the ultimate goal is to produce a permanent life-style change, the initial and primary focus should be on properly and thoroughly laying the foundation for a lifetime habit of exercising and fitness. Health-care professionals are strongly encouraged to consider the critical and primary importance of the behavior and habit of exercising, and to incorporate effective behavioral and programmatic strategies designed to prevent drop out and optimize adherence to a lifetime fitness program.

REFERENCES

1. Kentala E: Physical fitness and feasibility of physical rehabilitation after myocardial infarction in men of working age. *Ann Clin Res* 4(Suppl):1–84, 1972.
2. Martin JE, Dubbert PM: Behavioral management strategies for improving health and fitness. *J Cardiac Rehabil* 4:200–208, 1984.
3. Martin JE, Dubbert PM: Exercise applications and promotion in behavioral medicine. Current status and future directions. *J Consult Clin Psychol* 50:1004–1017, 1982.
4. Oldridge NB: Compliance and exercise in primary and secondary prevention of coronary heart disease: A review. *Prev Med* 11:56–70, 1982.
5. Martin JE, Dubbert PM: Adherence to exercise. In RJ Terjung (ed): *Exercise and Sport Sciences Reviews*. New York, MacMillan, 1985, p 137.
6. Martin JE, Dubbert PM, Katell AD, et al.: The behavioral control of exercise in sedentary adults: Studies 1 through 6. *J Consult Clin Psychol* 52:795–811, 1984.
7. Martin JE, Dubbert PM, Cushman WC: Controlled trial of aerobic exercise in hypertension. *Circulation* 72(Suppl III):III–13, 1985, (Abst).
8. Dishman RK: Compliance/adherence in health-related exercise. *Health Psychol* 1:237–267, 1982.
9. Andrew GM, Oldridge NB, Parker JO, et al.: Reasons for dropout from exercise programs in post-coronary patients. *Med Sci Sports Exerc* 13:164–168, 1981.
10. Thompson JK, Martin JE: Exercise in health modification: Assessment and training guidelines. *Behav Ther* 7:5–8, 1984.
11. McArdle WD, Katch FI, Katch VL: *Exercise Physiology*. Philadelphia, Lea & Febiger, 1981, p 1.
12. Montoye HD: *An Introduction to Measurement in Physical Education*. Boston, Allyn and Bacon, 1978.
13. Borg GV: Perceived exertion as an indicator of somatic stress. *Scand J Rehabil Med* 2:92–98, 1970.

Index

Page numbers in *italics* denote figures; those followed by "t" denote tables.